KEY THEMES IN PUBLIC HEALTH

Key Themes in Public Health comprises a series of introductory essays exploring key themes and concepts in public health.

Ranging from political and economic concern with improving population health and reducing health inequalities, to debates about how to protect populations from new health threats, as well as a concern with individual responsibility for lifestyles and behaviour, the themes discussed include: determinants of health, globalization, evidence, climate change, ethics, development, poverty, risk and prevention.

Presenting provocative ways of thinking about key ideas in a concise fashion, each essay provides a basic grounding in the relevant theme as well as a departure point for further study by:

- defining the theme in an accessible way;
- placing each idea in its particular social, political, economic and historical context;
- illustrating its application and significance for public health;
- identifying and exploring issues surrounding each of the themes.

This text provides an accessible overview for students new to public health who want to get to grips with the full range and complexity of this diverse and multidisciplinary field.

Miranda Thurston is Professor of Public Health at Hedmark University College, Norway.

'The growth of public health courses aimed at undergraduates has created a new need for textbooks that are appropriate and stimulating. Miranda Thurston has succeeded in producing something which strikes the right note. It is wide ranging in scope without being superficial and is accessible to the young learner. It is a sort of "Wiki". Just what the aspiring public health practitioner ordered.'

Professor John R. Ashton CBE, President of the UK Faculty of Public Health

KEY THEMES IN PUBLIC HEALTH

Miranda Thurston

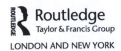

Routledge
Taylor & Francis Group

LONDON AND NEW YORK

First published 2014
by Routledge
2 Park Square, Milton Park, Abingdon, Oxon, OX14 4RN

and by Routledge
711 Third Avenue, New York, NY 10017

Routledge is an imprint of the Taylor & Francis Group, an informa business

© 2014 Miranda Thurston

British Library Cataloguing in Publication Data
A catalogue record for this book is available from the British Library

Library of Congress Cataloging-in-Publication Data

Thurston, Miranda, author.
Key themes in public health / Miranda Thurston.
p. ; cm.
Includes bibliographical references.

I. Title.
[DNLM: 1. Public Health. WA 100]
RA441
362.1–dc23
2013049204

ISBN13: 978-0-415-67381-5 (hbk)
ISBN13: 978-0-415-67382-2 (pbk)
ISBN13: 978-1-315-77010-9 (ebk)

Typeset in Sabon by
FiSH Books Ltd, Enfield

Printed and bound in the United States of America by Publishers Graphics, LLC on sustainably sourced paper.

To my parents, Mary and Victor

CONTENTS

ACKNOWLEDGEMENTS

Many people have served, directly and indirectly, as sources of inspiration for this book, including colleagues and students, past and present. There is one person without whom this book would not have been written, however, and who therefore needs particular mention. My partner, Ken Green, gave me the confidence to embark on the project as well as unwavering support throughout the whole process. He was also a challenging critical friend, honest and forthright, but always with the best of intentions. I must also acknowledge the help and support of Catherine Perry who commented critically on the draft manuscript with meticulous attention. In addition, I want to thank Hedmark University College for providing the time for me to complete this project, Gjensidigestiftelsen for funding my position and James Watson at Routledge for his faith and forebearance. My mother and father – Mary and Victor Thurston – have been a particularly constant source of inspiration and support throughout my entire life. This book is dedicated to them with love and deep gratitude. My guiding theme throughout has been (to invert one of my late father's many sayings) not to let a good story get in the way of the facts. I hope he would have approved.

ABBREVIATIONS

A&E	Accident and emergency department
ABCD	Asset-based community development
AIDS	Acquired immune deficiency syndrome
APHA	American Public Health Association
BRIC	Brazil, Russia, India and China
CEA	Cost-effectiveness analysis
CHD	Coronary heart disease
CSDH	Commission on the Social Determinants of Health
CUA	Cost utility analysis
CVD	Cardiovascular disease
DCLG	Department for Communities and Local Government
DH	Department of Health
DHSS	Department of Health and Social Security
EU	European Union
FCTC	Framework Convention on Tobacco Control
FPH	Faculty of Public Health
GAVI	Global Alliance for Vaccines and Immunization
GDP	Gross domestic product
GII	Gender Inequality Index
GIS	Geographical information systems
GNI	Gross national income
GP	General practitioner
HALS	Health Activities Literacy Scale
HAZ	Health action zones
HBAI	Households below average income
HBM	Health Belief Model
HDI	Human Development Index
HIA	Health Impact Assessment
HIV	Human immunodeficiency virus
HNA	Health needs assessment
HRA	Human Rights Act
IBA	Identification and brief advice
ICD	International Classification of diseases
IHR	International Health Regulations
IMD	Index (indices) of Multiple Deprivation
IMF	International Monetary Fund
IMR	Infant mortality rate

IPCC	International Panel on Climate Change
JRF	Joseph Rowntree Foundation
JSNA	Joint Strategic Needs Assessment
LDL	Low density lipoprotein
LSOA	Lower-layer Super Output Area
LSPs	Local Strategic Partnerships
MADD	Mothers Against Drunk Driving
MDGs	Millennium Development Goals
MI	Motivational interviewing
MMR	Measles, mumps, rubella (vaccine)
NCB	Nuffield Council on Bioethics
NHS	National Health Service
NICE	National Institute for Health and Clinical Excellence
NSMC	National Social Marketing Centre
NS-SEC	National Statistics Socio-Economic Classification
OECD	Organisation for Economic Co-operation and Development
ONS	Office for National Statistics
PHC	Primary health care
PRSPs	Poverty Reduction Strategy Papers
PSHE	Personal, social and health education
QALY	Quality adjusted life year
RA	Rapid appraisal
RCT	Randomized controlled trial
REALM	Rapid Estimate of Adult Literacy in Medicine
RGSC	Registrar General's Social Classes
RPA	Rapid participatory appraisal
SAPs	Structural Adjustment Programmes
SARS	Severe Acute Respiratory Syndrome
SEP	Socio-economic position
TB	Tuberculosis
TOFHLA	Test of Functional Health Literacy in Adults
TTM	Transtheoretical Model
UDHR	Universal Declaration of Human Rights
UK NSC	United Kingdom National Screening Committee
UN	United Nations
UNDP	United Nations Development Programme
UNFCCC	United Nations Framework Convention on Climate Change
UNICEF	United Nations Children's Fund
WHO	World Health Organization
WTO	World Trade Organization

INTRODUCTION

Key Themes in Public Health comprises a series of introductory chapters exploring various dimensions of public health. It is written in a context of expanding interest in public health, ranging from concern with the implications of climate change and ageing populations, through to the challenge of improving health for all at a time of global financial austerity, alongside new and enduring threats to health.

The book is intended primarily for those studying public health, in one form or another, at an introductory level and without specialist knowledge. It is, however, a student companion and reference book rather than a textbook. The aim of each essay is to inform students by providing a basic grounding in the relevant theme as well as a departure point for further study. Each theme is structured to furnish responses to questions such as 'What does this mean?', 'What are the central ideas and debates?' and 'How is this relevant to public health?' Each chapter begins with a comment on context in order to illustrate how ideas surface in particular social, political and economic milieux and have historical antecedents. From here, the theme is defined and explicated before its significance for public health is explored. Central ideas tend not to be premised on any assumed essence or value. Rather, the intention is to explore often competing ideas in order to reveal the complexity of issues. Some readers may be perturbed or frustrated by this approach on the basis that it rarely offers a definitive view, requiring instead that they themselves decide the adequacy and relevance of particular claims.

The length of each thematic chapter, as well as each section within a theme, differs, sometimes markedly so. These variations reflect, among other things, the complexity of the theme and its significance for public health. The chapter on inequalities in health, for example, is by far the longest. The theme also surfaces as a pertinent issue in many other chapters. This is necessitated by the centrality of the theme to public health policy and practice and the breadth and depth of the available research on inequalities in health, as well as its contentiousness among academics and policymakers in particular. In other themes – evaluation and social capital, for example – fairly extensive attention is giving to definitional issues as a basis for exploring more fully each theme's application to, and significance for, public health.

As the title of the book implies, the aim is to make sense of the broad field of public health by disentangling a number of individual 'stand-alone' themes. The intention in so doing is to seek clarity in a complex, expanding and contested field. The potential disadvantage of this approach is, however, that it tends to present component themes as distinct rather than as interrelated and often interdependent. The inclusion of some material under one specific theme rather than another reflects not only choices made in order to develop particular lines of argument, but also pragmatic decisions relating

1

to the desire to make complex material manageable and accessible to the reader within a concise format. Highlighting (emboldened) links to related themes as and when they first occur in a chapter goes some way towards overcoming the disadvantages of separating themes into distinct essays. Overlapping content across some themes also provides a partial solution to this issue.

The selection of key themes – which is, self-evidently, entirely mine – attempts to capture the contemporary public health field. Many, if not most of the themes will be familiar and their inclusion probably uncontentious, thereby reflecting the enduring concerns of public health policymakers, practitioners and academics alike. Behaviour change, for example, continues to occupy much of the policy and practice space in public health, despite evidence of the limited effectiveness of individually-oriented behaviour change strategies. Some readers might reasonably have expected particular themes to appear that, in fact, do not. In some cases, these topics materialize within other themes. The politics and economics of health, for example, appear as 'red threads' that run throughout the themes, reflecting their significance for public health. Other themes may seem out of place in a text on public health – socialization and education, for example. Their inclusion reflects the increasing recognition of the relevance of the wider, social determinants of health, as well as the life course (also included as a thematic chapter in its own right) in understanding long-term processes of health development.

A corollary to this approach is that the selection has eschewed an orthodox medical interpretation of public health. As a consequence, health care generally has a limited profile in the book. As many have noted, too often public health is conflated with health care, a tendency this text seeks to avoid. Medicine, as a major social institution, is included as a thematic chapter, reflecting its pivotal historical and contemporary relationship with public health. Few other medical or clinical ideas have, however, found their way into the text unless they relate directly to the prevention and health promotion domains of public health. Thus, chapters on screening and primary health care are both included. Adopting a thematic, rather than a topic- or issue-based approach, has also meant that subjects such as smoking and obesity are not included as themes per se. Rather, they appear within particular chapters as pertinent examples and illustrations of particular points. To some degree, identifying overarching themes forfeits some of the depth and debate surrounding particular issues, as well as the interrelatedness of themes. It does, however, allow better sense to be made of the vast public health research canvas.

Although written with an international audience in mind, examples from England provide many of the illustrations for each of the themes. To some extent this reflects the (re)emergence of public health as a major site of policy and practice activity over the past two decades or more, as well as the richness of public health research in England and the rest of the United Kingdom (UK: England, Scotland, Wales and Northern Ireland) more broadly. In this regard, the UK serves as a microcosm of trends unfolding in most high-income countries since the latter decades of the twentieth century. This makes it possible to identify a fair degree of commonality in the present-day characteristics of public health internationally in terms of issues, challenges and responses. Public health is, nonetheless, globalized in several respects. Thus, a number of themes (such as climate change and sustainable development) explicitly take a global perspective, exploring public health in low- and middle-income countries in particular.

A further point of reference is Scandinavia (Norway, Sweden and Denmark) and the Nordic countries (Scandinavia plus Finland, Iceland and associated territories) more broadly. Their seemingly enviable positions towards the top of a number of global health and development league tables have attracted considerable discussion and debate in the public health field in recent years. In a number of respects they provide a point of contrast to the main thrust of developments in other high-income countries. Drawing examples from these countries, therefore, provides a counterpoint to many of the debates emanating from elsewhere in the Western world. Of note, too, is the seemingly greater traction of public health as an aspect of an expanded welfare state in Nordic countries, at least for the time being.

The field of public health has benefited significantly in recent years from the increasing attention it has received from scholars working within a variety of academic fields, in particular from those working in the social sciences. In order to begin to understand the forces shaping public health the book draws on this rich disciplinary research base, incorporating theoretical ideas from across the sociological, psychological, physiological and epidemiological studies of public health as the subject matter of each particular theme requires. In so doing, the text seeks to develop a multidisciplinary perspective on each key theme. It falls short of offering an interdisciplinary perspective, the latter demanding greater integration and synthesis than has been possible within the constraints of the format used here. The text is especially informed by a broadly sociological perspective. Drawing on Mills' (1959) idea of the sociological imagination, the book endeavours to locate public health in its varied social contexts rather than treat it in narrow, individualistic terms. Such a perspective has the potential to reveal the ways in which, for example, unemployment, poverty and poor health are shared by many others and have their origins in the way society is organized. In other words, these phenomena occur in patterns, which are better understood as *public issues* rather than *personal* or *private problems* brought on by people's own inadequacies and failings. As Verweij and Dawson (2007: 29) note, however, describing something as 'a public health problem often serves implicit normative or political purposes'. Thus, public health is not a value-free activity or process.

Starting with contexts enables us to better understand the broad patterns of health and health inequalities as well as how health is shaped by, and contingent upon, a variety of global, national, local and familial determinants that are interrelated in dynamic ways. Notwithstanding the underlying genetic dimension to health and disease, the intention is to explore how health is socially constructed and socially produced. Such a perspective challenges the inevitability of patterns of health and disease. Using the example of the trend in childhood obesity in England over the last 30 years, a sociologically informed public health perspective would pose questions such as 'why here, why now, and why among these particular groups rather than others?' At the same time, however, the book attempts to avoid accusations of deterministic thinking in relation to deep-seated social forces. Rather, the book views people as interdependent with others in a range of settings, as well as with aspects of their physical and natural environments: to paraphrase Marx, individuals are thus viewed as 'free' to choose but seldom in conditions of their own choosing. Similarly, and as difficult as it can be at times, in analysing complex issues the aim has been to avoid advocacy. In common with many other policy arenas, much that is written about public health in policies, the media and even some academic work takes a polemical turn and uses the language of 'crisis', exhorting 'someone' to do 'something' about, what is taken to be, an agreed 'problem'. This is particularly pertinent to the field of public health, oriented as it is towards action. In the same vein, the book seeks to avoid assuming common agreement about issues. The aim throughout is on trying to develop an understanding of complex phenomena – often neglected in an action-oriented field such as public health – where 'understanding' can be equated with 'theoretical and abstract' and, therefore, insufficiently relevant to the 'real world' (Graham, 2007).

Public health: a word on terminology

Although all the themes in the book are initially defined and interpreted, the central term – public health – needs some discussion at the outset, not least because it has become a matter of some considerable controversy and dispute. Definitions continue to proliferate, expanding the meanings attached to the term to cover an ever-increasing number of issues. In addition, definitions frequently contain normative statements relating to what public health should do or be. These trends have, no doubt, contributed to the ambiguity surrounding public health; at times, public health seemingly includes everything but ceases to mean anything very much at all.

The term 'public health' combines two words, each of which can themselves be ambiguous. From a definitional point of view, the word 'public' is the more critical word, however. Verweij and Dawson (2007) argue that among the many definitions of public health, 'public' tends to be used in two different ways. In the most straight-forward interpretation, 'public' is an aggregate concept and equated with 'population'. In this sense, public health refers to the state of a population's health: that is, a population's (or population sub-group's) 'collective health' (Rose, 2008: 96). The notion of 'public' as applied to population or collective health has a *distributive* element that refers to the *pattern* of health in a population, as well as a *determinants* element that refers to the pattern of *causes* (Verweij and Dawson, 2007). The term 'public health' continues to be used in this way within and beyond the field to refer to a population's health and, sometimes, to patterns and variations within it. Thus, describing phenomena as 'public health issues' implies that they have consequences for the health of the public; in other words, they have implications for population health. The second interpretation of 'public' is in terms of *collective action* with specific (collective) goals in mind – to protect and promote a population's health alongside efforts to prevent illness and disease. The oft-quoted Acheson definition (1988: 4) expresses this interpretation, describing public health as the 'art and science of preventing disease, prolonging life and promoting health *through the organized efforts of society*' (emphasis added). Public health is thus a field of action and something that public health professionals (among others) 'do'. In England, it has become commonplace to discuss 'the public health function', particularly in relation to the activities of the specialist field of public health practice as well as the wider workforce. How public health policy and practice are interpreted and implemented takes many forms, however, varying by country as well as over time in terms of the particular emphasis and orientation of actions. Thus, pursuing a definitive answer to the question of 'what is public health?' can be a worthwhile process but an unproductive aim.

Historically, public health has been used in these two ways, that is to say, to signify collective actions as well as to describe the health of the population. The enactment of public health laws during mid-nineteenth century England as well as the more recent tobacco legislation in many countries, for example, involved collective efforts to improve the population's health. A third, more recent use of the term relates to public health as a theoretical field. Lang and Raynor (2012), for example, identify five models that have been more or less dominant during different historical periods, illustrating how the meanings attached to public health and its manifestation as a field of practice have shifted over time. They advocate an ecological model of public health, based on an understanding of the interdependence between human beings as well as between them and their environments. The implication of such a model is that social and environmental conditions allow, by degrees, health to flourish. The upshot of this is that health cannot be 'delivered' via services and professionals. In keeping with the ideas of Chadwick (a nineteenth century English social reformer associated with the development of public health) the model explains good health as flowing from the population to the individual, rather than the other way round. Beyond the academic field, however, progress has been slow and uneven in terms of adopting and integrating social and ecological models of public health into policy and practice. This trend reflects the broader point that the explicit use of theory (as well as evidence) remains relatively rare in public health.

Rather than offering a further definition of public health or selecting a preferred one, the foregoing discussion has sought to illustrate and clarify its multifaceted, contested and changing character. In so doing, it has also sought to provide some contours to the term as a basis for making better sense of what is covered in the ensuing chapters. Indeed, public health may more adequately be viewed as an epiphenomenon: that is to say, as a secondary phenomenon that occurs in one form or another alongside other, primary phenomena relating to broader social, political and economic processes. This means that how public health is conceptualized and operationalized in policy and practice shifts in relation to the dominant ideological values of the day. It also implies, however, possibilities for change.

Globally, the past decade has been a particularly turbulent period, characterized by a variety of economic, political and social upheavals as well as extreme climatic events, all with considerable implications for public health. During the writing of this book, a number of especially momentous events of significance for public health occurred. These instabilities will continue as an ever-present characteristic of life. This text thus provides an overview, a snapshot of public health at a particular historical period. In this respect, it inevitably represents an ongoing project.

ADVOCACY

Context

Public health has always been linked to action. John Snow advocated the removal of the handle of the Broad Street pump in Soho, London, in the middle of the nineteenth century because he considered it likely to be the source of the contaminated water that caused the cholera epidemics between 1853 and 1855. This classic example illustrates what is commonly understood by the term public health advocacy: constructing arguments designed to bring about a particular course of action, the ultimate purpose of which is to improve public health. Snow encountered much resistance to his advocacy from a variety of quarters. In part, this was because his theory of cholera transmission was at odds with the prevailing miasma theory (illness caused by breathing in bad air) of the time, but also because the vested interests of local councils and water companies made them resistant to his ideas and fearful of the cost implications of his analysis. Eventually, the pump handle was removed and the epidemic subsided. The pump remained in use, however, until some point in the 1880s. Although somewhat apocryphal, the Broad Street pump example illustrates the point that whether or not something is defined as an issue in need of resolution not only shifts over time – as it becomes more or less conspicuous in the media of the day – but also reflects the differing interests of particular groups and their varied public prominence.

Defining advocacy

Advocacy has been defined by Bassett (2003) in broad terms, as a process through which an issue is promoted by various forms of argumentation. Among the many definitions, some common ground can be identified: a focus on influencing laws, regulations and policies – sometimes at a global level – to bring about a desired change; an emphasis on forming coalitions and acting collectively to bring about maximum leverage; and an acknowledgement that, above all else, advocacy is a political process through which those with power – typically, governments and corporations, but also others with a vested interest in protecting their rights and liberties – are challenged. Definitions of public health advocacy tend to focus upon the overarching goal of creating environments that support **health**. Thus, advocacy can be viewed in terms of various activities that are pursued as a means towards a specified end. These dimensions are reflected in the definition proposed by the World Health Organization (WHO) (Nutbeam, 1998: 5): 'individual and social actions designed to gain political commitment, policy support, social acceptance and systems support for a particular health goal … taken by and/or on behalf of individuals and groups to create living conditions which are conducive to health'.

From these and other similar conceptions of advocacy, two overlapping definitional types can be discerned, each of which emphasizes a different level at which advocacy intentions originate and are directed. Some definitions emphasize **community**-level empowerment and mobilization, working in a so-called 'bottom-up' way, 'starting with the identification of the **health needs** and goals by the community members themselves' (Loue, 2006: 459). Carlisle (2000) argues that advocacy tends to be used in this sense when seeking to improve the lot of those who are vulnerable or otherwise disempowered, either through representing them as an individual (*case* advocacy) or lobbying on a specific issue (*cause* advocacy). This type of definition is particularly relevant to those working with individuals and community groups where capacity building (in relation to developing political advocacy skills, for example) and community activism are important.

Other definitions of advocacy emphasize wider social processes of change in which a broad coalition of interest groups come together over a specific issue. Chapman's (2004: 361) definition reflects this perspective, placing particular emphasis on the role of the media in the advocacy process: 'public health advocacy … is the strategic use of news media to advance a public policy initiative, often in the face of such opposition'. All told, advocacy is perhaps best defined as both a process and an outcome, as reflected in the definition offered by Christoffel (2000: 722) wherein 'advocacy is the application of information and resources (including finances, effort, and votes) to effect systematic changes that shape the way people in a community live'. In short, change at any level is the implicit and explicit purpose of advocacy.

The significance of advocacy for public health

The significance of advocacy as a core skill for those working in public health has been underscored in recent decades. In part, this is an aspect of a broader trend featuring the emergence of a number of health-related social movements, which have at their core the purpose of challenging the 'authority structures … of medicine, science, governments, and corporations' (Brown and Zavestoski, 2004: 679). Thus, advocates tend to question whose interests are being served by a particular law, regulation, policy or general situation. In so doing they seek to effect some form of re-patterning of a situation in order to better meet the needs of other groups. Advocacy is, therefore, less about mediation (in the sense of seeking to reconcile differences) and more concerned with opposition and activism in pursuit of a particular cause. In 1986, the *Ottawa Charter* identified advocacy as one of the three ways to achieve the conditions for good health and well-being. In the UK, the *Public Health Careers and Skills Framework* (Public Health Resource Unit/Skills for Health, [PHRU/SfH] 2008/2009) identifies advocacy as a key competence, particularly for those in leadership roles. The Framework states, for example, that the aims of public health will be achieved through 'acting as an advocate for the public's health' (PHRU/SfH, 2008/2009: 4) and that competence is needed to advocate for health and well-being and to reduce health **inequalities**. Professional organizations, such as the UK Faculty of Public Health (FPH) and the American Public Health Association (APHA) have also identified a role for advocacy in their organizations. Indeed, the APHA identifies itself as the 'primary voice for public health advocacy' in America, with the remit to 'protect all Americans and their communities from preventable, serious health threats' (www.apha.org/advocacy). This role may well involve drawing attention to the negative impact of various corporate practices on population health – so-called 'corporate disease promotion' (Freudenberg, 2005: 298). In the USA, the potential for public health practitioners to contribute to the criminal justice process by influencing how courts approach issues relevant to public health has also become apparent (Kromm *et al.*, 2009). In relation to substance use and domestic violence, for example, public health practitioners might help courts decide on the appropriate balance of **prevention**, rehabilitation and punishment.

Advocacy is seen by some as an obligation and as much a part of public health practice as science (see, for example, Weed and McKeown, 2003). However, Chapman (2004) argues that advocacy is rarely prioritized by those working in public health. This may be due to a perceived lack of skills as well as limited opportunities for their development. Gomm *et al.* (2006) identify three core skills necessary to work effectively as an advocate: working collaboratively with multiple stakeholders, building effective alliances and coalitions; using media strategically; and, thinking analytically and strategically about policy solutions. These so-called 'higher order' skills tend not to be the focus of the **education** and training of public health practitioners. Chapman (2001) argues that few public health practitioners are skilled in translating research findings into policy and practice and managing the (often prolonged) ensuing process of argumentation.

Weed and Mink (2002) and Chapman (2001) focus on the potential role and responsibilities of epidemiologists in the advocacy process. They see epidemiological **evidence** as the foundation of advocacy not least because it can provide descriptive data related to particular phenomena as well as evidence relating to **causality**. Advocacy thus begins (but does not end) with specific facts – for example, about deaths due to smoking or speeding drivers. All argue that some of the reluctance to engage with the advocacy process lies in the perceived tension between scientific objectivity and the political character of public health policy making. They conclude, however, that a role in advocacy is compatible and consistent with the public stewardship responsibilities of epidemiologists working in public health.

By its very nature, advocacy involves trying to influence policy, be that at an organizational, local or national government level. Many of those working in public health outside academia are government officials who may see advocacy as a form of criticism of their employers. Some have argued that those working in public health should only engage in advocacy independently of their official role and within the confines of their organizational values and philosophies (Regidor *et al.*, 2007). This might have the effect of limiting the public stewardship roles of those with leadership responsibilities, such as directors of public health in England, as well as aspects of the community development roles of, for example, public health nurses. In the case of child poverty, research suggests that while public health nurses tend to be attuned to the impact of poverty on child and family health their public health role can often be constrained by the organizations within which they work (Cohen and McKay, 2010). Nevertheless, in a climate of increasing professional regulation and surveillance – a process that has been accelerated by the growing involvement of private sector organizations in the delivery of **health promotion** and public health work – it is likely that the political character of advocacy will lead to a marginalization of this type of work among some occupational groups. There may, nonetheless, be greater scope for advocacy through voluntary sector organizations, which have traditionally used their client- and community-centred role to 'give a voice' to marginalized groups. However, the recent trend towards the commissioning of services, in countries such as England, may limit the advocacy role of voluntary organizations because contractually-agreed outcomes take priority.

Successful advocacy often requires strategic planning in order to maximize support and pressure for a particular argument and action in order to bring about a specific outcome (Chapman, 2001, 2004). This usually begins with the 'framing' of an issue, specifically in relation to what is at stake and what needs to be done. Chapman (2001) argues that framing is important due to the differing perspectives on what precisely is at issue in any given event. Framing takes place, therefore, in a complex, shifting and often controversial context and necessarily involves rebutting and *re*framing opponents' arguments. Framing involves the presentation of an issue not so much as an individual, personal matter but rather as a public problem (Mills, 1959), shifting responsibility away from the individual towards those with power to bring about social change. It also involves presenting policy alternatives as solutions, which, crucially, have practical appeal (Gomm *et al.*, 2006). An example of a grassroots approach to advocacy is Mothers Against Drunk Driving (MADD; www.madd.org) in the USA, which began through the efforts of one mother whose 13-year-old daughter was killed as a result of an accident involving a drunken driver (Loue, 2006). As a not-for-profit organization, MADD has been successful in engaging members of the public, the media and legislators in its campaigns, bringing about a number of changes in the law (for example, mandatory jail sentences for drunk driving and increasing to 21 the minimum legal age for drinking in the USA).

Advocacy is, then, not simply a technical issue involving the presentation of information; values lie at the heart of advocacy and are the source of protracted debates. All analyses of both advocates' and opponents' positions are ultimately reducible to their underpinning values (Chapman, 2004). The history of debates around gun and tobacco control illustrates this point. The advocacy process underscores the values inherent in such debates and reveals which values tend to take precedence. Central to these debates are matters relating to the economic and social costs of particular actions and inactions. An intervention will be deemed more or less justifiable depending upon the particular values of the interested parties, including the general public. In many cases, whether or not action is the outcome of advocacy (as in the case of gun control) will depend more on values than any assessment of **risk** (Chapman, 2001). For example, even though the probability of being killed by gunshot is low, the value attributed to the potential to save lives through stricter gun control is judged to be 'worth' the specific infringement of some individuals' freedom to own and use a gun, at least in some countries.

By definition, values are emotionally loaded because they are an expression of the things that matter to people. This might explain why some who work in public health may be reluctant to engage in advocacy, preferring what they see as a more detached, neutral and scientific approach to the interpretation and use of evidence. However, the controversial character of many public health debates (for example, second-hand cigarette smoke) suggests that the 'facts' are 'interpreted' differently by particular interest groups because of their varying value positions. This explains why 'communities can become outraged by low risk issues' (Chapman, 2001: 1230).

Media advocacy has emerged as a tool in the advocacy process in recent years. It tends to be used to frame particular stories about issues and exert pressure on individuals and organizations. Building extensive support and sustaining interest in an issue has been enabled through the development and use of social media and mobile phone technology over the last decade or so. Subsequently, a number of 'advocacy coalitions' (Buse *et al.*, 2005: 132) have emerged, which use a variety of media to form virtual communities that have the merit of being both flexible and quickly mobilized in response to issues. Such media may also overcome some of the difficulties of mobilizing collective action among those who share particular beliefs (Sabatier, 1998).

Examples include the UK-based 38degrees, MoveOn in the USA, GetUp in Australia and the transnational community Avaaz (voice). Such virtual networks tend to be founded by small groups of activists and volunteers who not only share particular values and beliefs, but also operate on a not-for-profit basis and remain independent of political party allegiance or corporate sponsorship (often being funded through donations). Their stated aims tend to involve, among other things, the democratization of decision-making. A variety of issues are chosen for campaigns (influenced by members) including the environment, human rights, corruption, access to health care and media freedom. Such advocacy communities can be seen as having the potential to influence many of the wider **determinants** of health although that may not be their primary concern. For these reasons, it is important not to underestimate the role of the media in advocacy. Most people obtain their information about health issues, including public health issues, from news and other social media. Chapman (2004) argues that most public health reforms have been preceded by protracted periods of news coverage of debates for and against changes. However, use of the media in public health advocacy tends to be different from its use in **health education** and **social marketing**. These latter approaches focus more on the provision of information intended to persuade individuals to alter their behaviour in some way.

The sheer complexity of the social world makes it difficult to attribute cause and effect in the advocacy world. This is especially the case when the timescale over which the advocacy process takes place is protracted – as in the case of tobacco control. There are a number of examples, nevertheless, where changes have been made to policies, laws and regulations following concerted public health advocacy campaigns: examples include the adoption of municipal smoking bylaws in Canada (Asbridge, 2004) and cycle helmet laws in New Zealand and some parts of Canada. In recent years the virtual advocacy coalition model has been shown to be a particularly effective means of advocating change. A campaign led by 38degrees, for instance, is widely credited with halting the proposed sale of state-owned ancient forests in the UK in 2012. This is noteworthy given the research suggesting that the advocacy model works less well in closed centralized political systems such as the UK (Buse *et al.*, 2005).

Sometimes the state itself may use a public health advocacy approach in order to influence how citizens act. In 1997, the Swedish Government introduced Vision Zero (www.swedishtrade.se/usa/visionzero) to reduce traffic fatalities on Sweden's roads to zero by 2020; by 2009, Sweden had the lowest per capita traffic fatalities in the world. The Vision Zero approach involved a variety of measures, including changes to the road infrastructure to minimize the likelihood of human error, safety improvements to vehicle technology, speed limit control, surveillance and associated penalties. Other Scandinavian countries such as Norway have implemented similar policies.

As indicated above, much public health advocacy has involved focusing on a single issue. However, advocacy approaches have been increasingly used in relation to health inequalities. The collection and publication of data showing the social and geographical patterning of health and health behaviours has been used to argue that health inequalities are unfair, unjust and should be narrowed. While something of a consensus has developed around the perceived need to narrow, if not eliminate, such inequalities, how to achieve this goal remains contentious. It is possible, however, to discern a growing pressure on politicians to act on the basis of social justice, rather than, for example, the values of the market (Dorfman *et al.*, 2005).

Conclusion

Although advocacy involves bridging the gap between knowledge and action, this is only part of the story. Advocacy involves challenging the status quo and the use of power to achieve a particular (public health) end. This can mean that advocacy does not always sit well with some public health practitioners who view their practice as predominantly underpinned by the values of scientific competence, accountability and high ethical standards, not political involvement or controversy. However, advocacy has the potential to lead to forms of transformational change of the kind required to narrow health inequalities. In this regard, Popay *et al.* (2010) argue that public health practitioners have a duty to draw attention to the health consequences of social injustice and articulate a vision for a fairer society.

BEHAVIOUR CHANGE

Context

Behaviour change – as both an idea and a goal – has a rich but somewhat chequered history in the field of public health. Nonetheless, how people behave is an important **determinant** of their **health** as well as having implications for the health of others. Worldwide, smoking and alcohol consumption (so-called 'modifiable behaviours'), for example, account for a significant proportion of premature death and disability (Kaner and McGovern, 2013). Research suggests, however, that while the number of people attempting to change some aspect of their behaviour is high, the proportion achieving sustainable change is low. Understanding how people develop particular patterns of behaviour is, therefore, a central endeavour of public health. How such patterns are explained has considerable implications for policy and practice.

Defining behaviour change

Definitions of behaviour change are sparse. The root of the term lies in the field of behavioural psychology (or behaviourism), which views behaviour – people's overt, observable actions – as acquired through a process of conditioning. People's responses to stimuli in the environment are seen as shaping behaviours. Underlying biological and psychological processes such as cognition, motivation, emotion and so on are viewed as relatively unimportant. According to this view, behaviours can be trained and changed through the use of reinforcement and punishment, for example. Behaviourism, as a theory of learning, has, however, been criticized on the grounds that it does not take account of internal mental states or the notion of free will. Neither does it explain how learning takes please without the use of reinforcement or punishment. However, concepts central to this perspective continue to influence, to varying degrees, a number of psychological models of health behaviour change that have emerged in recent years.

In the public health field, behaviour *change* refers to the explicit intention to shift behaviours in a more 'desirable' direction, away from health damaging towards more health enhancing forms. Change might be directed at behaviours towards health services (for example, taking up an invitation for **screening**) or a particular habit (such as smoking or being physically inactive). More recently attention has focused on changing more complex behaviour such as that relating to modes of travel (Goodwin, 2008) and various kinds of pro-environmental behaviours such as household recycling (Fornara *et al.*, 2011). Interest has also grown regarding how to change the behaviours of health professionals and practitioners. Changing doctors' prescribing behaviours, encouraging health professionals to use **evidence**-based guidelines as well as integrate **health promotion** and **prevention** into the primary care setting are examples of recent topics of interest in this area.

The significance of behaviour change for public health

There has been a resurgence of interest in behaviour change in a number of countries following the publication in 2008 of Thaler and Sunstein's book entitled *Nudge: Improving Decisions About Health, Wealth and Happiness* (see nudges.org). In the UK, the coalition government established a *Behavioural Insights Team* (the 'Nudge' Unit) in 2010, to which Thaler was appointed an adviser (Pykett *et al.*, 2011). The 2010 White Paper on public health in England (Secretary of State for Health, 2010) – *Healthy Lives, Healthy People* – made frequent reference to supporting innovative approaches to behaviour change, such as nudging. Behavioural economics (nudging) is but the latest reincarnation of psychological approaches to behaviour change that have been popular in public health over several decades. The 'nudge' approach is based on the premise that behaviours are never entirely rationally-based and that people need help in making better health choices. Referred to as libertarian paternalism (Thaler and Sunstein, 2008), strategies based on the concept of nudging seek to protect individual freedom of choice while at the same time instituting a supportive system of government (Vallgårda, 2012). 'Choice architecture' – the environment in which people make choices – is a key idea, the aim of strategies being to craft the environment to shift choices in a particular (health enhancing) direction. Strategies might include institutions imposing small costs on those who depart from healthy options, altering the design of public spaces or using psychological prompts (framing and wording options) to promote 'citizenly' behaviour (Pykett *et al.*, 2011). Although presented as pragmatic common sense, Pykett *et al.* (2011) point out that priming people to behave in ways desired by the government through subtle means can still amount to coercion. The application of behavioural economics to cancer screening programmes (in order to increase uptake) has been viewed as especially problematic, given the potential to compromise the process of informed consent (Ploug *et al.*, 2012). The **ethics** of behavioural economics therefore raise particular issues.

Despite such criticisms, a behavioural economics approach has been applied to a range of health issues. In particular, financial incentives (penalties and rewards) have been used in a number of low- and high-income countries to promote behaviour change in a wide variety of health arenas. The idea here is that small, frequent, immediate payments increase and reinforce motivation to change some aspect of behaviour. Small financial incentives have met with a degree of success in increasing the uptake of HIV testing and counselling in Malawi as well as encouraging safe sex practices (to prevent the spread of HIV/AIDS) in Tanzania (De Walque *et al.*, 2012). In the Tanzanian study, however, those offered a smaller financial incentive ($10 rather than $20) showed no change in behaviour. Schemes of this type have also been used in the USA to increase the uptake of health checks and educational activities among low-income families

(Morris *et al.*, 2012), to promote smoking cessation among pregnant women, mediation adherence and weight management, with some degree of success (Loewenstein *et al.*, 2012). All such schemes treat the behavioural *symptoms* of more deep-seated structural problems and are likely therefore to be of limited success, particularly in the longer term. However, the appeal of behavioural economics to policymakers who prefer a 'light touch' to government intervention has meant that less regard has been given to evidence of effectiveness or adequacy of theoretical premises (Lowenstein *et al.*, 2012).

Beyond behavioural economics, several psychological models of behaviour change have been developed and tested out in the health field. Models can be useful devices for identifying the relevant constructs that describe and, to varying degrees, explain the phenomenon under study, particularly with a view to predicting what the behavioural outcome might be. Over the past few decades four models in particular have been applied fairly extensively to a range of health behaviours including screening, alcohol consumption, smoking, exercise, dental flossing and breastfeeding (Mielewczyk and Willig, 2007): the transtheoretical model (TTM), also referred to as the stages of change model (Prochaska and Diclemente, 1983); the health belief model (HBM) (Rosenstock,1974; Becker, 1974); protection motivation theory (Rogers, 1983); and the theory of reasoned action (Fishbein and Ajzen, 1975), together with its extension, the theory of planned behaviour (Ajzen, 1985).

Beliefs, attitudes and motivation towards a specific behaviour are central constructs in these models, which also emphasize, to varying degrees, the influence of social norms and 'significant others' (those whose views matter and influence a person's intention to act). There has, nevertheless, been extensive criticism of these models. Much of the criticism stems from the findings of empirical studies that give limited support for the models in terms of their power to explain and predict changes in behaviour. West (2005: 1038), for example, described the TTM as 'little more than a security blanket for researchers and clinicians', accounting for its popularity among professionals in terms of its intuitive appeal as representing a cognitive reality – that is, that people move through a series of stages in a linear fashion, one stage leading to another. Mielewczyk and Willig (2007: 811) argue that social cognition models in general have a 'major conceptual flaw' based as they are on a predominantly rational conceptualization of health behaviour. Although studies have found that providing people with information and advice can change beliefs, attitudes and even intentions, changes in behaviour do not necessarily follow. West, for example, argues that people's expressed intentions to stop smoking are unstable over short periods of time and are dependent on what else is happening in their lives; that is, they reflect the 'moment-to-moment balance of motives' (West, 2005: 1038).

This lack of congruence between key constructs and behavioural outcomes has given rise to critical reviews of, and revisions to, the theoretical basis of many models. These revisions appear, however, to have achieved relatively little in terms of increasing their explanatory power or deflecting further criticism. Most psychological models tend to place undue emphasis on rationality and the conscious weighing up of costs and benefits in decision-making. Psychological approaches have also been criticized for paying less attention to processes of primary and secondary **socialization** through which habits and predispositions to act are developed. Such approaches also tend to neglect the emotional, and sometimes spontaneous, dimensions of behaviour, particularly relevant in the health field, in which vicarious enjoyment and fun play a part. People tend to act in customary, habitual ways, and/or ways that fulfil some kind of emotional need, such as a desire to repeat satisfying experiences. Established patterns of behaviour are thus relatively stable and hence difficult to change (Prättälä and Puska, 2012). The influence of addiction – particularly influential in behaviours such as smoking (West, 2005) – is also neglected in many models. In this regard, behavioural economics represents a more adequate appreciation of the reality of health decision-making.

Because psychological models tend to describe behaviour in isolation and without reference to the social and cultural context within which it is embedded, they have been labelled 'reductionist' in that the behaviour itself is the focus. Research in other disciplinary fields such as social anthropology and sociology gives primacy to contextual factors in understanding behaviours. Not only are there multiple contextual influences, these vary in their significance over time and **place**. That behaviour is complex and contingent on other factors raises significant issues about the extent to which it is possible to develop a model with strong explanatory power for all behaviours and all situations. More fundamentally, Mielewczyk and Willig (2007: 824) question the use of the term 'health behaviour' arguing that 'it would make more sense to conceptualize such behaviours as constituent parts of complex practices and consider the possibility that their meanings and the reasons for their occurrence vary across contexts'. Graham's qualitative research (1989) on women and smoking illustrates this point. Her research showed that smoking was bound into women's everyday experience of caring for children in a low-income household in that it was part of the way in which they structured their caring role and coped when things were stressful or went wrong. Significantly, women were aware of the harms of smoking and often tried to cut back. Moreover, these caring practices and the place of smoking within them were shaped by broader material circumstances of living in poverty. Viewing actions as embedded in broader social practices – such as caring for children – not only reveals the complexity and fluidity of actions, but also challenges the very meaning of the term 'health behaviour'. Broadening the focus from the individual to the social also brings into view how social norms within groups influence patterns of behaviour over time and place. Shared expectations – among women caring for children in circumstances of poverty, for example – influence social practices such that, as in this case, smoking becomes normative – that is to say, compliant with expectations. In a similar vein, Marston and King's (2006) qualitative systematic review revealed a variety of social and cultural influences that explained why young people sometimes engaged in unsafe sex. They concluded that providing young people with information and free condoms alone was unlikely to lead to changes in how they approached having sex.

The emphasis on psychological models in public health policy has direct implications for the type of public health interventions advocated. Psychological constructs, such as motivation and cognition, have been used to inform strategies for behaviour change. In England, brief advice, brief interventions and motivational interviewing (MI) have been promoted by successive governments as offering relatively simple ways for health professionals to integrate health issues into every contact regardless of a person's presenting issue. In England, identification and brief advice (IBA) has been the main approach advocated to address alcohol-related harm. MI – 'a directive, client-centred counselling style for eliciting behaviour change by helping clients to explore and resolve ambivalence' (Rollnick and Miller, 1995: 325) – has become especially popular as an alternative to brief advice, for which there is limited evidence of effectiveness (Rollnick *et al.*, 2010). MI (including its condensed form, behaviour change counselling) may hold intuitive appeal to policymakers and practitioners in that it has some congruence with traditional clinical encounters in which clinicians respond to the kinds of issues patients often bring (Miller and Rollnick, 2012). Evidence of its effectiveness is mixed, however, particularly with regard to the sustainability of changes. Critical factors in MI are the collaborative style of the practitioner, the demonstration of empathic understanding, acceptance of resistance and relapse, and support for self-efficacy (Wilson and Schlam, 2004). The extent to which practitioners who are not trained within the psychotherapeutic tradition can embrace these ways of working is a moot point. Training **primary health care** staff to increase their confidence, competence, effectiveness and inclination to use MI and other similar techniques, however, may well be limited (Butler *et al.*, 2013). This finding reinforces the point that behaviour change is difficult, and no less so for health professionals. Encouraging primary health care professionals to address prevention through **lifestyle** advice and behaviour modification ('making every contact count') is likely to be no less difficult than changing patients' behaviour.

Conclusion

Approaches to behaviour change based on the provision of information are likely to be favoured over and above those that focus on the conditions that encourage and support particular forms of behaviour, in spite of their limited evidence of effectiveness (House of Lords Science and Technology Select Committee, 2011). International evidence suggests, however, that there are relatively high levels of public support for a full range of interventions – not just individual-level psychological ones – to change behaviour (Branson *et al.*, 2012). Change is possible, as illustrated by studies that have tracked improvements in smoking, healthy eating and traffic safety during periods of social and economic change (Prättälä and Puska, 2012). However, of particular concern in public health is the extent to which behaviour change interventions may widen **inequalities** in health. As Graham (2007: 43) points out 'those born into privilege are more likely to experience themselves as agents of their own destiny; the sense of driving one's own life is harder to secure and to sustain for those struggling against disadvantage'.

CAUSALITY

Context

Causality – that is to say, understanding how putative causes (antecedents) might be related to specific effects – has always been a primary concern of **epidemiology** and public health. Epidemiological research on disease aetiology (the study of factors that cause disease) – such as the work of Doll and Hill (1954, 1964) and others, elucidating the link between tobacco smoke and lung cancer – has played a major role in the development of **prevention** strategies and **advocacy**. This work has contributed significantly to our understanding of cardiovascular disease and cancers in particular. Interest in cause and effect relationships has increased in recent years, not only within epidemiology and public health but also within the social sciences. In part, this reflects the growth of research into the wider, social **determinants** of **health** which has shifted the focus away from single factor exposures and specific diseases towards more complex issues, such as the link between poverty or class and life expectancy.

In public health, as well as other fields such as social **policy** and criminal justice, there has also been a growth of interest in understanding the impact of interventions. This has involved a shift from the more traditional medical interests of epidemiology – associated with trialling the impact of drugs, vaccines and other, primarily clinical, interventions – towards the **evaluation** of often quite complex social interventions. The burgeoning interest in cause and effect relationships reflects wider developments in the policy and practice field: the requirement to evaluate interventions to see 'what works'; the increasing importance attached to defining and measuring outcomes; the emphasis on using **evidence** to inform policy and practice; and, the use of commissioning to provide services that achieve specified outcomes. All these developments require knowledge about cause and effect relationships.

It should be noted at the outset, however, that in most public health situations establishing evidence of causation is methodologically and cognitively complex. Questions relating to the potential harms of regular consumption of alcohol during pregnancy, the clustering of cases of childhood leukaemia around power stations or the potential role of St John's Wort in the treatment of depression pose considerable challenges for researchers. Furthermore, heated debate about the meaning of 'cause' has generated a confusing vocabulary for those not familiar with the logic of science and philosophy. For those working in public health, nevertheless, it is necessary to have some appreciation of causality in order to make sense of claims about 'cause and effect' and appraise the relevance of these to public health policy and practice. As Tam and Lopman (2003: 477) point out, 'how we view causation influences (whether consciously or not) the way in which we frame research questions and analyse and interpret epidemiological data'.

Defining causality

A useful starting point for thinking about 'cause' is to distinguish it from the concept of association (or correlation). At times, there is a tendency to conflate the two, using the words interchangeably. Porta (2008: 8) defines association in terms of 'statistical dependence between two or more events, characteristics, or other variables': in other words, two things that tend to go together. Variables that are linked to certain disease outcomes in this statistical way are referred to as '**risk** factors'. Associations can be described as 'positive' if an increase in one variable is accompanied by an increase in another. Thus, a high level of low-density lipoprotein cholesterol (LDL) has been identified as a risk factor for coronary heart disease (CHD) in that it is associated with an increased risk of developing the disease. Establishing this association is the starting point for thinking about whether or not high LDL has a *causal* role in CHD. An association is, however, a statistical rather than a biological phenomenon, the latter being of critical importance if causality is to be attributed. Associations can also be described as 'negative' if an increase in a variable is accompanied by a decrease in another. Subjective well-being, for example, is negatively associated with obesity (Bökerman *et al.*, 2013).

An association may be due to chance; it may, in other words, be fortuitous. However, statistically significant associations (that is, those that are unlikely to be due to chance) require careful interpretation as they may be due to bias or confounding. In epidemiology, bias refers to errors that create false patterns, indicating differences between groups where there are, in fact, none, or conversely failing to detect real differences (Bhopal, 2008). Bias as a possible explanation for an association needs, therefore, to be excluded. Confounding refers to the presence of a third factor – a confounder – that confuses the observed association because it is itself associated with the exposure of interest and is also a risk factor for the disease. It leads to a spurious (not genuine) association. Taking account of a confounding factor is important because it accounts for some or all of the association. Matthews (2000) illustrates how associations can be problematic by reporting the results of a correlation study of stork pairs against the number of births in each of 17 countries (r=0.62, p=0.008). This statistically significant association is evidently non-causal and likely to be, according to Matthews, explained by a confounding variable. In the history of epidemiology there are many associations that, on closer inspection have been found to be due to confounding. The departure point for thinking about causality comes once chance, bias and confounding have been excluded (Constantine, 2012).

Within epidemiology there are very many definitions of 'cause'. However, two kinds of definition can be discerned, namely deterministic and probabilistic (Parascandola and Weed, 2001). Drawing on Galileo's descriptions for causes in the experimental sciences (Porta, 2008), definitions based on a deterministic concept of cause tend to be couched in terms of necessary and/or sufficient causes. A cause is described as *necessary* if the effect cannot occur without it and *sufficient* if it always produces that effect. Thus, a cause may be necessary and sufficient, necessary but not sufficient, sufficient but not necessary, and, neither necessary nor sufficient. Applying this thinking to infectious diseases makes it possible to conclude that microorganisms are necessary causes of disease but rarely sufficient. Tuberculosis (TB) for example, requires exposure to the tubercle bacterium (*Mycobacterium tuberculosis*) but disease ensues only if the host is susceptible. The basis of host susceptibility relates to factors such as poverty, malnutrition and overcrowding, as well as genetic factors and previous exposure. There is an important interplay here between the host, agent and environment. The component causes model, for example, is a deterministic model that has been extensively applied in epidemiology in order to identify individual risk factors for disease. Tam and Lopman (2003: 477) explain how 'a person, through exposure to various risk factors, eventually accumulates a combination of contributing exposures that constitute a sufficient cause and that, under identical conditions, invariably lead to disease'.

Definitions of causation have developed in response to the rise of chronic degenerative diseases as the major causes of mortality and morbidity where, as Susser (2001) points out, most causes are neither necessary nor sufficient but contributory. Hence, multifactorial models of causation – reflected in the metaphor of the 'web of causation' – have been developed to account for the complex set of factors and interactions that can be enabling, predisposing, precipitating or reinforcing. A definition based on a *probabilistic* concept of causation is provided by Bhopal (2008: 125): 'a cause can be considered to be something that alters the frequency of disease, health status, or associated factors in a population'.

The significance of causality for public health

There has been considerable criticism of multifactorial risk factor models of causation (the metaphor of the web) in recent years on two points. First, this form of model represents a 'black box' way of thinking, which overlooks mechanisms that connect causes with effects (Parascandola and Weed, 2001; Susser, 1998). Second, all exposures tend to be treated as if they are on the same level (Krieger, 2008). Part of the debate relates to the extent to which epidemiology as a population science has moved towards individualized understandings of causes. Traditional risk factor models tend to explain the social determinants of disease in terms of **lifestyle** behavioural factors and their biological consequences. The list of risk factors identified for CHD through the Framingham study illustrates this issue. Krieger (2008: 223) argues that 'societal patterns of disease represent the biological consequence of the ways of living and working differentially afforded to the social groups produced by each society's economy and political priorities'. The challenge is to find a way of conceptualizing and incorporating these patterns into a theory of causation. Susser (1998) uses the metaphor of Chinese boxes to present causes co-existing at the same level and Campaner (2011) the idea of multiple webs within which contributing and counteracting mechanisms play out over time. Krieger (2008) and Susser (1998) have coined the terms 'ecosocial epidemiology' and 'ecoepi-demiology' respectively, to represent a paradigm that seeks to connect biological consequences with social experiences and structural factors.

Bringing together the biological, statistical, psychological and social into a coherent reasoning process can be facilitated by using the Hill (1965) criteria, or viewpoints as he preferred to call them. This process is often referred to as the method of causal inference, central to which is the application of judgement. The nine criteria (temporality; strength of association; dose-response relationship; consistency; specificity; biological plausibility; coherence; analogy; and, experiment) are used to help develop an explanatory account for moving from the observed statistical association to a conclusion of causality. Temporality – that the exposure *always* precedes the outcome – is the only essential feature of causality. These criteria can be easily integrated into a probabilistic model of cause but less so a deterministic model. However, although the Hill criteria have been widely accepted within epidemiology they have attracted controversy on the grounds that they overlap, are obscurely described, lack internal coherence based as they are on different models of causality, and are irrelevant in some circumstances (Thygesen *et al.*, 2005). Nonetheless, for the novice they can provide a useful starting point for integrating and evaluating evidence relating to causes.

Although empirical data form the basis of the process of causal inference it is worth remembering that in all sciences it is impossible to observe directly a cause and effect relationship. This means that 'Causation is always attributed *theoretically*, as the best possible explanation of the available evidence' (Roberts, 2009: 30) (emphasis added). In epidemiology, theoretical generalizations about causation relate to the population level and cannot be used to provide explanations for each individual. Vineis (1997: 11) illustrates this point by arguing that 'although eliminating smoking cannot predict the individual risk closely, it will eliminate more than 90 per cent of lung cancers at the population level'. Thus, conclusions about cause and effect relationships are always provisional and, by degrees, uncertain; they cannot be proven, hence why discussions about causes – disputes about smoking and lung cancer and, more recently, income inequality and health – generate considerable debate.

Discussions about causation have assumed particular significance in recent years in the field of the social determinants of health, particularly in relation to the specific issue of the relationship between income inequality and health. Through a series of cross-sectional studies, Wilkinson and Pickett (2010) explored the relationship between income inequality and 12 different health (life expectancy and infant mortality, for example) and social (such as teenage births and imprisonment rates) phenomena, comparing countries as well as states within the USA. Their analysis showed that those countries where the gap between rich and poor was smaller (low income inequality), such as in Norway and Japan, were more likely to have fewer social problems and better health and well-being than those countries where the gap was larger (for example, the USA, the UK and Portugal). Drawing on the Hill (1965) criteria, they considered the causal role of income inequality (as an indicator of social class inequality) using the process outlined above, moving from statistical associations to considering alternative explanations before moving on to proposing a theory of causation by drawing on evidence from a diverse range of disciplines. Wilkinson and Pickett proposed that income inequality and low social status are linked to health and social phenomena via psychosocial pathways that have biological consequences. Stress has been implicated as an important variable in this mechanism (Brunner, 1997). It explains how social organization influences human biology in a way that can predispose towards poorer health, as Krieger (1999) and others have argued.

Conclusion

It may be that the continuing presence of a narrow deterministic definition of cause in some quarters reflects a desire to insist that epidemiology is scientific. In public health, however, a broader view of causation has emerged, based on Rose's concept of 'the causes of the causes … the determinants of exposure' (2008: 133). According to this view, exposures to risks (proximal or 'downstream' factors that relate closely to the disease) are shaped by distal (or 'upstream') factors relating to the social, political and economic context. This broader and more complex conceptualization has been pre-eminent in explaining health **inequalities** in recent years. A number of challenges remain, however, particularly in relation to communicating such complex theoretical ideas to both policy makers and lay audiences. In these circumstances, the tendency to over-simplify problems and solutions is likely to prevail.

CLIMATE CHANGE (AND SUSTAINABLE DEVELOPMENT)

Context

The first World Climate Conference took place in 1979. It is only in the relatively recent past, however, that a degree of scientific consensus has emerged regarding the **evidence** for climate change as well as its likely impact on **health**. Scientific consensus notwith-standing, there continues to be disagreement about the severity of climate change, likely future scenarios, the level of urgency required, and the readiness and scope to mitigate the consequences (Costello *et al.*, 2009). Such tensions are commonplace in the field of public health but are particularly noteworthy in the case of climate change not least because they obfuscate an already complex field and delay potential action. As Giddens (2008) points out, the sceptics (primarily non-scientists) are a significant group and get a significant hearing. This much seems evident from the protracted timescale within which a framework for global co-operation on climate change – largely driven by the United Nations (UN) – has emerged. In 1987, the Brundtland Report (World Commission on Environment and Development) drew attention to the ways in which **economic development** was generating considerable global environmental degradation, threatening biodiversity and human health and well-being, as well as impacting on climate change. The term 'sustainable development' was used to reflect the interdependencies between humans and the environment and the necessity of integrating economic aims with social, human and environmental goals if human and natural capital were not be to compromised for future generations. The report also raised questions about the need to manage **risk**, uncertainty and irreversibility, concluding that in relation to climate change there might be little time for corrective action. Since then, the UN has generated a modicum of momentum and commitment to these ideas through the Rio Earth Summit (UN, 1992), the UN Framework Convention on Climate Change (UNFCCC, 1992), the Kyoto Protocol (1995) and the UN Human Development Report on Sustainability and Equity (Klugman, 2011).

Social **inequalities**, health inequalities, social justice and the form that economic development has taken over many years have increasingly been a feature of climate change discussions. Greenhouse gas emissions per capita are higher in economically advanced countries (more than four times the carbon dioxide emissions and about twice the methane and nitrous oxide emissions) compared to those less advanced, yet it is disadvantaged people who experience the worse effects of climate change (Klugman, 2011). Floods, high winds and landslides resulting from extreme weather events are more likely to affect the poor, children, women and the elderly. Furthermore, poorer nations are apprehensive that their economic development will be limited while more powerful, richer nations such as the USA refuse to control their own emissions. The USA is responsible for approximately 25 per cent of global carbon emissions but is yet to ratify the Kyoto Protocol (December, 2012). The convergence of these complex agendas provides both opportunities and challenges for public health. It has been argued recently, for example, that actions to address climate change, can, if carefully considered, of themselves give rise to multiple health benefits (Watts, 2009).

Defining climate change

Although extreme *weather* events are said to be one manifestation of *climate* change it is important to distinguish between these two inter-related concepts. Weather refers to the day-to-day state of the atmosphere and its short-term variation. Climate, on the other hand, refers to statistical weather information typically averaged over a 30-year period. Hence, climate change relates to shifts in the pattern of weather over the longer term. Although there are many influences on the earth's climate, a distinction is made between 'natural' influences (volcanic eruptions and solar flares, for example) and 'anthropogenic' (human-induced) influences. Global warming is one aspect of climate change that refers specifically to the increase in global average temperature near the earth's surface. Over the last century this has risen by 0.74°C, more than half of which

(0.4°C) has occurred since 1979 (Intergovernmental Panel on Climate Change [IPCC], 2007). The emerging scientific consensus is that global warming, particularly since the 1970s, is anthropogenic – resulting from the burning of fossil fuels and the release of so-called greenhouse gases such as carbon dioxide and methane – and is a primary driver of climate change. Definitions of climate change tend to differ in relation to how the natural and anthropogenic causes are framed. The UNFCCC (1992: 3) focuses upon the latter: 'a change in climate which is attributed directly or indirectly to human activity that alters the composition of the global atmosphere and which is in addition to natural climate variability observed over comparable time periods'. This differs from that of the IPCC which gives recognition to both: 'a change in the state of the climate that can be identified (by using statistical tests) by changes in the mean and/or the variability of its properties and that persists for an extended period, typically decades or longer'. Climate change, the IPCC adds, 'may be due to natural internal processes or external forcings, or to persistent anthropogenic changes in the composition of the atmosphere or in land use' (IPCC, 2012: 3). The emphasis given to anthropogenic activities is one of the most controversial aspects of the climate change debate.

The significance of climate change for public health

The idea of 'ecological public health' has emerged in recent years, reflecting the shifting character of contemporary public health issues. As a concept, ecological public health is predicated on the premise that human beings and the environment are interdependent in a multitude of complex ways. Furthermore, these interdependencies are viewed as having consequences for the health both of humans and the environment (Lang and Raynor, 2012). Climate change provides a particularly apposite illustration of these interdependencies. Although the world ecosystem has considerable absorptive and regenerative capacities, the extent and character of human intervention in nature appears to have jeopardized the stability and productivity of the ecosystem, giving rise to a number of interrelated problems with far-reaching consequences for public health.

The health consequences of climate change are largely mediated through changes to regional and local weather, as well as rises in sea level (Haines and Patz, 2004). In terms of changes in the weather, increases in temperature and the intensity of precipitation, as well as the frequency of extreme weather events can have direct and indirect effects on individual and population health. Thermal stress, due to an increase in the number of hot days as well as rises in the frequency of heat waves can directly increase deaths due to cardiovascular, cerebrovascular and respiratory disease in older people and those with existing disease (Costello *et al.*, 2009). Extreme weather events involving intense precipitation, high winds or prolonged drought, can also lead directly to death and injury. Such events also give rise to a number of indirect effects through the devastation of local and regional environments. Floods, and the landslides that often accompany them, can wipe out settlements, destroying people's livelihoods and incomes, as well as the infrastructure of their communities. Concerns about water quality and the integrity of sanitation systems always attend such extreme events creating the conditions for the emergence of major outbreaks of epidemic disease. Food production is also threatened by drought, which jeopardizes soil quality and thus fertility, reducing crop yields and raising prices. The knock-on effects of diminishing precipitation in some food-growing parts of the world increases the irrigation requirements placing further pressures on freshwater supplies. Food security generally has become more of a pressing global concern. Flooding combined with rising sea levels can cause considerable damage to coastal and island communities, which tend to be settled by indigenous people who rely on natural resources. Demand for food and water can give rise to migration, increasing pressure on resources elsewhere. A tipping point may be reached insofar as civil unrest and perhaps armed conflict emerge as consequences of the pressures on resources. Increasingly, however, high-income countries – and especially the people who are disadvantaged within those countries – experience the devastation caused by extreme weather events, such as Hurricane Sandy in New York in 2012, heat waves in Europe in 2003 and in Australia in 2009 and 2012.

Rising temperatures, increases in precipitation and humidity and sea level rises are also likely to lead to alterations in the distribution of infectious diseases. Vector-borne and rodent-borne diseases are especially likely to increase. Malaria, tick-borne encephalitis and dengue fever may well become increasingly widespread (Costello *et al.*, 2009). Animal infections will be similarly affected by climate change. Precisely how vectors and pathogens will respond to climate change is uncertain, particularly because they are in dynamic interaction with their hosts. In all probability, more populations will be at risk from a number of infectious diseases, the outcome of infection may be more severe given their limited resistance and health system responses will come under greater strain.

Ultimately, climate change can, of course, threaten the very existence of the human and natural world, creating the conditions in which people's basic necessities – food, water, shelter, livelihood and so on – are threatened. Climate change is, however, unfolding in a global context of environments that have already become fragile through many years of economic exploitation through overgrazing, deforestation, desertification and mineral extraction; globally, approximately 40 per cent of land is degraded (Klugman, 2011). Added to this is the issue of women's limited reproductive rights in many parts of the world and the attendant population growth (the estimated population in 2011 was 7 billion), which puts considerable pressure on resources. In this regard, Klugman (2011: 10) observes that 'If all women could exercise reproductive choice, population growth would slow enough to bring greenhouse gas emissions below current levels. Meeting unmet need for family planning by 2050 would lower the world's carbon emissions an estimated 17 per cent below what they are today.'

The UN and some governments have identified a need to re-consider the form economic growth takes as a fundamental issue to address. The UN has coined the term 'climate-resilient economic development'. Norway, for example, argues for a greener global economy, one that, interrelatedly, addresses poverty and protects the environment (Norwegian Ministry of Foreign Affairs, 2011) and is aiming to be carbon-neutral by 2050. The UN goal is to reduce greenhouse gas emissions in an effort to keep global warming at two degrees above the period average. The UN Kyoto Protocol provides the global framework of legally binding commitments to emission reduction targets. However, actions are required at the national level if progress is to be made. In 2008, the UK Government passed the *Climate Change Act*, which set legally binding targets for reducing greenhouse gas emissions by at least 34 per cent by 2020 and 80 per cent by 2050 (using 1990 as the baseline). Enacting legislation improves the likelihood of being able to take a long-term view and sustain progress if there is a change of government. The UK exceeded its targets in 2012; this was probably due to a blend of milder weather, an increase in renewable energy generation, and the financial downturn (Harvey, 2012).

The idea of climate-proofing or sustainability-proofing *all* policies has been discussed. This has much in common with Milio's idea of health in *all* policies and the benefits of inter-sectoral action (Milio, 1981). Giddens (2008) for example, discusses the greening of fiscal systems through developing environmental taxes that incentivize environmentally friendly activities, such as transferring to renewable energy.

Strategies that aim to reduce emissions of greenhouse gases have the potential to benefit public health, a message that has, hitherto, been somewhat obscured (Watts, 2009). This introduces a new perspective into thinking about climate change. For example, the introduction of low-emission cookstoves into households in India would improve substantially indoor air quality, decreasing the risk of respiratory tract infections in children and chronic respiratory and heart disease among adults (Wilkinson *et al.*, 2009). In London, decreasing emissions through a decline in motor car use alongside an increase in walking and cycling have been estimated to lead to substantial health benefits through declines in heart disease, stroke, breast cancer, dementia and depression (Woodcock *et al.*, 2009). Changes to agricultural practices to reduce greenhouse gas emissions, such as reducing livestock numbers, might lead to a shift in dietary intake away from animal saturated fats, with subsequent reductions in heart disease (Friel *et al.*, 2009). Reductions in short-lived greenhouse pollutants from fuel combustion, such as methane and nitrogen oxide which generate ozone, would reduce mortality and morbidity due to cardiopulmonary toxicity (Smith *et al.*, 2009b).

There is some evidence that scientists are becoming radicalized as robust data on climate change accumulates. Stern – the author of the UK government-commissioned review of climate change (2006) – has subsequently stated that he underestimated the risks and should have been more forthright in articulating the threats posed by climate change (Stewart and Elliott, 2013). However, there remains a substantial gulf between scientists and the public and politicians especially, although within all groups there is a spectrum of beliefs about climate change and its implications. Some have argued that those working in public health should adopt an **advocacy** role in this regard, working to shift opinions towards acceptance of the scientific evidence and the need for concerted action (Yarlagadda *et al.*, 2012) as well as draw attention to the health benefits of climate change mitigation policies (Smith *et al.*, 2009b). In a similar vein, Klugman (2011) argues for the greater involvement of women in decision-making positions given their tendency to be more pro-environment than men.

Conclusion

Climate change poses considerable threats to health. However, mitigation strategies that protect the environment offer the promise of improving health through a variety of pathways, while reducing social and health inequalities. In common with most public health issues, although it has proved necessary to establish the scientific basis of climate change, solutions ultimately lie in the political and economic realm. Climate change, as a global **determinant** of health, links the global economy with the environment and health, illustrating the necessity for global governance. Trade liberalization – and the deregulation and privatization that have accompanied it – has led to extensive environmental degradation: deforestation in Indonesia (one million hectares per year) for the paper and palm oil industry, for example (Walt, 1998). Extreme weather conditions (heat waves that lead to fires and drought for example) that have human and environmental costs also challenge the notion of a 'natural' disaster. The environmental movement has had some success in getting climate change and other related issues onto the agenda of international agencies such as the World Trade Organization (WTO) (Yach and Bettcher, 1998) and this may be a way of furthering the **global health** agenda more broadly. On the basis of considerable analysis of the latest data, the IPCC's 2013 report concludes unequivocally that the climate system is warming, that changes since 1950 are unprecedented and, moreover, human influence has played a key role. If these changes are to be limited, then sustained reductions in greenhouse emissions are required. Time, however, may well be running out.

COMMUNITY

Context

In many **policy** areas, including public health, there has been a long history of focusing on 'communities', a tendency that gathered momentum in the latter decades of the twentieth century in the UK as elsewhere. Under the UK Labour governments of 1997– 2010 this was especially the case with a resurgence of interest in 'community' rather than 'society' (Levitas, 2000). During this time many communities were considered 'problematic' insofar as they were fragmented, weak and detached from mainstream society. Despite this, communities were also viewed as a means of 'reconstructing civil society' (Crawshaw *et al.*, 2003: 37). In this sense, the term community was interwoven with other policy ideas relating to social inclusion (see **deprivation**), **social capital**, responsibility, opportunity and civic engagement. Despite a change of government in the UK, these ideas persist, re-packaged using the language of 'localism' and the 'big society' and emphasizing self-help, self-reliance and social obligations. The attractiveness – to those on both sides of the political spectrum – of framing policy in terms of community may lie in its apparent neutrality, which, on the face of it, depoliticizes problems and solutions (Mowbray, 2005). Discussions about communities, however, are always politically charged and hence should always be treated sceptically.

Defining community

Despite its political currency, there is some consensus that the term community has been overused in recent years giving it a vagueness and ambiguity that reduces its value as a concept (Roberts, 2009). In public health, the term community is most frequently applied to a geographic area, **place**, neighbourhood or administrative unit. Area-based initiatives such as health action zones (HAZs) illustrate this trend. Social scientists, however, tend to think about communities in terms of social relations, such as those relating to occupational, faith or sexuality networks (the 'gay community', for example). Roberts (2009: 40) offers a fairly restricted definition that illustrates this approach, defining a community as 'a group that is wider than an extended family, but whose members are bound by kin-type relationships, among whom there is a sense of belonging, and a shared identity'. Based on this definition, even relatively small geographic areas may well comprize a number of different communities. Defining community in this way also implies that people are likely to be members of several communities, reflecting the varied ways in which their identities and their sense of belonging is constituted in relation to the diverse realms of their lives. There may also be limitations in thinking that communities can be strengthened – made more stable and socially cohesive – by creating strong bonds between people. Rather, it may be more realistic to think in terms of communities as dynamic and fluid, where people move between identities and have a number of weak ties with others in a variety of different **settings** (Taylor, 2000). Thus territory-based conceptualizations of community (such as neighbourhood) are limited as a working model because they tend to underestimate the heterogeneity and fluidity of small populations.

Community is, nevertheless, a concept that has a constellation of positive connotations, that is to say, it implies positive and wholesome attributes such as inclusivity and belonging (Mowbray, 2005). Defining communities in terms of values and identities inevitably throws into sharp relief the significance of power and its distribution in communities. Not only can power be used to include or exclude people (Levitas, 2000) on the basis of certain characteristics, it can also be a source of tension and conflict.

The significance of community for public health

Community-based initiatives – relating to **health**, **education**, regeneration, crime reduction, employment, sport – have become one of *the* defining features of public health and social policy in the past 40 years or so. In keeping with the political and professional ascendancy of the notion of (territory-based) communities, working *in* communities has become the predominant way of organizing public health in recent years. To some degree this represents an acknowledgement of the spatial distribution of health and deprivation (Taylor, 2000), with the worst health and deprivation tending to occur together. In the UK and elsewhere, the development of 'local community health profiles' to describe small populations and the production of regular local 'needs assessments' have been promoted as providing a rationale for deciding where, when and how to concentrate resources. In public health the predominant approach to working in deprived communities has been endeavouring to improve service provision in light of the fact that the quality and quantity of services in more deprived areas tend to be poorer (fewer doctors as well as less well-qualified teachers, for example) (Dorling, 2010). National programmes such as HAZs, Sure Start programmes and Total Place have focused on improving local services, as well as their co-ordination, and encouraging innovation. A particular feature of these initiatives has been community involvement. In the case of HAZs, Crawshaw *et al.* (2003: 37) argue that 'experts guide the community in becoming responsible for their own health ... not just so that the individual can manage their own well-being, but also so that they have a duty to participate in the well-being of their community'. However, targeting the most deprived areas tends to miss some of the most deprived individuals (Powell and Moon, 2001).

Although approaches based on community participation are more likely to be successful, particularly in terms of sustainability, they raise important issues relating to balances of power and control. While the rhetoric may be couched in terms of 'putting communities in the driving seat', the reality seems quite different. Taking HAZs as an example, Crawshaw *et al.* (2003) found that community involvement and represen-tation were at best problematic. Not only did control of decision-making reside with the local authority, there was also tension between local and national priorities. The notion that community-based programmes are about self-determination appears, therefore, to be somewhat illusory (Mowbray, 2005). The potentially exploitative character of initiatives has also been noted. Community participation has been predicated on the idea of voluntarism. Unpaid work, however, is a matter of some significance given the levels of poverty in deprived communities targeted by initiatives (Levitas, 2000). Participation also tends to involve particular people and the burden on them can be considerable given the plethora of community-based initiatives (Taylor, 2000). Perhaps more fundamentally, community-level approaches leave untouched the structural factors that are the root causes of social **inequalities** and poor health (Crawshaw *et al.*, 2003). The ideological rhetoric implies that if communities show sufficient collective resolve they will be able to swim against the tide that had previously engulfed them and, by extension, if they are unsuccessful in meeting this challenge they will only have themselves to blame.

Just as community-based initiatives are not new, neither are the criticisms. The community development movement that emerged in the 1950s in a number of low-income countries in an effort to counter some of the consequences of decolonization, became a global phenomenon particularly associated with urban and peri-urban renewal (du Sautoy, 1966). Community development emerged as an activity supported by professionals (community development officers) as well as an academic field of study. It was defined by the UN (1948) as a process designed to create the conditions for economic and social progress for the whole community with its active participation and fullest possible reliance upon the community's initiative (cited in Head, 1979). According to this view, participation is linked to transformative, community-directed – that is, initiated and built from the bottom up – social and economic change. The idea of collaborating *with*, rather than acting *on*, local people has much in common with the ideas of Freire (1972). He emphasized empowerment through a process of 'conscientisacion' – developing understanding about the roots of oppression through a process of respectful dialogue (Blackburn, 2000; Smith, 1997/2002). Freire's idea of praxis – theoretically informed action linked to certain values, such as social justice – has implications for those working with communities in the field, who become required to disempower themselves 'in order to provide the empowerment space which the oppressed require' (Blackburn, 2000: 13). Although there have been a number of criticisms of Freire's ideas (Taylor, 1993), they shed light on why community-based approaches have varying degrees of success. In countries such as the USA, there has been a greater emphasis on community *mobilization* – getting people doing things and using community resources – rather than *participation* – giving people the power to choose how, when and in relation to what they should be involved. This illustrates the varied ways in which community development can be operationalized, either as a utilitarian effort to get a project done at lower costs or in terms of empowerment where participation is an end in itself (Labonté and Laverack, 2001; Morgan, 2001). In the field of **health promotion**, community participation based on an empowerment model is articulated in the *Ottawa Charter* (WHO, 1986) through community action, signalling the intrinsic value that is attached to the process of empowerment itself.

Projects based on an empowerment model can, nevertheless, have a number of unintended consequences. Although participation can benefit physical and mental health it can also lead to feelings of stress, burnout and disappointment, for example (Attree *et al.*, 2011). The use of microfinancing (provision of small loans) via the Grameen Bank in Bangladesh was a community-based strategy that aimed to empower women through increasing their control over decisions relating to finance. Although successful – insofar as there was a high rate of loan repayment (Laverack, 2001) – many women (63 percent) claimed to have little control over their own loan and to be under pressure to repay it. As a consequence, this strategy produced new forms of dominance and violence for women (Rahman, 1999). Elsewhere however, community development female empowerment programmes have had wider positive impacts including among non-participants (Kandpal *et al.*, 2012).

Its widespread use notwithstanding, the term 'community development' appears to have fallen out of favour in UK and US policy circles in recent years. Increasingly, building **social capital** and community capacity are the terms used to describe community-based work. Capacity building, however, has been criticized for its tendency to focus on 'deficits' – the problems and needs of communities – rather than its 'assets'. Such an approach can lead to dependency on services that are developed in order to meet perceived needs (Foot and Hopkins, 2010). The asset-based community development (ABCD) model of Kretzmann and McKnight (1993; Kretzmann *et al.*, 2005) emerged in the USA and has informed asset transfer approaches in the UK and elsewhere (O'Leary *et al.*, 2011). The Marmot Review (2010) in England also gave some impetus to asset-based approaches involving local participatory decision-making. Communities are reconceptualized in terms of having a number of tangible and intangible assets, of which people's knowledge, skills and enthusiasms are a central part. The language of 'co-production' is used to indicate the building of working relationships between and among local residents, local associations and local government and public sector organizations to solve locally determined issues. This implies that those working in these organizations should re-frame their role in terms of enabler, catalyst and alliance builder (Ashton, 2010), a move that is likely to require extensive professional development (Taylor, 2000). In particular, professionals are likely to need considerable political acumen to negotiate conflict and work in an **advocacy** role (Mowbray, 2005). Community ownership requires self-determination; this can lead to the identification of issues that differ from those of local or national health services or councils (Foot and Hopkins, 2010). Power sharing is also a complex, iterative and time-consuming process (Carr-West, 2010). Asset-based approaches, however, are presented as a way of building a pathway out of poverty and social exclusion rather than ameliorating their consequences (Burkett, 2011). Such approaches, therefore, generate the same kind of questions and criticisms alluded to earlier in relation to the structural causes of poverty (DeFilippis, 2001).

Conclusion

The language of community-based work can be confusing, not just because many terms are contested. Much of the rhetoric refers to giving people choice and control at a community level. Although community participation offers an approach that seeks to transform existing power relations, communities remain on the margins of power in most **partnership** programmes (Taylor, 2000). Furthermore, the add-on character of community-based approaches tends not to disrupt the main thrust of much mainstream service provision. Last but by no means least is the structural issue. How is it that communities are considered able to solve problems that successive governments have failed to do resolve?

DEMOGRAPHY

Context

Demography, alongside **epidemiology**, has a well-established role in public health, describing as it does key features of population dynamics in relation to mortality, fertility and migration. Epidemiology is dependent upon good demographic information but demography is of much wider relevance to public health. Concerned with charting trends in population size and structure, demography has become especially relevant to understanding the **health** implications of population growth and contraction, migration and population ageing. The links between health, **economic development** and population dynamics have been particularly debated. Shifts in population size and structure also generate and reflect differing **health needs**. Most regions and countries of the world are experiencing unprecedented and often rapid demographic change, with considerable implications for population health. As such, demography occupies a central position in contemporary public health debates.

Defining demography

Demography is defined as 'the study of human populations – their size, growth, density and distribution' (Leone, 2010: 1). Its development as a discipline during the nineteenth century reflected the needs of emerging nation states for information about their populations, essential for, among other things, developing a system of taxation and determining the adequacy of military capacity (Ribbens *et al.*, 2011). Its development has thus paralleled the emergence of formal systems for the collection of **official statistics**. Malthus (1766–1834) – often described as the founder of modern demography – is widely viewed as stimulating (controversial) debate about the relationship between population growth, health and poverty, ideas that remain relevant today, particularly in relation to **global health**. Descriptions of population composition in relation to age, sex, ethnicity, disability, class, marital status and family composition provide the basis for documenting patterns of health and disease and trends over time, **place** and sub-group. It is therefore a core discipline in public health with its population-based approach to the study of patterns of health and disease.

The significance of demography for public health

In England, Malthus' ideas are generally accepted as having accelerated the passing of the Census Act in 1800. The census – an enumeration of a given population – is a central tool of demography because it attempts to record information on all persons in every household – age/date of birth, sex, occupation, national origin, language, marital status and income – as well as information at the household level (Porta, 2008). The world's first formal census was carried out in the USA in 1790. In Britain, the first census was carried out in 1801, the next in 1841, with many countries following suit over the course of the nineteenth century. The scale and complexity of the census has increased considerably in recent years in most high-income countries, with additional questions added from time to time. In the 2011 census for England and Wales a number of health-related questions were included (for example, 'How is your health in general?', www.ons.gov.uk/census2011). Although participation is compulsory in the UK, 100 per cent coverage is rarely achieved. In the 2011 census the person response rate varied by local authority area from 82 per cent to 98 per cent. In Australia, financial penalties are incurred for failing to complete and return census documents. Here, the non-response rate in 2011 was 3.7 per cent (www.abs.gov.au/websitebs/censushome). Overall, the value of the census in providing population statistics with a high degree of accuracy is generally considered to outweigh the costs of conducting such a large-scale initiative. Not only does the census provide information for government purposes, it also provides a rich data source for researchers, providing long time-series data and information on population sub-groups.

Population size is estimated through the census, normally at 10-year intervals. Size is determined by the interplay between mortality (the number of deaths), fertility (the number of live births) and migration (the movement of people from one population to another). Systems for collecting data on deaths, births and migration have been established in high-income countries. These 'vital statistics' provide the basis on which changes in population size can be monitored between census points. In many low-income countries these systems are lacking or fragile, making it difficult to monitor population size. The calculation of mortality and birth rates is also made problematic because of the requirement for not only an accurate numerator (number of deaths or live births) but also a denominator – usually estimated as the mid-year population. 'Crude' (unadjusted) rates are important because they reflect the actual experience of a population. 'Adjusted' rates (standardized for age and sex) although artificial, enable meaningful comparisons across populations and over time.

In high-income countries death certification (by a doctor) is a legal requirement. The certificate records cause of death as well as other socio-demographic information such as the name, sex, date of birth, places of residence and death, occupation and whether the deceased had been medically attended before death. All causes should be listed and coded. Causes are defined in the tenth (1990) version of the *International Classification of Diseases and Related Health Problems* (ICD-10) (WHO, 2012). The cause of death is defined as all those diseases, morbid conditions, or injuries that either resulted in or contributed to death and the circumstances of the accident or violence that produced any such injuries. The underlying cause of death is defined as 'the disease or injury that initiated the train of events leading to death or the circumstances of the accident or violence that produced the fatal injury' (Porta, 2008: 60). The WHO describes the ICD as the 'global standard for mortality and morbidity statistics' (www.int/classifications/icd/factsheet/en/index.html). The system is used by more than 100 countries to report mortality data, used as a primary indicator of population health. In the UK, however, the system of death certification has come under recent public scrutiny and there have been enduring questions relating to the accuracy of death certification with errors being common (Tuffin *et al.*, 2009), particularly in the elderly, where post-mortems are rare.

However, in many low-income countries mortality statistics are not routinely available.

Fertility refers to the actual production of live offspring, the rate of which also influences population size. A system of birth certification provides the legal basis for recording all live births. The birth certificate typically contains information on name, date, place, identity of parents and sometimes additional information such as birth weight. It provides the denominator for the infant mortality rate (IMR – deaths during the first year of life) and certain other vital rates such as the neonatal mortality rate (the number of deaths in the first 28 days of life per 1000 live births in a given year). Both the IMR and the neonatal mortality rate are particularly sensitive indicators of maternal, newborn and infant health as well as the care they have received. Under-reporting and misclassification of deaths in the early period of life are common, however, particularly in countries where rates are high. Reducing child mortality was identified as Goal 4 of the Millennium Development Goals (MDGs) (UN, 2010). Globally, a 60-fold difference in IMR has been reported, from a high of 182/1000 live births in Sierra Leone to 3/1000 in Sweden (Schell *et al.*, 2007). In sub-Saharan Africa in 2008 one in seven children died before their fifth birthday. Three socio-economic variables predicted 92 per cent of national IMR: gross national income per capita, female illiteracy rate and income distribution (Schell *et al.*, 2007). Access to effective contraception and safe abortion services also remain key concerns if women are to be enabled to restrict their family size. Population growth in low-income regions remains an important factor slowing down progress towards all MDGs as well as limiting food security and contributing to environmental pressures (Leone, 2010).

Migration also influences population size. Population flows reflect the impact of 'push' factors (such as famine and war) as well as 'pull' factors (freedom from persecution and the opportunity to gain employment and a better standard of living, for example) (Roberts, 2009). Calculating migration rates is difficult, however, because following people's movements is problematic. This is particularly the case for tracking the flow of people who move within their own country, which accounts for the majority of movements (United Nations Development Programme (UNDP), 2009). The demographic trend towards ageing populations combined with better employment opportunities (including those for low skilled workers) in many high-income countries, has created a 'demand' for migration (UNDP, 2009). Nonetheless, in spite of migration contributing positively to the economy of many countries, it remains a politically charged issue.

At a global level, countries differ quite markedly in terms of whether or not their populations are expanding, contracting or static. Understanding these trends is central to health policy development and planning in relation to the assessment of health needs (including the assessment of future needs for school places, jobs, care for the elderly, and so on) and allocation of resources. Recent developments in demography associated with the use of modelling software allow predictions of future population growth and size, as well as the pressures that are likely to ensue. Population growth in low-income regions of the world has been estimated as 1.4 per cent per year, in spite of high mortality from HIV/AIDS and high maternal mortality more generally (Leone, 2010). In these regions, health tends to be poor, particularly among children. By contrast, countries that were once part of the Soviet Union have experienced population decline in recent years due to emigration, increases in death rates (particularly related to alcohol consumption among middle-aged men) and sub-replacement fertility. China has become noted for including population control as a key aspect of its economic reforms, introducing the one child **policy** in 1979. Whilst this has given rise to smaller family size, it has also resulted in an imbalance in the sex ratio: in 2001 there were 32 million more men under 20 years of age than women, with some predicting that the ratio is likely to worsen in the future (Ding and Hesketh, 2006). The social consequences of these developments are potentially considerable.

Demographic transition theory describes a country's shift from high fertility and mortality levels (stage one), towards a decline in mortality and fertility (stage two), through to low fertility and mortality (stage 3). All high-income countries have been through this transition. The demographic transition leads to a change in the age structure of a population, which is primarily influenced by declines in fertility. As birth rate declines, the proportion of children and young adults declines; as death rates decline (including among infants and children usually) the proportion of older people increases. Population pyramids visually present an overview of the age and sex profile of a specified population. A pyramid with a wide base and a narrow top – indicating a high birth rate and a young population, with lower life expectancy and few people in older age groups – is a pattern typical of low-income countries. This picture contrasts with that of a pyramid from a high-income country such as Switzerland, which has a narrower base and a wider top, illustrative of a lower birth rate, higher life expectancy and larger numbers of people in older age groups.

In high-income countries, population ageing (reflected in an increase in the average (median) age of the population alongside an increase in the number and proportion of older people in the population, especially those over the age of 60–65 years) and population shrinkage have emerged as major public health concerns. Both reflect long-term trends in fertility, mortality and migration. Global projections suggest that the number of older people will exceed the number of children for the first time in 2047 (Leone, 2010). Japan, Germany (among many European countries) and Russia, for example, all have declining, as well as ageing populations. According to a UN forecast, almost every third person will be 65 or over by 2040 (Persson, 2006). Life expectancy – which has increased over the past 140 years in many countries – is unlikely to have yet reached its biological maximum.

Other demographic trends with significant health implications relate to women not only having fewer children, but having them later and spacing them further apart. There has also been a trend towards an increase in couples with no children and an increase in divorce rates in many countries (Persson, 2006). The emergence of new family structures due to high divorce rates and increasing numbers of children born outside marriage also have implications for population health. Impacts of these trends can work via poverty generation. In most high-income countries, for example, children of single mothers have a much higher poverty rate compared to those in two parent families (Heuveline and Weinshenker, 2008). If these trends continue, not only will many people live alone in old age, they may also be poor. The impact on informal caring arrangements as well as on the formal health and social care systems is likely to be significant. Ageing puts pressure on health and social care systems, although this may well have been overstated in extent (Leone, 2010). A smaller proportion of working-age people will need to support an increasing proportion of elderly (and very elderly) people. Furthermore, while life expectancy has increased, it has not necessarily led to better quality of life during the later years of life. Chronic disease management is likely to be a central aspect of meeting the needs of an ageing population.

There has been much debate about the range and significance of factors driving declines in fertility and mortality (Caldwell, 1986). With regard to declines in fertility, reduced dependence on family labour for survival, increased investment in individual children and women's alternative employment choices have been identified (Ribbens *et al.*, 2011). As far as the role of women is concerned, in addition to improvements in female literacy, access to effective contraception and equality legislation have contributed significantly to women's empowerment, enabling them to have more control over their family size in particular, as well as their lives more generally. The decline in death rates reflects, in part, an epidemiological transition away from fewer infectious disease pandemics towards increases in chronic degenerative diseases as the major causes of death. Public health measures, improvements in nutrition, as well as medical interventions in recent years have been important drivers of declines in death rates. Of particular concern for many low-income countries, however, is the co-existence of both chronic degenerative (such as obesity and diabetes) and infectious diseases (TB, for example) as fertility rates decline alongside increases in life expectancy (Leone, 2010).

Conclusion

Population dynamics in relation to size and structure continue to vary across countries with differing implications for public health policy and planning. Population ageing appears likely to dominate the thinking of many politicians in high-income countries in future decades. This demographic feature, however, reflects long-term improvements in the social and economic living conditions of populations. In other words, it is a reflection of improved standards of living and a longer life. Alongside these concerns are those that relate to population growth in many low-income countries. Not only does a demographic perspective reveal such **inequalities**, it also points towards a better understanding of the implications of continued global population growth for the environment, **climate change**, food security, the economy, and so on, as well as population health and longevity.

DEPRIVATION AND POVERTY

Context

Historically, poverty has been the main concept for making sense of the **health** consequences of being economically poor. In England, some of the earliest social survey research carried out by nineteenth century reformers such as William Booth (in London) and Seebohm Rowntree (in York) examined the relationship between income and living conditions during a period of **economic development** driven by the Industrial Revolution (Fraser, 2009). In both cities approximately a third of the populations studied were living around the subsistence poverty line, lacking the necessities to maintain a healthy life. Booth and Rowntree concluded that this level of poverty was not due to individual 'idleness' or 'fecklessness' but unemployment and low wages, exacerbated by large families (Roberts, 2009). These conclusions resonate with and reflect enduring political debates in many high-income countries with expanded **welfare states**. Yet, media representations of those living in poverty as 'deserving' or 'undeserving' can undermine attempts to understand the causes and consequences of deprivation (Seymour, 2009). Associated as they are with **inequalities** in health, poverty and deprivation continue to be politically charged social facts, particularly in the UK, one of the richest countries in the world.

Defining deprivation and poverty

In public health, it has become commonplace to use the term 'deprivation' rather than poverty and the UK uses measures of deprivation to monitor its progress in reducing child poverty (Berthoud and Bryan, 2011; Department for Work and Pensions, 2012). Townsend (1987) was a key proponent of the need to define and operationalize the concept of deprivation coherently and scientifically (in the sense that a specific level could be identified below which a family would be defined as 'deprived') as a basis for allocating resources to areas. He argued that both deprivation and poverty were relevant to analysing social conditions and were related but conceptually distinct. Accordingly, he defined deprivation as 'the level of conditions or activities experienced' and poverty as 'the incomes and other resources directly available' (140). Subsistence or absolute poverty – defined by the World Bank as living on less than US$1.25 per day – tends to be used in low-income countries. In the European Union, where welfare states seek to ensure that there is little, if any, absolute poverty of the kind found in low-income countries (or that seen during the time of Booth's and Rowntree's research in England), poverty is defined in relative terms. Relative income poverty involves comparing a household's income, adjusted for family size, to the median income of the population; those with incomes below 60 per cent of the median are viewed as in relative poverty (Seymour, 2009). In the UK, households below average income (HBAI) is treated by the government as the key indicator for monitoring income poverty. According to Townsend's distinction, people might be deprived but not in poverty. He argued, however, that where people experience 'multiple or severe single forms of deprivation' (Townsend, 1987: 131) they were likely to have very little income and few other resources. This suggests that low income is a valid proxy measure for deprivation and is increasingly used as such.

Overall, defining poverty in relation to income, and deprivation in relation to material and social conditions that relate to levels of income, provides a degree of conceptual clarity. In recent years, however, there has been a tendency to expand the concept of poverty to refer to more than income, limiting its usefulness (Roberts, 2009). Tomlinson *et al.* (2008) for example, describe poverty as a multidimensional concept of which material deprivation is a part. An alternative view on both poverty and deprivation has been provided by Sen (1983) with the concept of 'capabilities' – a person's capability to function – and, relatedly, 'entitlements', which he argues better conceptualizes standards of living. There has, nevertheless, been considerable criticism of Sen's approach (Townsend, 1985; Friedli, 2012) on the grounds that it tends to individualize poverty and deprivation rather than viewing them as socially created. Nonetheless, the capabilities approach has been used extensively in an **economic development** context, where poverty is understood as being deprived of the capability to lead a good life and development is understood as capability expansion.

The significance of deprivation and poverty for public health

Having an adequate income is important because it represents being under fewer constraints; it thus broadens the possibilities for being able to develop a reasonable standard of living. What constitutes the 'necessities for a decent life' continues to be a source of considerable controversy, however. The 1983 *Breadline Britain* survey was one of the earliest attempts to establish what an acceptable standard of living was by asking people not only about the basic essentials (such as food), but also about participation in society (Pantazis *et al.*, 1999). Deprivation was thus seen as having multiple dimensions: housing and household facilities, food, clothing, **education**, working and social conditions, and so on. A key distinction was made between people's material (goods and services) and social (activities and relationships) conditions. The 60 per cent of median income threshold reflects an assessment of what level of income is required to be able to afford the necessities for a decent life – in other words, to meet material *and* social conditions – relative to societal norms.

The appearance of the term 'social exclusion' in the late twentieth century emphasized the social dimensions of deprivation rather than the material. In so doing, social exclusion downplays the significance of income poverty for deprivation. Social participation was central to Townsend's definition of deprivation and he argued that 'people may be said to be deprived if they do not have, at all, or sufficiently, the conditions of life ... which allow them to play the roles, participate in the relationships and follow the customary behaviour which is expected of them by virtue of their membership of society' (Townsend, 1987: 130). From this perspective, deprivation is also more adequately conceptualized as *relative*. The *Breadline Britain* survey revealed that the majority of people judged a wide range of goods, services and activities as necessary for a minimum standard of living. This subjective collective view has been used in work by the Joseph Rowntree Foundation (JRF) to develop a 'minimum income standard' for the UK (Davis *et al.*, 2012). This study concluded that two parents with two children needed to earn at least £18,400 to support their family. This figure included, among many other things, a computer and access to the internet, viewed as necessities for all working-age families. McKay (2004), however, argues that income use reflects patterns of spending based on choice and rationality rather than contextual constraint. Because deprivation includes an individual subjective dimension – a feeling of not having something that one would like – the interaction between choice and constraint is complex and not easily unravelled. Some explanations for health **inequalities** centre on relative deprivation, emphasizing individual perceptions and social comparisons (Bernburg, 2010).

In the UK, indices of deprivation have been used extensively in public health, particularly for planning and resource allocation purposes. Two of the earliest indices developed – the Carstairs Index (Carstairs, 1995) and the Townsend Index (Townsend, 1987) – have been applied to health inequalities research. Both indices are derived by combining four variables, three of which are the same in each index: the percentage of (i) those of economically active age who are unemployed (direct measure of deprivation); (ii) households lacking a car (income indicator); and (iii) households overcrowded (direct measure of deprivation). The fourth variable in the Carstairs Index is low social class, whereas the Townsend Index uses households not owner-occupied. Their main limitation is that they are both based on infrequently updated census variables (Morgan and Baker, 2006). Approaches to measuring deprivation have, however, been refined over a number of years, predominantly by adding variables, made possible by the increasing availability of local-level administrative data. The English Index of Multiple Deprivation (IMD) 2010 comprizes 38 indicators organized across seven distinct domains: income, employment, health and disability, education, access to housing and other services, crime, and living environment (Department for Communities and Local Government (DCLG), 2011). Each domain has its own score. An overall IMD score is also calculated for each Lower-layer Super Output Area (LSOA – small areas of around 1,500 people: in England there are 32,482 LSOAs). The score reflects the experiences of those who live in an area. A high area deprivation score indicates that a large proportion of people living in the LSOA experience various forms of deprivation and are therefore classed as deprived (DCLG, 2011). On the basis of the IMD score, each LSOA can be ranked, with '1' representing the most deprived area. Thus, the IMD measures *relative* deprivation. Some people living in an area with a high deprivation score may not experience deprivation and, similarly, not all those deprived live in a deprived area. In England, IMD scores have been used as a basis for identifying where initiatives to address deprivation (or specific aspects relating to particular domains) should be located. They are likely to be used increasingly to understand community needs and guide service commissioning. Similar indices of deprivation have been developed for areas beyond the UK (in South Africa, for example).

Deprivation consistently has been shown to be associated with poorer health, including life expectancy and self-reported health (Blane *et al.*, 1996; Kondo *et al.*, 2008; Phillimore *et al.*, 1994; Sloggett and Joshi, 1998). Thus, area-based health initiatives targeted at areas of high deprivation have become common **policy** options in many countries in recent years. However, the association between deprivation and poor health raises contentious questions of **causality**. Do statistical associations reflect the characteristics of individuals and households (the population *composition* of an area) or characteristics of the **place** itself (that is, the context)? Several studies have used multiple logistic regression techniques to separate out neighbourhood from individual-level effects. Framing questions in these dichotomous terms, however, tends to obscure complex interrelationships between people and their neighbourhoods (Cummins *et al.*, 2007). **Evidence** increasingly suggests that the key explanatory variable in the relationship between deprivation and health is poor socio-economic circumstances coupled with low educational attainment, which limits life chances (Kiernan, 1995; Sloggett and Joshi, 1998). Thus, excess mortality in deprived areas can be explained by the concentration in those areas of individuals with adverse personal or household socio-economic factors (Slater, 2013). However, the area people live in may well play a secondary role.

The geographical segregation of rich and poor has been well-documented in a number of countries, including the UK (Atkinson and Kintrea, 2001; Dorling *et al.*, 2007; Wilkinson and Pickett, 2010). Poor people tend to live in poor neighbourhoods because of lower house prices and the availability of social housing. Affordability is reflected in limited population turnover in areas of deprivation with movement tending to be within the area rather than outside (Bailey and Livingston, 2007). Even when areas are 'gentrified', poor people are displaced rather than remaining and benefiting from any residential improvements (Slater, 2013). Seeking 'neighbourhood effects' and targeting interventions at areas of deprivation obscures how individuals and areas are linked to the wider macroeconomic system. The extent to which these are adequate strategies for ameliorating poverty and deprivation is questionable since, 'the problems in the neighbourhood are rarely problems of the neighbourhood' (Andersson and Musterd, 2005: 386).

Deprivation and poverty can lock families into a 'cycle' of disadvantageous circumstances from which it is difficult to escape (Welshman, 2008). More recently the term 'intergenerational mobility' has been used to convey a similar idea. A study in Sweden, for example, found that the neighbourhood in which children lived with their parents was strongly related to the kind of neighbourhood they lived in 5, 12 and 18 years later. Thus, children living with their parents in a neighbourhood of high poverty concentration were very likely to end up in a similar area much later in life (Ham *et al.*, 2012). Considerable attention has been given to trying to understand the mechanisms through which being born into disadvantageous circumstances can be perpetuated. Understandings of parenting in conditions of socio-economic deprivation and the consequences for children's development have become more nuanced in recent years through linking macro-level effects and micro-level processes relating to **socialization,** normalization and stigmatization (Andersson and Musterd, 2005). These kinds of explanations also draw on the notion of a 'culture of poverty', used to emphasize how being resource-poor can generate beliefs about the world that limit people's horizons. Being unemployed, for example, can lead to feelings of hopelessness about finding work and resignation about the future; feelings that can be amplified in certain neighbourhoods and networks and can be transmitted inter-generationally. Possible consequences of this are limited aspirations and even dependency on state welfare. Children brought up in these circumstances often fail to develop the predispositions necessary to do well at school. Intergenerational mobility is less likely in Britain and the USA compared to Canada and the Nordic countries, however (Blanden *et al.*, 2005). A critical factor in mobility is educational attainment. However, how well children do at school may increasingly be related to income because of parent's ability to buy in support and enrichment of various kinds (Ball, 2010).

Conclusion

Deprivation and poverty remain significant issues for public health. For children, growing up in deprived circumstances can be particularly corrosive in relation to their developmental health and well-being. Given that poverty and unemployment have structural origins – the economy and the labour market – little will change until these are addressed. Even when people move in and out of poverty there is not always a corresponding fall in deprivation (Berthoud and Bryan, 2011). Long-term low income tends to be associated with long-term deprivation, suggesting that it is not easy to change living conditions even if income temporarily rises. Deprivation thus differentiates more clearly between those who can and cannot afford necessities than a classification based on low income (Saunders and Naidoo, 2009).

DETERMINANTS OF HEALTH

Context

Concerned as it is with **prevention**, public health has always been preoccupied with the determinants of **health**. In England, the public health movement emerged out of concern with the environmental determinants of health such as clean water and air. The rise of **medicine** and the expansion of health care, however, shifted attention towards individual-level biological and behavioural determinants. Since the 1970s, there has been a resurgence of interest in the wider social, economic and cultural determinants of health. Two recent reports – *Closing the Gap in a Generation: Health Equity Through Action on the Social Determinants of Health* (Commission on the Social Determinants of Health (CSDH), 2008) and *Fair Society, Healthy Lives: The Marmot Review* (Marmot, 2010) – synthesized **evidence** on the social determinants of health and made recommendations for how they could be addressed, particularly with the goal of social justice in mind. Together these reports present an extensive evidence-base on the determinants of health and health **inequalities** throughout the lifespan. To date, however, relatively slow progress has been made on implementing recommendations from either report.

Defining the determinants of health

Porta (2008: 65) defines a determinant of health as 'any factor that brings about change in a health condition or other defined characteristic'. Thus, determinants of health occupy a central place in theories about health production and disease causation (see **causality**). In the human sciences, however, the notion of a 'determinant' tends to be underpinned by a probabilistic model of health and disease rather than a deterministic one. According to this view a determinant is one that increases the likelihood of health (or disease) being produced but may be neither necessary (the change cannot happen without it) nor sufficient (the determinant is enough to bring about the change on its own). The WHO defines social determinants as 'social and economic conditions under which people live which determine their health. These circumstances are shaped by the distribution of money, power and resources at global, national and local levels' (www.who.int/social_determinants/en/).

The significance of the determinants of health for public health

'Tackling' the determinants of health has become a major feature of public health **policy** in many countries. There is some concensus that addressing the *wider* social determinants of health is central to improving overall population health and to reducing health inequalities. In order to provide a framework for considering how and where to intervene a number of models have been developed, perhaps the most widely cited of which is that of Dahlgren and Whitehead (1991). All models are representations of reality, necessarily simplifying phenomena by including some elements over others and reflecting some relationships between particular elements rather than others. Thus, models are constructed to be both descriptive – identifying relevant elements – as well as explanatory – representing how the different elements identified relate to one other. Dahlgren and Whitehead's model represents individuals (in terms of their age, sex and genes – constitutional determinants of health that cannot be altered to any degree) at the centre of four concentric 'layers of influence'. Individual **lifestyle** factors represent the innermost layer. These types of factors, along with their biological consequences, are often referred to as proximal (or downstream) determinants, in other words, those that are closer in time or distance to the health outcome of interest, making it easier to trace the links between the determinant and the outcome. Social and **community** influences, living and working conditions, and general socio-economic, cultural and environmental conditions represent three additional layers of influence. Distal (upstream) determinants – such as the global ecosystem or the macroeconomic environment – are those influences that are more remote in time or position to the outcome of concern and more difficult to link together, even though they may be no less influential (Porta, 2008). The model presents health production (or disease causation) in terms of the outcome of complex layers of interacting influences that operate at proximal and distal levels. Barton and Grant (2006) have extended Dahlgren and Whitehead's model to produce a similar 'health map' that focuses on the global ecosystem and the natural and built environments, seeking to convey their impact on human health and well-being in neighbourhoods through similar interacting layers of influence. Models developed in the Marmot Review (2010) and the CSDH (2008) have been presented in terms of a **lifecourse** dimension indicating that some periods, such as childhood, may be more sensitive to social and other influences than others.

Models of increasing sophistication have been developed in relation to the social determinants of health, emphasizing the social production of health through, for example, levels of income and **education**, type of employment, quality of material environment, forms of lifestyle, and so on. The explanatory power of such models lies in the extent to which they can account for patterns of health. This necessarily involves theorizing – that is to say, explaining speculatively – how social phenomena might have biological consequences. Krieger (2001) proposes an ecosocial approach, which seeks to integrate social and biological reasoning to explain how the circumstances in which people are born, grow up and live affect not only their mental and physical health and well-being but also their life expectancy. The interactions between the layers of influence underscore how particular conditions make some health-related outcomes more likely than others. Krieger's ecosocial approach has much in common with that of Durkheim's work on social dynamics and suicide, from which he concluded that suicide was not an isolated individual tragedy but a reflection of social conditions (Durkheim, 1987, 1970). Evidence increasingly indicates that social determinants might act via psycho-physiological pathways involving chronic stress (Brunner, 1997). Civil servants in the UK with greater exposure to job strain and lower job control, for example, had higher levels of fibrinogen in their blood, increasing their **risk** of coronary heart disease (Blane *et al.*, 1996). Similarly, depression – mediated through disadvantaged living conditions – has been linked with immunological dysfunction (Chandola and Marmot, 2004).

Although critical of Dahlgren and Whitehead's model on the basis that it does not fully explore generative mechanisms, Williams argues that a central explanatory feature is its 'porosity, its receptivity to the complex interactions and relationships between economic conditions, social structure, social relationships and networks, individual behaviour and psychosocial factors' (Williams, 2003: 139). Thus, a macroeconomic system based on the ideology of neo-liberalism (that is to say having a minimum of regulation of labour and financial markets for profit maximization and low taxation) has influenced the most recent economic downturn (Krugman, 2013). This, in turn, has had consequences for the labour market: rising unemployment, increased competition for jobs and an increasing proportion of low quality jobs – part-time, temporary, low wages and with poor promotion prospects – making it more likely that people will be locked into a working life of job insecurity (Taylor, 2011). These developments in the labour market mean that in-work poverty has increased (Aldridge *et al.*, 2012). Because young people tend to be especially adversely affected by economic recessions relative to older people they are at risk of experiencing the enduring scars of unemployment, including poverty and material **deprivation**, with consequences for their physical health and mental well-being. Suicide has been linked to unemployment, with rates tending to rise during periods of economic recession (Stuckler *et al.*, 2011). The combined effect of economic hardship and social dislocation (such as that likely to be experienced whilst unemployed) has been found to increase the risk of poor health (Ahnquist *et al.*, 2012). This example illustrates how consequences cascade from broad global events and national policies to influence individual biographies (Williams, 2003). This has been described as understanding the causes of the causes (Rose, 2008).

Graham (2004) offers an overview of models, referring to their core elements as: social structure; social position; social/material environment; behavioural/physiological factors; illness and injury; and, their social consequences. More fundamentally, Graham differentiates the social determinants of health from the social processes that give rise to the unequal distribution of social (health) determinants – something implicit in the models discussed above. An example from Bangladesh illustrates the distinction drawn by Graham. In Bangladesh, a large majority of people are poor in both income and health terms, a key determinant of which is access to sufficient, nutritious food. The unequal distribution of privately owned land limits the extent to which many families can provide food for themselves: the wealthiest 16 per cent of the rural Bangladeshi population own approximately 66 per cent of the land. What social processes have given rise to this unequal distribution of land ownership? Navarro (2009) explains it in terms of power differentials between and among classes – in this case between the elite landowners and the poor – and their influence over the state. In Bangladesh 75 per cent of the members of parliament are landowners with a vested interest in utilizing their political power to ensure that income, food and health inequalities are maintained. Thus, *social position* is key because it 'marks the point in the model where societal-level resources enter and affect the lives of individuals ... [and] shapes access and exposure to a set of intermediate factors' (Graham, 2004: 107). Consequently, resources such as land, food and income flow into people's lives unequally, enabling those who command more resources to have the greater number of options for avoiding risks (Graham, 2004). Power imbalances manifested in social position – be that in relation to class, ethnicity, gender, disability and so on – have been described as 'the fundamental social cause of health' (Link and Phelan, 1995: 80). The social processes through which power is generated and distributed are, unsurprisingly, viewed by many commentators as pivotal to understanding social and health inequalities.

At a global level, the fundamental determinants of health (what might be termed the prerequisites for survival) remain unmet for very many people: 'roughly one third of all human deaths – 18 million annually – are due to poverty-related causes, straightforwardly preventable through better nutrition, safe drinking water, cheap re-hydration packs, vaccines, antibiotics and other medicines' (Thomas Pogge, cited in Mooney, 2012: 3). The default response of high-income nations to famine, disease outbreaks and other disasters in low-income countries (including outbreaks of war) has become the deployment of emergency aid rather than a concerted focus on the root causes (determinants) of these events. In London, during the nineteenth century, the class structure that emerged during industrialization meant that not all were equally affected by the squalor and poor living conditions that bred epidemics. Those groups with lower status, less power and inadequate income were more likely to be exposed to health hazards and so carried a heavier burden of ill-health. Differential exposure – both then and now – is not, however, inevitable. Rather, it relates to social arrangements (the enduring structures of society) and requires political will if such arrangements are to alter. Navarro (2009) has criticized the CSDH (2008) on the basis that its recommendations neglect the critical issue of power. In other words, the CSDH focussed principally on the social determinants of health rather than the determinants of social inequality. A focus on the latter implies a need for more far-reaching policies – relating to employment and fiscal policy, the public provision of education, housing, social security, and so on – of the kind countries such as Sweden and other Nordic countries have been seeking to implement (Diderichsen *et al.*, 2012).

Conclusion

Individual-level factors in the form of genetic determinants of health, illness and disease have re-emerged as a central concern of public health. A range of questions have, however, been raised about the appropriateness of relying on sophisticated biomedical and technological approaches to health improvement when basic prerequisites for health in many parts of the world remain unmet. The extent to which genomic solutions might exacerbate inequalities, given their likely costs, is also a concern. Furthermore, the promise that the human genome project will create sufficient knowledge and understanding of the genetic sequencing of human chromosomes to lead to the development of personalized drugs and treatments for contemporary diseases and illnesses has yet to be realized (Pang and Weatherall, 2012). Against this background, the importance of action on the social processes that give rise to the unequal pattern of determinants of health remains a priority if health at a global level is to improve.

ECONOMIC AND HUMAN DEVELOPMENT

Context

The concept of 'development' has historically (and somewhat ambiguously) been used to refer to some form of social progress, transition or advancement in a country. Yet the conventional orthodoxy has been to discuss a country's level of development in economic terms. In recent years, however, the UN has been influential in promoting a broader view of development based on human (abilities, skills, knowledge and other capabilities) as well as economic capital. According to the UN, human development represents progress in terms of the extent to which a country provides people with choices and freedoms, including those relating to their **health** and welfare. This broader view of development reflects a growing appreciation of the complex relationship between economic growth, human development, and population health. The 18 MDGs (adopted by 189 nations during the UN Millennium Summit in September 2000) reflect this interdependence by focusing efforts on goals that relate to fundamental development domains, such as poverty reduction, literacy, reproductive choices and so forth.

Defining economic and human development

Economic development has traditionally been strongly linked with economic growth, which has been the predominant marker for tracking a country's advancement. The term refers to qualitative shifts in a country's economy towards increases in economic productivity. The conventional specific indicator of economic development has been gross domestic product (GDP), defined as the market value of all goods and services produced within a country in a given period of time. GDP per capita (person) has often been used as an indicator of the standard of living in a country. In recent years, the World Bank has categorized countries as low-, middle-, or high-income (on the basis of the related measure of gross national income (GNI) per capita – gross national income converted to international dollars, using purchasing parity rates). Until relatively recently, development defined in these economic terms was viewed as the foundation for social development and improvements in health and welfare.

Mounting criticism of the economic approach, however, led the UN to publish its first human development report in 1990. In this report, human development was defined as 'a process of enlarging people's choices … for people to lead a long and healthy life, to acquire knowledge and to have access to resources needed for a decent standard of living' (UNDP, 1990: 10). Since then, the UN, as well as academics working in relevant fields, has elaborated the notion of human development in terms of people's capabilities (see for example, Nussbaum, 2011). Economic prosperity is thus viewed as conceptually distinct from human development. The Human Development Index (HDI) was developed by the UN to provide a composite measure of the core dimensions of human development represented in the definition cited above: health (life expectancy), **education** (attainment) and standard of living (income). Paralleling the economic approach, the UN categorizes countries on the basis of their HDI score into low (zero), medium, high, and very high (1.0) human development. Accordingly, in the very high category, Norway is ranked first out of 186 countries (HDI 0.955), the UK 26th (HDI 0.875) and Niger 186th (HDI 0.304). Those in the low category are predominantly from the African subcontinent (http://hdr.undp.org). Two measures have subsequently been added to extend the HDI: a gender-related development index measuring gender inequality in economic and political terms (GII), and a human poverty index as a multidimensional measure of poverty (Bettcher and Lee, 2002). The GII reflects **inequalities** in achievement between men and women using three indicators: reproductive health, empowerment and labour market participation (ranging from zero – women fare equally – through to 1.0 – women fare poorly). In 2013, Norway was ranked fifth out of 186 countries (GII of 0.065), the UK 34th (GII of 0.205) and Niger 146th (GII 0.707) (Malik, 2013).

The significance of economic and human development for public health

The significance of a country's economic resources for health has been extensively explored (Ranis *et al.*, 2000). Since the 1970s, studies have shown that life expectancy increases rapidly in poorer countries during the early phases of economic development (Preston, 2007). Increasing GDP per capita by relatively small amounts has the potential to lift substantial proportions of people out of poverty, giving rise to a decline in childhood mortality and increasing life expectancy (Gordon, 2010). Many consider poverty (the international poverty line set by the World Bank is $1.25 a day) – which is most dense in low-income countries, particularly those that are indebted – to be one of the most pressing global public health issues of contemporary times. Living in poverty in a low-income country means that even the most basic living conditions are unmet: estimates suggest, for example, that there are one billion slum dwellers and 780 million without access to clean water worldwide (UN, 2010). These conditions create highly inauspicious circumstances for health, illustrated by the associated high rates of infant and maternal mortality and short life expectancies (48 years in Middle Africa compared with 81 years on average in the 19 'longest lived' populations). In these circumstances health tends to be further compromised by limited access to food of at least reasonable quality. In 2010, about one in four children were underweight and approximately 925 million people suffered from chronic hunger (UN, 2012). Some 222 million women lack access to modern contraceptives, putting families further under strain (Greene *et al.*, 2012). Poverty, and the high infant and child mortality rates it tends to give rise to, continues to be a major contributor to high fertility rates (Kibirige, 1997; Bongaarts, 2009). These conditions significantly restrict the possibilities for human development.

As GDP per capita increases further, however, improvements in life expectancy begin to tail off (at about $5,000 per capita in 2006) and eventually plateau, with 'diminishing returns' from increased per capita income (Preston, 2007: 488). This suggests that the relationship between economic development and life expectancy is less straightforward for those countries aligned along the plateau, many of which (but not all) are high-income countries such as Norway, the USA and Japan (see Wilkinson and Pickett, 2010). Although GDP is generally viewed as a reasonable indicator of living standards in a country, it provides no basis for understanding how economic resources are used (Preston, 2007). The varying life expectancies at any given level of national income per capita may, at least in part, reflect differences in how resources are used within a country. Cuba and Costa Rica have life expectancies that exceed what might be predicted from their relatively low GDP per capita, for example. This is reflected in each country's HDI values – both categorized as high by the UN: Cuba ranked 59th (HDI 0.780) and Costa Rica ranked 62nd (HDI 0.773) (Malik, 2013). Conversely, some countries achieve reasonable economic growth but fare less well in terms of human development (Jolly *et al.*, 2009). Then again, the Bahamas and New Zealand have similar levels of GDP per capita but markedly different life expectancies and years of schooling, resulting in being ranked 49th and 6th respectively in their HDI value. In discussing the improvements in HDI values among a number of countries in the southern hemisphere in recent years (Brazil, Mexico, India, for example), Malik (2013) argues that these countries have, in varying ways, accelerated human development through a proactive developmental state, tapping into global markets alongside sustained social policies and innovation. According to this view, economic growth is a means to an end, the end in this case being improved human development.

Eradicating poverty and hunger are two of the eight MDGs (www.un.org/millenni-umgoals). Although precisely establishing levels of poverty is difficult, recent estimates suggest that they are falling in all regions of the world, driven largely by improvements in China and India (Chandy and Gertz, 2011). Notwithstanding these trends, estimates in 2011 indicated that there were just under 900 million people still living in poverty. Furthermore, recent analyses of the impact of the global financial crisis on some of the world's poorest people suggest that any progress may be short lived; the UN estimates that 64 million more people will be pushed into extreme poverty (UN, 2012). Advances are fragile because poverty and poor health are entrenched in spite of aid programmes. Poverty Reduction Strategy Papers (PSRPs) have become the primary vehicle for delivering aid to countries, following on from Structural Adjustment Programmes (SAPs), which became largely discredited in the 1990s (Lazarus, 2008). A strong criticism of SAPs was that loans were given under specific conditions that reflected the dominant neo-liberal ideology (free market economics) of the World Bank, International Monetary Fund (IMF) and its donors (primarily the USA, UK, Canada and Japan) (Larkin, 1999). Thus, high-income countries prescribed **policy** direction in recipient countries in relation to trade liberalization, privatization of state assets, currency devaluation and the introduction of user fees for health and education, shaping their economic development according to the neo-liberal model. This hegemony – the domination of one set of ideas over another to such an extent that no alternatives are considered (Roberts, 2009) – illustrates not only how countries are interdependent but also the differential consequences of being interdependent, which are most favourable to those with more economic and political power. Not only did SAPs fail to alleviate poverty, they tended to exacerbate problems. Food price increases, for example, had severe implications for the adequacy of children's nutrition (Verheul and Rowson, 2001).

SAPs and PSRPs have come to be viewed as largely serving the interests of donor countries and, in particular, their multinational corporations by, for example, creating access to cheap labour in environments with limited regulatory requirements, as well as to valuable natural resources. Although PSRPs were designed to address many of the criticisms of SAPs (primarily by requiring that countries develop their own strategy for poverty reduction through a process of democratic participation to engender 'ownership') (www.imf.org/external/np/exr/facts/prsp.htm), participation has been problematic in many countries (Lazarus, 2008). Overall economic growth – the hallmark of adjustment programmes – has been negligible. Even in democratic low-income countries, PSRPs lead to a skewed income distribution, widening within-country income and health inequalities (Bjørnskov, 2010). India, the ninth largest global economy (Global Health Strategies Initiatives, 2012), not only has the highest levels of child malnutrition in the world (38.4 per cent of children under 3 years old are stunted) (Rao, 2012) but is also projected to have nearly 80 million people with diabetes by 2030 (Fried *et al.*, 2010). Economic growth on its own will not be sufficient to improve population health and reduce inequalities because the poor tend to benefit least from economic growth unless other policies are put in place (Schrecker *et al.*, 2008). In other words, there is little or no spin-off or trickle-down effect from economic growth.

Poverty reduction strategies are more likely to achieve their objectives if they are multifaceted and focus on the root causes. Protecting women's reproductive rights, for example, enabling their access to free education, and improving child survival have long been advocated as central to reducing poverty because they support reductions in fertility (Greene *et al.*, 2012; Lithell *et al.*, 1992). Reducing maternal mortality also directly influences child survival as motherless children are 10 times more likely to die prematurely compared to those with a mother (UN, 2010). Policies that invest in health can also directly benefit the economy. Poor health limits the size of the available workforce as well as limiting its knowledge and skills through impeding access to education (Martin *et al.*, 2012). In short, poverty stands in the way of meeting human and economic development goals.

Unrestrained forms of economic growth tend to compromise sustained economic *and* human development, with a variety of negative consequences for health (Szreter, 1997). In particular, unregulated forms of economic growth are likely to lead to widening social **inequalities in health**. A recent report reveals economic inequality in the UK to be the highest in recorded history and the UK to be one of the most unequal high-income places in the world (Shaheen, 2011). Furthermore, as Szreter (1997) argues, economic development can be disruptive, leading to the emergence of new patterns of disease. As countries make the transition towards a globalized economy, chronic degenerative diseases such as cardiovascular diseases emerge (Narayan *et al.*, 2010). Low- and middle-income countries increasingly face the dual burden of coping with a complex mix of infectious and chronic degenerative diseases.

Conclusion

Some consensus has emerged in recent years – at least among some academics – that there is a complex and reciprocal relationship between economic development and human development, improvements in each making the other more likely. Yet questions remain, particularly in relation to whether policies should pursue economic growth or health investment first (Husain, 2010). Their interdependence, however, suggests that both must be pursued as part of a regulated macroeconomic policy (Jolly *et al.*, 2009). However, the human development approach has yet to be accepted within the UN itself, let alone elsewhere. Nonetheless, because health and development are inextricably linked, new ways of approaching development have considerable potential to improve the health and economies of populations, making a major contribution to global public health.

EDUCATION

Context

The relationship between education and **health** has received considerable research attention in recent years. Longitudinal studies have been particularly important in advancing knowledge and understanding of this complex relationship. Educational opportunities, however, vary considerably both within and between countries. In 2010, the UN estimated that 39 million school-age children were not in school, with girls being somewhat less likely to receive any form of education compared to boys in some areas. Even in countries where free universal education is enshrined in law, children do not benefit equally from schooling. Education is thus a core dimension of inequality and a key **determinant** of health. It is, therefore, an important **policy** domain for addressing social **inequalities** in health, especially if policies focus on equalizing educational attainment across social groups (Graham, 2007).

Defining education

Education is a form of (secondary) **socialization,** which takes place through a variety of social institutions, such as schools, colleges and universities. What distinguishes education from other forms of socialization (including indoctrination) is an intention to transform people's understanding of the world and thus enhance their capacity to act upon it as rational, self-governing individuals. In this respect it is more open-ended and diffuse than the notion of 'training', in which skills are taught for a specific end (Roberts, 2009). Conventionally, educational philosophers of the liberal tradition have viewed education as fundamentally concerned with *valuable* knowledge – theoretical and practical. However, while the liberal tradition of education might reflect the preferred view of what education *should* be, it is now generally accepted that it is better to view education as a normative practice – that is to say, as it is carried out in day-to-day life. The normative perspective is based on the premise that the aims and purposes of education shift over time and **place**, shaped by a variety of historical, cultural and political factors.

Contemporary views of education tend to emphasize the preparation of young people for adult life in their society. How the curriculum is constituted and which subjects are included – statutory and non-statutory – reflect the judgements made, for example, by policymakers regarding what is desirable knowledge for young people. In many high-income countries, such as England, there has been an increasing emphasis on assessment and testing in a relatively narrow range of subjects, with the needs of employers and the economy in mind. According to some, this has given rise to a neglect of the broader aims of education, such as those relating to human well-being and the enrichment of society, eliding the ways in which education might lead to a more equitable society (Pring, 2011). This view of the purpose of education has resonance for understanding social inequalities in health. Shifts towards more utilitarian views of the social role of education reflect the changing values and priorities of governments with considerable power and control over state education in many countries. By way of illustration, the position of personal, social and **health education** within the curriculum (including sex and relationships education) in England and the USA has varied over time and place, reflecting the ideological views of government about what is desirable for children and young people to know, when they should know it and how this might be differentiated by gender, religious denomination and so on.

In health inequalities research, education is measured in terms of years of full-time education or, increasingly, highest educational qualification, which seems to be the critical factor in understanding associations between education and health (Graham, 2007). As a measure, its main advantage is that it remains stable even if health status changes, which may not be the case for income and occupation. It is also moderately stable across adulthood. Questions about education are also relatively straightforward to ask and more likely to be answered compared to questions relating to income (Shaw *et al.*, 2007). Its main limitation is that level of education *predicts* socio-economic status, rather than *representing* it (Graham, 2007).

The significance of education for public health

In high- middle- and low-income countries there is an education gradient in health. Adults with a lower level of education tend to die earlier and have a higher prevalence of most kinds of health problems (Mackenbach, 2006; Marmot, 2005). In high-income countries, such as England, those with a higher level of education are more likely to have better self-reported health, be more satisfied with their lives and have higher levels of happiness and well-being (Graham, 2007). They are also more likely to smoke less, be physically active and drink moderately (Cutler and Lleras-Muney, 2010; Ross and Wu, 1995). In countries such as the USA, these patterns appear to have strengthened in recent times, with a higher level of education protecting against both the onset of disease as well as promoting better health outcomes among those with a disease (Goldman and Smith, 2011). The protective effect of education is particularly well-illustrated by an analysis of adult mortality in the Russian Federation during the social and political upheavals of the 1990s. Although mortality increased dramatically during this period, those with the lowest level of education were the most affected while those with a university-level education were not affected at all. Alcohol consumption accounted for some but not all of the observed differences (Plavinski *et al.*, 2003). Overall, the **evidence** suggests that educational achievement is a fundamental prerequisite for health.

Considerable attention has been directed at understanding the pathways that connect level of education to health, which are likely to be complex and multidimensional. Socio-economic position (SEP) is an overarching term that refers to the social and economic factors that influence a person's or group's position in society and has been the preferred term in health research. Although there are a large number of ways of measuring SEP (see, for example, Shaw *et al.*, 2007) income, occupation and education are most frequently used, particularly when discussing inequalities in health. Although interrelated, each probably reflects different influences on health (Winkleby *et al.*, 1992). Social class tends to be the concept used in the social sciences to imply that groups share social, cultural, political, economic, educational and occupational features (Roberts, 2009). Social class, it seems, is particularly pertinent to understanding the relationship between education and health.

Despite formal equal educational opportunities in high-income countries such as England (where attendance at school between the ages of 5 and 16 years is compulsory), social class inequalities in educational achievement at age 16 have increased since 1989 (Graham, 2007). Yet, in the UK, more young people from all social classes are spending longer in full-time education than at any previous point. Family background, including family poverty, has been found to be a particularly significant influence on educational achievement (McCulloch and Joshi, 2001). Thus, childhood disadvantage is linked to adult disadvantage because 'class origins influence educational trajectories and educational trajectories influence class destinations' (Graham, 2007: 128).

Family background is particularly important for understanding how children develop the capacity to learn and benefit from school. Parenting styles, which themselves are shaped by parents' socialization experiences as well as their access to resources, nurture different types of cognitive and linguistic skills and competences (Chambers, 2012). While parenting is generally challenging, middle class parents are better positioned and resourced to negotiate these challenges, in part because their households appear more likely to comprise two parents of similar social background. They are also more likely to have the financial, interpersonal and psychological resources to provide a safe and secure home and a stimulating learning environment. Children's physiological responses to these aspects of the family home environment are likely to be positive in that they influence memory, attention and problem-solving (through the release of dopamine) in a way that enhances cognitive development (Wilkinson and Pickett, 2010). Middle-class parents are also better positioned to provide the necessary financial, intellectual and cultural support their children need as they move through the school system (Reay, 2004, 2006). Such parental engagement is more likely if parents have a higher income and more education themselves (Ball, 2010).

Rather than compensating for disadvantaged family background it seems that schools often exacerbate social class differences. Cognitive abilities, for example, diverge as children progress through school, widening rather than reducing school entry differences (Graham and Power, 2004). Micro-interactional processes between teachers and children, as well as between teachers and parents, are important in explaining this phenomenon. Middle-class children have the kinds of attributes that are valued and nurtured in most schools; as Reay puts it 'class is lived in classrooms' (2006: 288). This means that not all children are encouraged to develop ambition, self-esteem and self-worth – key factors in educational success. Thus, rather than acting as a mechanism for social mobility education often reproduces social class (and probably other) inequalities across generations. This is particularly the case with regard to access to higher education, which has conventionally been seen as a key factor in reducing class inequalities. Indeed, the expansion of higher education in many high-income countries in recent years seems to have disproportionately benefited children from well-off families rather than the most able, strengthening the links between educational achievement and social class (Machin and Vignoles, 2004). Interestingly, in recent years Britain and the USA have become significantly less mobile compared to Nordic countries. In Britain, at least part of the explanation for this lies in the strengthening relationship between family income and educational attainment as well as labour market success (Machin and Vignobles, 2004). In the UK, the proportions of those children who stay on at school after the compulsory leaving age and then go on to university is strongly income-related (Reay *et al.*, 2010).

Educational achievement in the form of qualifications is a key determinant of young people's position in the labour market and thus their occupation and income in adulthood (Graham, 2007). A number of implications for health flow from this. Quality of life, especially the quality of working life, is likely to be better for those with a high level of education. This includes having a more secure, satisfying and subjectively rewarding job, with more prospects for career and salary progression. The corollary to this is that life tends to have fewer stresses and anxieties relating to the likelihood of being unemployed, or in part-time, routine or casual work (Ross and Wu, 1995). Furthermore, increasing level of education can lead to different forms of thinking, use of knowledge and decision-making patterns that may directly relate to specific health-related behaviours in some contexts (Cutler and Lleras-Muney, 2010). Research in Ghana, for example, suggests that those with a higher educational level were more likely to take steps to protect themselves against HIV compared to those with similar levels of knowledge but lower educational qualifications (Peters *et al.*, 2010).

Educational achievement is also an important determinant of women's reproductive choices (Martin, 1995). The trend towards delayed cohabitation and parenthood since the 1970s in most high-income countries has been particularly apparent in those from higher social classes and with a higher level of education. Early pregnancy and childbirth, particularly in the teenage years, remains more prevalent among those living in poorer circumstances and with fewer qualifications or educational prospects. Although patterns vary, teenage pregnancy and birth rates have declined over the past 40 years in several high-income countries (Singh *et al.*, 2009) and may be related to increases in women's educational attainments and entry into higher education. Neighbourhood and area disadvantage also increase the chances that motherhood will be experienced early. When educational and economic opportunities are limited, early entry into motherhood can be a route to a valued identity, generational inclusiveness and an alternative route to perceived fulfilment (Graham, 2007). Increasing the educational success particularly of boys and girls living in areas of disadvantage is a public health strategy that has the potential to contribute to a decline in teenage pregnancy rates, among many other things.

Generally, the longer young people stay in education, the better their health and life chances. Improving access to education and limiting drop-out, particularly for girls, continues to be a key priority for the UN in many low-income countries. There is some consensus that educating girls is one of the most cost-effective ways of spurring economic development through women's entry into the labour market, delaying and limiting child-bearing and yielding significant intergenerational gains. In rural parts of Pakistan, girls were shown to be less likely to drop out of school if their mother had attended school or were in a better-off family (Lloyd *et al.*, 2009). Women's empowerment, including their sexual empowerment and right to control their reproduction, is interdependent with their educational success. A study in Ghana found that increased contraceptive use was associated with having a formal education, increased wealth and being in an unmarried partnership (Crissman *et al.*, 2012). Fundamentally, this suggests that creating the preconditions within which contraceptive use is more likely requires access to formal education for men, as well as for women in particular.

Conclusion

Education, it seems, is a fundamental determinant of better health and a longer life. The Marmot Review (2010) placed particular emphasis on education as a determinant of health. It made a number of recommendations relating to improving the quality of education, particularly in the early years, and especially through supporting parents as the primary agents of children's **socialization**. Policy responses such as Head Start in the USA and Sure Start in the UK used multifaceted **community**-based programmes delivered in deprived areas in order to focus on preventing developmental delay in children. **Evaluation** of Head Start has provided strong evidence of its effectiveness and cost-effectiveness (Anderson *et al.*, 2003). Sure Start local programmes were, however, fundamentally modified before evidence of their impact could be produced (Glass, 2006). Nonetheless, investment in the early years is a preventive strategy that is likely to have considerable public health benefits (Hertzman *et al.*, 2010). The provision of free universal education – as articulated in MDG number two – is therefore a necessary precondition for improving population health and reducing social inequalities in health. It seems, however, that class, ethnicity and gender remain important in explaining patterns of educational success in those countries where education is available to all.

EPIDEMIOLOGY

Context

Historically, the epidemiological approach to the study of **health** and disease has played a central role in the emergence of public health. John Snow is often described as the first 'shoe-leather' epidemiologist, a phrase used to convey his first-hand observational approach to the study of epidemics. His work on cholera in London during the mid-nineteenth century influenced the development of the public health movement and the passing of the first public health acts in England. Epidemiology's association with public health has continued to the present day, following the rapid expansion of the discipline following the Second World War. It is often described as *the* core discipline in public health, providing the 'science' (rather than the 'art') underpinning efforts to improve health and prevent disease.

In recent years, however, there has been considerable criticism of epidemiology from several quarters including from within public health (Ness and Rothenberg, 2007). Some have questioned the scientific credentials of epidemiology, arguing that its methodological weaknesses limit its powers of prediction to the point where its conclusions are of little value. The emphasis in epidemiology on methodology and empirical observations has also led to charges of the discipline being 'atheoretical'. Others have questioned the increasing reliance of epidemiology on statistics and statistical modelling, approaches that tend to fragment, decontextualize and individualize complex health-related phenomena. The emergence of genetic and molecular epidemiology has accelerated these tendencies by shifting the focus away from the environment. This mounting criticism led McPherson (1998) to conclude that if epidemiology was to provide a constructive basis for modern public health then it was in need of a fundamental re-think. In order to be able to evaluate these arguments some understanding of the character and purposes of epidemiology and its relationship with public health is required.

Defining epidemiology

There is some degree of randomness to health and disease, including, for example, a person's genetic endowment and the circumstances into which s/he is born. That said, epidemiology is underpinned by the idea that 'once the dice are thrown' the occurrence of health and disease is much less a matter of chance but, rather, has causes. The epidemiological question is thus not why an individual person is unwell but, rather, why a specific population has a particular level and distribution of disease (Rose, 2008).

This reflects epidemiology's core concern with populations and population sub-groups. Establishing causes requires careful quantification – counting the number of deaths or cases of disease, for example – and comparison in relation to time, **place** and persons. Why, for example, has obesity increased in many populations over the last thirty years (time)? Why does life expectancy vary by country (place)? Why are some people more likely to develop lung cancer than others (persons)? The fundamental premise of epidemiology is that by asking questions about the occurrence of health and disease in populations, patterns can be revealed and **determinants of health** identified. Porta's definition of epidemiology reflects these core features (2008: 81): 'the study of the occurrence and distribution of health-related states or events in defined populations or societies, including the study of the determinants influencing such states, and the application of this knowledge in order to control the health problems'. What Porta implicitly points to here is the primary purpose of epidemiology, namely, to generate knowledge that can be used in **prevention** as well as to promote health.

The significance of epidemiology for public health

In recent years there has been a proliferation of branches or sub-specialities of epidemiology, differentiated on the basis of either methodology (for example, **lifecourse** epidemiology), disease focus (cancer epidemiology, cardiovascular disease epidemiology) and/or the level at which determinants of health and disease are investigated (molecular epidemiology, nutritional epidemiology, social epidemiology). Diversification within disciplines is an inevitable aspect of their development and reflects various influences over time. One such influence has been the shift away from infectious diseases towards chronic degenerative diseases as the main causes of mortality and morbidity in high-income countries. Although somewhat of an over-simplification, this 'epidemiological transition' accompanies a country's economic and social development and reflects increases in life expectancy. The rise of chronic degenerative diseases – themselves a manifestation of living longer – has been accompanied by a shift in focus within epidemiology towards the study of individual **risk** factors: genetic, biological and behavioural. Traditionally, risk factors have been seen in terms of 'exposures' – for example, exposure to an infectious agent, atmospheric pollution, an occupational hazard, tobacco smoke, and so on – and the measurement of exposure has been an important feature of the epidemiological approach.

There may, however, be significant limitations to conceptualizing many social determinants of health in terms of exposure, an issue that has fuelled debates about the character and purpose of epidemiology and the need to frame the discipline in unambiguously social terms. According to Krieger, *social* epidemiology focuses on 'explicitly investigating the social determinants of population distributions of health, disease and well-being, rather than treating such determinants as mere background to biological phenomena' (Krieger, 2001: 693). In other words, social epidemiology seeks to (re)focus attention on the environment, in this case the social environment. In this regard, the current challenge for epidemiology is the development of explanatory models that integrate the different levels of analysis into a more complex and coherent whole.

The various branches of epidemiology notwithstanding, most epidemiologists draw on similar study designs and methods, adapting each to the specific focus of study. There are many different ways of classifying epidemiological study designs and the terminology can be confusing. All study designs operate at the level of populations and, to varying degrees, measure disease burden and distribution (in other words they are descriptive) and explore causal relations (they are analytic). Epidemiological approaches are underpinned by a reasoning process that ultimately enables judgements to be made about **causality**. The relative emphasis on descriptive and analytic purposes and approaches varies, however. In broad terms, studies are either observational or experimental. Observational studies (cross-sectional, case-control and cohort studies) as the name suggests, involve examining events as they unfold (Bhopal, 2008). All make use of the survey as a study design for systematically collecting information about the study population. Cross-sectional studies involve taking a snapshot (rather than following a population into the future as a longitudinal design would), aiming to measure the burden of disease, usually in terms of prevalence (the total number of people with a disease or health-related state) in a population at a particular place and time. Socio-demographic and person-level information, including that relating to relevant exposures, is also collected. This allows comparisons of population sub-groups to be made. The main purpose is not only to describe the patterns of disease but to use descriptions to generate hypotheses that might account for the observed distribution. John Snow's work on mapping cholera outbreaks in London is often described as a classic example of a cross-sectional study used (alongside other information) to formulate a hypothesis about causes. The strengths of a cross-sectional study design lie in the fact that they provide a good measure of disease burden as well as facilitating the collection of data on a number of other variables. Such studies tend to be cheap and relatively quick to carry out, particularly if they make use of existing secondary sources of data such as medical records, registers and other routinely collected **official statistics**. They can also be used to study multiple outcomes at the same time. However, they are limited in the degree to which any one study can explore causal relations. Associations can be generated but because cross-sectional studies collect data on risk factors and outcomes at the same point in time they cannot comment on whether the former (risk factor) precedes the latter (outcome).

The utility of cross-sectional studies is illustrated by the work of Wilkinson and Pickett (2010) in *The Spirit Level*. This work collated a large amount of research in order to develop the proposition that income inequality correlates, often strongly, with various health and social problems. The authors develop a causal explanation – drawing on a range of biological, psychological, sociological and epidemiological research – for how income inequality might *cause* these problems. The analysis and conclusions presented in the book stimulated considerable debate and criticism, particularly from those to the right of the political spectrum (Noble, 2011). The criticism centred on the extensive use of cross-sectional data, the calculation of correlation coefficients (measures of statistical association) and statistical significance testing (to eliminate chance as an explanation for associations described) on data sets from a large number of countries as the basis for reaching conclusions on causality.

Sometimes a series of cross-sectional studies, often conducted retrospectively, might be carried out over time to develop an understanding of trends. This approach can be particularly valuable when some kind of change is introduced at a population level. A recent study reported on the impact of smoke-free legislation in Scotland on pregnancy outcomes, specifically in relation to pre-term delivery and small-for-gestational-age babies (Mackay *et al.*, 2012). Mackay *et al.* used measured rates of these two outcomes using routinely collected pregnancy data before and after the legislation came into effect. They found fewer premature births following the smoking ban in Scotland, although noted that this had begun three months prior to the ban. They concluded that while all retrospective studies are limited because of the problems of ruling out other factors, the findings could be taken to suggest an overall beneficial effect of the legislation on outcomes.

The development and use of case-control and cohort studies emerged during the post-war period in an effort to build stronger study designs for investigating causality. Both types of study set out to establish if there is an association between a disease and a certain exposure and calculate the strength of that association. The work of Doll and Hill (1950, 1954, 1964) on lung cancer was stimulated, at least in part, by large post-war increases in the disease, which were thought to have an environmental cause, possibly air pollution (Saracci, 2010). Their first study was a case-control study, the 'cases' being those with lung cancer and the 'controls' a matched group (for sex and similar age) without the disease who were in the same hospital at about the same time as the cases (Doll and Hill, 1950). Both cases and controls were interviewed and asked the same questions about their smoking habits (quantity, frequency, age when they started/stopped, and so on); that is, they looked back into the past (hence the term retrospective studies) of cases and controls to explore rates of exposure in the two groups. Case-control studies tend to be cheaper than cohort studies because they start with those who have the disease. They are also useful for studying rare diseases and conditions. Case-control studies suffer, however, from a number of biases (for example, recall bias) and confounding, and various strategies have been developed to minimize each of these. Despite this, they can be used to further develop and explore a hypothesis that might have originated from a cross-sectional study.

In 1951, Doll and Hill followed their case-control study with a prospective cohort study, in order to overcome some of the problems inherent in case-control studies. All members of the British Medical Association (the cohort) were sent a questionnaire containing questions about their smoking habits. Cohort studies compare disease rates in those 'exposed' – in this case, smokers – to those 'unexposed' – non-smokers, which form a type of control group within the study. The cohort was followed over time, with cause of death extracted from death certificates. As this example, illustrates, cohort studies are invaluable for exploring exposures in real life situations, and which cannot be explored through experimental studies for ethical reasons. They can also explore several outcomes at the same time. However, the major advantage of cohort studies over case-control studies is that because they include people who do not have the outcome under investigation at the outset, the time sequence between cause and effect can be explored leading to clearer conclusions about causality. A major disadvantage of cohort studies is the effort and costs of follow-up. They too suffer from various forms of bias and confounding.

Experimental studies are better able to test hypotheses than observational studies and can provide stronger **evidence** of causality if properly carried out with sufficiently large sample sizes to detect real differences between groups studied (that is, with sufficient statistical power). The use of the randomized controlled trial (RCT) – a classic experimental study design – has been extensive in the clinical environment in recent years. Cochrane (1972) argued that medical procedures and treatments should be subjected to rigorous **evaluation** through the use of RCTs. The use of randomization to allocate trial participants to either intervention group or control group minimizes various forms of bias and confounding, both of which can beset observational studies. In public health, ethical and practical concerns have limited the use of RCTs. Nonetheless, their use in the evaluation of public health interventions has grown in recent years. In England the Medical Research Council (MRC) launched a randomized double-blind prevention trial to test the idea that folic acid supplementation pre-conceptionally and during the first trimester might protect women with a prior pregnancy affected by a neural tube defect from a recurrence (MRC Vitamin Study Research Group, 1991). Folic acid was shown to have a 72 per cent protective effect. In 1996, the US Food and Drug administration required almost all flour to be fortified with folic acid. While this lead to a number of countries following suit, others (in Scandinavia and much of Europe) did not (www.ffinetwork.org/country_profiles/index.php). This illustrates the varied ways in which epidemiological evidence is used to inform public health **policy**, even when evidence has been generated from experimental studies.

Conducting experimental studies in everyday environments is particularly challenging. The North Karelia project (launched in east Finland in 1972) was a multifaceted public health intervention designed to reduce levels of cardiovascular disease (CVD). At that time, North Karelia had the highest CVD rates in the world (Puska, 2008). Evaluation of the intervention was based on a 'before and after' study design with a comparative control group comprising an adjacent population, so did not involve randomization. The subsequent evaluation concluded that the intervention had a 'small but real program effect on health-related behaviours and risk factor levels' (Wagner, 1982: 52). However, the finding that there were also improvements in the control population on a range of measures illustrates the difficulties of separating out the impact of the intervention from broader secular trends. This example also illustrates the impracticality of controlling the diffusion of ideas and practices from the intervention to the control population.

Conclusion

Public health continues to be beset by debate over the quality of epidemiological studies and the data they generate. However, if well executed, some research designs have greater power to elucidate the determinants of health and the effectiveness of interventions than others. Nevertheless, questions continue to be raised regarding the extent to which epidemiology on its own, particularly in its individually focused risk factor incarnation, can contribute knowledge and understanding of value to contemporary public health problems. For some, social epidemiology is part of the solution. Kaplan (2004), for example, argues that epidemiology must see all that it does as embedded in the social world and is sceptical about simplistic calls for better statistical techniques. In a similar vein, Krieger (2001) advocates the inclusion of social science perspectives, particularly in relation to theory development. Both perspectives emphasize an interpretation of 'public' (in public health) as 'social configurations of subjects that interact' (Van der Maesen and Nijhuis 2000: 139) rather than simply an aggregate variable equated with the concept of population. There are, however, limits to any discipline's contribution to knowledge. In part, such debates relate to broader concerns about the need to develop public health as an interdisciplinary field – one that includes qualitative research and participatory approaches and is salutogenic in orientation – stimulated through, and involving dialogue with, other disciplines (Long, 1997). Such developments, first articulated nearly 20 years ago, remain especially pertinent given that the hope of improving health and controlling disease promised by the human genome project appear unlikely to be delivered in the foreseeable future (Davey Smith and Ebrahim, 2001).

ETHICS

Context

Ethics provides a framework for considering the kinds of issues raised by public health action and inaction. In this regard, governments play a significant role in protecting and improving **health** and preventing disease. When and how governments should intervene are matters of some debate, however, given that their role implies both obligations and power (Thomas *et al.*, 2002). In pursuing population-level health benefits the state must pay due regard to the rights, liberties and interests of individuals. Balancing these interests makes decision making far from straightforward. This is particularly the case when their actions seek to restrict people's behaviours or infringe their civil liberties. Recent debates about the availability and price of alcohol, parents' responsibility for their children's vaccination status, restrictions on smoking in public spaces and corporate social responsibilities for health illustrate the potentially contested character of state actions.

Defining ethics

There is a tendency in some literature to use the terms 'ethics' and 'morals' inter-changeably. There are advantages, however, in distinguishing between them. Ethics provides a systematic theoretical framework that can be used to understand the basis on which certain actions might be judged right or wrong, good or bad, acceptable or unacceptable, justified or unjustified. Such frameworks are based on principles that reflect particular values (typically, respect for autonomy, the primacy of avoiding harm and creating benefits that outweigh potential harms, and justice) and rules (more specific in content and scope than principles) and express standards for human actions. In this way, ethics can help clarify issues and assist in answering such questions as 'what should be done here?' Morality, on the other hand, refers to 'norms about right and wrong human conduct that are so widely shared that they form a stable (although incomplete) social agreement' (Beauchamp and Childress, 2009: 2).

From an ethical perspective, public health can be understood as consequentialist or end-oriented as well as beneficence-oriented as the promotion of health and welfare of the population is its primary goal (Childress *et al.*, 2002). In this regard the Nuffield Council on Bioethics (NCB, 2007) advocates a stewardship model for public health based on the view that the state has a responsibility to provide the conditions under which people can lead healthy lives if they so wish, while at the same time avoiding 'unnecessary' coercion and restrictions on personal freedoms. The Council describes the stewardship model as 'prioritarian' (NCB, 2007: xvi) in that it focuses on strategies to improve health among the most disadvantaged groups. In the same vein, Faden and

Shebaya (2010: 1) emphasize social justice in their definition of public health ethics: 'while balancing individuals' liberties with promoting social goods is one area of concern, it is embedded within a broader commitment to secure a sufficient level of health for all and to narrow unjust inequalities'. Such a view implies that public health ethics involves weighing up general considerations in the context of specific policies and practices in order to provide justifications for certain actions, as well as asking specific questions about systematic disadvantage. These perspectives reflect contemporary concerns relating to social **inequalities** in health.

The significance of ethics for public health

In considering the significance of ethics to contemporary public health issues the overarching question is how action (or inaction) by the state can be defended? Childress *et al.* (2002: 171) argue that 'In a liberal pluralist democracy, the justification of coercive policies, as well as other policies, must rest on moral reasons that the public in whose name the policies are carried out could reasonably be expected to accept'. They propose a number of justificatory conditions – effectiveness, proportionality, necessity, least infringement, public justification – intended to help determine whether promoting public health warrants overriding such values as individual liberty or justice *in specific instances*. Nonetheless, all ethical decisions are based on judgements that reflect the value apportioned to these different conditions and, consequently, will, to varying degrees, generate disagreement and debate. The population perspective of public health – rather than the individual perspective of **medicine** and health care – is, however, the predominant reason why some have argued that there is a need to 'articulate a distinct ethic for public health' (Thomas *et al.*, 2002: 1057).

Since the emergence of public health as a social movement in the mid-nineteenth century in England, the state has used legislation and other actions to protect and promote people's health. The first public health reforms in England relating to the provision of safe drinking water and the development of an effective sewerage system have tended to be seen as universally beneficial. This type of public health action is often referred to as a 'collective' or 'social' good because it seeks to improve the health of the whole population as well as prevent illness and disease in ways that may well have been unlikely if left to others (Childress *et al.*, 2002). Skrabanek (1990) points out, however, that the scientific basis for a population-based approach may be limited, particularly in terms of the benefits that might be accrued relative to harms.

How governments interpret their role in public health will vary according to the normative political philosophies of the elected government – that is to say, ideological views regarding how society could and should be organized and how power might be used to achieve particular ends. Those with a liberal predisposition will seek to preserve certain freedoms on the (ideological) grounds that restrictions on autonomy must always be examined and justified. Governments of a more social democratic persuasion tend, however, to view the state apparatus as an important vehicle for achieving certain social goals, including those relating to public health. Governments that act in ways that may be seen as limiting individual freedoms (on the grounds that they are endeavouring to protect their citizens from harm) are often referred to as paternalistic and tend to be described (somewhat disparagingly) as 'nanny states'. Ideologies are underpinned by particular values: that is to say, beliefs about those things that have worth or significance for people and which are seen as good and desirable in themselves – such as freedom, social justice and the right to be heard. In contemporary society, the political make-up of most elected governments is complex. Hence, decisions about how to proceed in relation to issues such as public health are often the subject of intense debate. A central aspect of such deliberations is the extent to which individuals can be viewed as free to act given circumstances that may not be of their own choosing (McKee and Raine, 2005).

The value accorded to health in contemporary society is reflected in debates surrounding the 'right' to health articulated in a number of international documents, which place certain obligations on signatory states. In 1948, the *United Nations Universal Declaration of Human Rights* (UDHR) articulated a comprehensive range of rights and freedoms applicable to everyone (www.un.org/en/documents/udhr/). Article 25 specifically referred to the right to a standard of living adequate for health and well-being. While the UDHR identifies general principles of human rights, the *United Nations International Covenant of Economic, Social and Cultural Rights,* effective from 1976, sets out binding commitments in respect of economic, social and cultural rights. Article 12 specifically recognizes the ostensible right of everyone to the 'enjoyment of the highest attainable standard of physical and mental health' (www2.ohchr.org/english/law/cescr.htm). The *Covenant* also sets out rights in relation to a number of the social **determinants** of health. In the UK, *The Human Rights Act* (HRA, 1998) enshrined in law some (but not all) of the international rights to which it was a signatory. The right to health is also enshrined in the WHO's constitution, which states that the enjoyment of the highest attainable standard of health is one of the fundamental rights of every human being (http://apps.who.int/gb/bd/PDF/bd47/EN/constitution-en.pdf).

The efforts of the UN and the WHO in developing international commitments towards the notion of a 'right to health' illustrate how rights are socially constructed – rather than God-given or natural – and reflect particular values. It is noteworthy that the movement to develop an international framework of human rights came in the early post-war period following the revelations of Nazi atrocities during the Second World War. If rights are to mean anything, governments must grant and protect them through their constitutions and various forms of legislation. The corollary to this is that rights adopted by international bodies such as the UN only become effective when they are endorsed and enforced by national governments (Roberts, 2009). A right to health has yet to be enshrined in the HRA (Keen, 2012). Some argue that free market economies are themselves harmful to health equity and challenge the right to rights. As Schrecker *et al.* (2010) point out, human rights are fundamentally egalitarian; therefore there can be no trade-off between the rising wealth of middle classes if poverty persists.

Such reservations notwithstanding, the international human rights framework has the potential to be used as a vehicle for progress on health equality (Schrecker *et al.,* 2010) and, in recent years, some have used the 'language, institutions and procedures of human rights' in their **advocacy** (Reubi, 2011: 625). Advocates in the field of HIV/AIDS as well as tobacco control have used this approach. There have, nonetheless, been a number of criticisms of rights-based advocacy on the grounds that rights are only one aspect of a broader argument about what makes a claim – such as a right to health – valid (Beauchamp and Childress, 2009). Referring specifically to health, Beauchamp and Childress argue that social ideals and principles of obligation relating to group interests and communal values 'are as critical to social morality as rights and none are dispensable' (Beauchamp and Childress, 2009: 355).

The 'right' to health is directly linked to arguments about social justice. From an ethical standpoint, justice implies that 'each person in society ought to receive his [or her] due and that the burdens and benefits of society should be fairly and equitably distributed' (Beauchamp, 1976: 102). If social inequalities in health are viewed as the product of a free market economy then such markets are, by definition, unjust. Accordingly, collective actions are required to mitigate the effects of the socio-economic and political environment. One implication of this argument is that public health action 'should not be narrowly conceived as an instrumental or technical activity … [but rather as] a way of doing justice, a way of asserting the value and priority of all human life' (Beauchamp, 1976: 108). Because people's values vary, however, so too will their ideas on whether particular practices and outcomes are just (Roberts, 2009).

Policies to improve population health and reduce health inequalities raise questions about what degree of intervention might be acceptable to the public. Some actions provoke little public reaction and may even go unnoticed if they are limited in the extent to which they intrude into people's lives. The 1998 UK legislation to limit the size of packs of some analgesics available over-the-counter to reduce suicide **risk** is such an example (Hawton, 2002). Proposals to fluoridate the water in some regions of the UK, however, met with (local) public outcry. Yet adding fluoride to drinking water is a public health measure directed at improving dental health by protecting against tooth decay; not only does it positively affect tooth mineralization it also has anti-bacterial properties (NCB, 2007). Furthermore, because dental health varies by social class in the UK it has the potential to reduce inequalities in dental health among a potentially vulnerable group – children (McGrady *et al.*, 2012). The study of water fluoridation, however, illustrates the tension between balancing benefits against potential harms in a situation in which a whole population is affected and when individuals cannot give their consent or easily 'opt-out'. Water fluoridation thus represents an intervention that effectively eliminates any individual choice and is, therefore, highly intrusive. The benefits that accrue from water fluoridation are also unclear. A systematic review concluded that it was difficult to quantify how much water fluoridation reduced the prevalence of dental caries, which was already at a historically low point in the UK (McDonagh *et al.*, 2000). Consumption of fluoridated water is also not without some harm, of which the most extensively studied has been fluorosis – visible markings on the teeth (McGrady *et al.*, 2012). Drinking fluoridated water has also been associated with bone fractures and some cancers. In circumstances where **evidence** of benefits is weak, uncertainties remain over harms, and alternatives (fluoride toothpaste, for example) are available, the NCB (2007) argues that the state should seek the views of the public in order to provide a mandate for, or against, action such as fluoridation. If this course of action is pursued, the provision of unbiased, accessible information is critical.

Compulsion through law has also been used to prevent and control the spread of some infectious diseases. Here, the main ethical concern is how to reconcile individual consent with **community** benefits (NCB, 2007). In the case of vaccination, high 'herd immunity' (the proportion of people with immunity in a community) leads to large population benefits. Governments vary in the extent to which they have made vaccination programmes mandatory, however. In the USA, for example, children are required to be vaccinated before they enter school (with some exemptions) and in Australia, certain welfare payments have been linked to vaccination compliance. In the UK, vaccination is voluntary but there have been recent calls to make some childhood vaccinations compulsory following outbreaks of measles (Bosley, 2009). Laws have also been passed in some countries that compel individuals to be treated if infected. In New York City, the Department of Health passed a raft of measures in relation to treatment for TB, including directly observed therapy (watching patients take medication) (Bayer, 2008).

In some cases, the main opposition to a legislative compulsion may come from commercial and corporate interests. Once again in New York City, the Department of Health sought to ban the use of artificial transfats in food served in the city's cafés and restaurants (as well as place calorie information on menus) in an attempt to reduce the high rates of heart disease. These measures were enforceable through fines (Mello, 2009). The New York State Restaurant Association sued the Department but a court ruling eventually affirmed the right of the Department to compel restaurants to comply, thereby confirming the responsibilities of third parties – particularly corporations – towards the public and their health. In the UK, this issue has been debated in the context of the development of a 'public health responsibility deal', in which representatives from the food and alcohol industries (and other businesses and organizations) have been invited to work in **'partnership'** with the government in order to promote the public's health (http://responsibilitydeal.dh.gov.uk/). The emphasis has been on businesses making voluntary pledges and committing themselves to self-regulation. This approach has provoked considerable criticism from those within public health, predominantly on the grounds that there is a fundamental conflict of interest between the profit-oriented goals of industry representatives and their supposed interest in promoting the health of the population. Thus, it is unlikely that self-regulation and voluntariness will work in the best interests of public health (House of Lords Science and Technology Select Committee, 2011).

Legislation that seeks to protect individuals from harm by directly restricting their personal behaviour also raises ethical issues. Examples here include the compulsory wearing of car seat belts and motorcycle helmets, gun control and restrictions on the speed of car travel. Recently, Austrian provinces have made it compulsory for children under 16 years old to wear helmets while skiing or snowboarding. These examples effectively eliminate individual choice. Actions of this type, however, are generally justified in public health on the basis of bringing benefits not only to individuals but also others – they represent a 'collective good' in other words. Public acceptability is likely to be higher the more strongly justified the case for action and the less intrusive it is in restricting individual behaviour. The wearing of car seat belts falls into this category. Nonetheless, such actions are often described as paternalistic, in that the state is seen as coercing individuals to lead healthy, responsible lives.

A number of ethical issues are raised by the use of financial disincentives and incentives to influence behaviours. Disincentivizing consumption of alcohol and tobacco by raising prices through the tax system is regularly used by governments. The main ethical concern here is that it may be unfair if the same tax is applied to all because of differences in disposable income and health behaviours (NCB, 2007). According to Bayer (2008), however, excise taxes are always regressive, burdening the consumption options of the poor more than the well-off. Such levies tend to generate inequality rather than bring about fairness because those on better incomes can absorb increases more easily. Particular behaviours such as cycling to work have been incentivized by providing tax-breaks for the purchase of a bike. This, alongside traffic congestion charging in some cities, can encourage active travel. These examples are perhaps less controversial as they constitute enabling strategies and are, by degrees, less coercive.

In addition to scrutinizing the role of the state, there are several issues to note related to the everyday work of public health practitioners with obligations as well as power relating to their duty of care for the well-being of individuals and communities (Mann, 1997; Thomas *et al.*, 2002). There is a duty, for example, to avoid stigmatization and victim-blaming (Bayer, 2008). This might also entail ensuring that communities are provided with information about local issues and extend to advocating on their behalf. According to this view, public health professionals and practitioners have obligations towards improving social and community conditions.

Conclusion

Ethical issues have surfaced throughout the history of public health. Concerned as it is with promoting and protecting the health of populations through collective actions, public health has had a traditional concern with balancing personal liberties alongside promoting social goods. In recent years, however, there has been something of a shift towards a broader commitment to health for all and narrowing social inequalities in health. This commitment has been articulated explicitly in terms of global equity, fairness and social justice. Paralleling this shift has been an expansion of neo-liberal ideology among many governments as well as a number of global institutions. Justice-based obligations relating to improving the conditions of everyday life for those most disadvantaged are unlikely to hold sway when the dominant ideology emphasizes personal freedoms and choices. Nonetheless, public health ethics provides a framework for evaluating these different arguments and actions.

EVALUATION

Context

Efforts to gauge the impact of policies, programmes and services – in general terms, interventions – have become relatively commonplace in most, if not all, **policy** arenas. How deeply embedded an evaluation culture is, however, varies by country and sector. The USA, for example, established a public system for generating and disseminating public health evaluation **evidence** in the 1960s, through the US Centre for Disease Control Task Force on Community Preventive Services. In the UK, the evaluation culture expanded throughout the Labour government's period of office (1997–2010), during which time considerable resources were committed to national and local evaluation studies of major government initiatives, ostensibly to find out 'what works'. An aspect of this expansion was the establishment in 1999 of the National Institute for Health and Clinical Excellence (NICE) – comparable in some ways to the US system referred to above (Kelly *et al.*, 2010). The role of NICE was to advise the UK government on how to maximize population **health** using the best available evidence and given specified resources. In the first instance, NICE focused on health care in general and therapeutic drugs in particular. Its role widened in 2005 to include advice relating to **health promotion** and disease **prevention**.

The expansion of evaluation has generated a considerable body of evidence in the form of peer-reviewed articles, formal published reports, informal documents (grey literature), as well as various types of 'evidence synthesis' (such as systematic reviews and meta-analyses). Nonetheless, policymakers lament the continuing lack of robust evidence regarding 'what works' in public health. Thus, in the short to medium term at least, evaluation in its various forms appears here to stay. Nevertheless, despite the rhetoric of evidence driving policy decisions in public health, the reality may be somewhat different. Being alert to these issues can offer some insight into how politics shapes the conduct and uses of evaluation.

Defining evaluation

In public health, evaluation is concerned with trying to assess change at the population or sub-group level rather than at the individual level. Many approaches to evaluation are based on a quantitative scientific paradigm, often drawing substantively on ideas relating to experimental study designs as well as **epidemiology** more generally. These scientific ideas are reflected in Porta's definition of evaluation as 'a process that attempts to determine as systematically and objectively as possible the relevance, effectiveness and impact of activities in the light of their objectives' (Porta, 2008: 86). This definition highlights the conventional emphasis in evaluation on judging the impact of interventions in relation to their goals – that is, whether they achieved what they set out to achieve. The concept of 'effectiveness' captures this idea specifically insofar as it refers to 'the extent to which a specific intervention ... when deployed in the field in the usual circumstances, does what it is intended to do for a specified population' (Porta, 2008: 76). Effectiveness is differentiated from the term 'efficacy', which is used to refer to an assessment of effectiveness under ideal conditions, typically assessed through an RCT (Porta, 2008). Effectiveness and efficacy both centre on the issue of **causality** or attribution, in that they seek to link the intervention to the attainment of certain outcomes. Thus, 'what works' is conceptualized in terms of the degree to which specified outcomes have been achieved.

The assessment of impact has conventionally involved the use of RCTs. This methodological approach has been applied extensively in public health to assess the value of therapeutic drug use (such as aspirin and anti-hypertensive drugs for the prevention of cardiovascular disease), **screening** programmes (for breast and colon cancer, for example), and other preventive interventions such as **community**-based smoking cessation programmes. However, evaluation of more complex, multifaceted public health programmes has stimulated considerable debate about the extent to which the RCT in particular, as well as the scientific methodological paradigm in general, can yield valid and reliable evidence of success. Perhaps more fundamentally, criticism has been directed at the scientifically informed definitions of evaluation (such as that of Porta cited above) that imply that it is possible to obtain a certain degree of consensus about the goals of an intervention as well as the appropriate way to conduct evaluation.

These debates have emerged within the field of health promotion in particular, where a social model of health and well-being, (underpinned by values such as participation and equity), is advocated. Definitions of evaluation in this field tend to focus on programmes or projects, which are viewed as dynamic entities, comprising activities and services put together to address a problem in a given context with a specific population (Rootman *et al.*, 2001). This means viewing programmes as a process of social change rather than a one-off 'dose' or 'treatment' (Springett, 2001) and, furthermore, one which may have unplanned, as well as planned outcomes. In this vein, Rootman *et al.* (2001: 26) define evaluation as 'the systematic examination and assessment of features of a programme or other intervention in order to produce knowledge that different stakeholders can use for a variety of purposes.' In shifting the emphasis away from effectiveness, evaluation approaches based on this definition allow issues of acceptability and equity to be explored. These differing definitions illustrate a spectrum of approaches to evaluation, from those relatively narrowly conceptualized and based on the assessment of pre-determined goals through to more open-ended models that are receptive to the possibility of unplanned and unintended consequences (Green and South, 2006).

Evaluation is often linked to the concept of 'monitoring', which typically involves the systematic collection of routine data to keep track of organizational and programme activities. In this way, monitoring is often used to support evaluation. However, the terms differ in their meaning: monitoring is descriptive, whereas evaluation, as the term implies, involves judgement. The rise in both evaluation and monitoring activities reflects a trend towards greater accountability and performance management in the public sector in many countries. The use of indicators as 'targets' has, however, had a number of unintended consequences, not least of which has been the emergence of the phenomenon of 'gaming'. Given the pressure to meet targets, strategies are employed that ensure they can be reported as having been met (Hood, 2006). In other words, the process of monitoring and evaluating a system usually disturbs it in some way (Allen *et al.*, 2001). The use of targets to monitor the English health **inequalities** strategy has been shown to have influenced General Practitioners' (GPs) behaviours towards pharmacological interventions in order to be able to demonstrate progress over a relatively short timescale (Blackman *et al.*, 2009). The conclusion from this and other research is that if indicators become targets they cease to be good measures – Strathern's re-statement of Goodhart's Law (Elton, 2004).

The significance of evaluation for public health

It has become commonplace in public health to use the term 'wicked issues' to refer to entrenched problems that require complex multilevel interventions involving many different agencies and activities (Petticrew *et al.*, 2009). In a number of countries, area-based initiatives have been introduced in areas of disadvantage to address such issues. HAZs, Sure Start, New Deal for Communities and healthy living centres, for example, were introduced during the late 1990s and early 2000s in England as key dimensions of the Labour government's health strategy to improve health alongside narrowing health inequalities. These types of interventions were complex in character, not simply in organizational terms but rather because they sought to bring about change at a number of levels – individual, family, systems of provision, **community**, area, and so on – as well as in relation to a variety of social and behavioural outcomes (Barnes *et al.*, 2003).

The considerable methodological challenges these complex, multilevel community-based interventions raise for evaluators have been debated at length. Some consensus has emerged that an exclusive focus on RCTs is inappropriate, not just on ethical, methodological or practical grounds but also, more fundamentally, in terms of internal attribution. Referring to these initiatives as 'programmes' rather than 'interventions' signals their multifaceted and dynamic character, as well as how they are mediated through human interactions over time. Consequently, the diversity of elements, the complexity with which they relate to one another as well as the multi-layered context within which they are embedded are viewed as generating multiple pathways through which changes might occur. For evaluators, this poses difficulties in discerning how change is mediated and which characteristics of a programme are influential. A 'theory of change' perspective (Connell and Kubisch, 1998; Weiss, 1995) and 'realist evaluation' (Pawson and Tilley, 1997) have emerged as a response to these challenges. Although different in a number of ways, both seek to understand *how* complex interventions produce outcomes over time – sometimes referred to as the programme logic – by studying the links between programme elements, outcomes and contexts (Connell and Kubisch, 1998). The theory of change 'unpacks' the intervention – often viewed as a black box (Pawson and Sridharan, 2010) – to bring to the surface and articulate a causal explanation (a theory) for how the intervention, delivered in a particular context to a specific group of people, will bring about change. Realist evaluators emphasize that many such 'theories' emerge, with the evaluator selecting a subset that appears to be most promising. The evaluation then focuses on testing these theories out in various ways, the ultimate aim of which is to identify possible causal pathways, which may, by degrees, be transferable to other situations (Blamey and Mackenzie, 2007). Both realist and theories of change approaches seek to understand social processes – referred to as generative mechanisms in realist evaluation – that give rise to varying outcomes, depending on people's circumstances.

In relation to their application to complex community programmes, both theories of change and realist evaluation have been subjected to criticism on a number of levels. The former is viewed as too simplistic and the latter too linear, while both approaches are criticized for tending to view the programmes as separate from, rather than a part of, the context (Barnes *et al.*, 2003). Some also view such approaches as descriptive rather than explanatory and therefore relatively silent on 'what works' in relation to the achievement of outcomes. Although RCTs have continued to occupy a pre-eminent place in evaluation, alternative approaches such as theories of change have been increasingly embraced by researchers in recent years. Process evaluation (focusing on how programmes are delivered) has been incorporated into RCTs to explore questions relating to implementation. Focussing on the process has the potential to generate a better understanding of how programmes built on a sound theory may or may not achieve their desired outcomes because of difficulties inherent in implementing complex programmes. Oakley *et al.* (2006) integrated process evaluation into an RCT to explore the effectiveness of peer-delivered sex **education** relative to teacher-delivered sessions. They concluded that integrating process and outcome data 'revealed the circumstances in which peer led sex education was most effective' adding that 'the peer led approach is not a straightforward answer to the problem of school disengagement' (Oakley *et al.*, 2006: 414). The latest guidance on evaluation published by the UK Medical Research Council emphasizes the importance of developing a programme theory of change at the development stage of an intervention, to be used in subsequent evaluation, as well as incorporating a process evaluation element (Craig *et al.*, 2008), a trend seen in some other countries (Rogers *et al.*, 2000).

A particularly significant development within the field of public health has been the use of economic evaluation. The aim of this approach is to systematically 'identify, measure and compare the costs and outcomes of alternative interventions' (Sefton *et al.*, 2002: 7). Economic evaluation has been used extensively in **medicine**, health care and social welfare to provide an ostensibly rational and transparent basis for making the best use of limited resources. The concept of efficiency is used to refer to the relationship between the outcomes and costs: an efficient allocation of resources maximizes the benefits of an intervention for a given cost (Sefton *et al.*, 2002). Cost-effectiveness analysis (CEA) is a particular type of economic evaluation that has been used in the health field. Cost utility analysis (CUA) is a particular type of CEA used by NICE to generate a cost per quality adjusted life year (QALY). The QALY is a widely used measure of 'utility' or well-being and is used to measure health improvement based on the duration of life and the health-related quality of life (Rawlins and Culyer, 2004). CUA has also been used in the public health field. Such economic approaches have shown that public health interventions can be cost-saving, as in the case of universal influenza immunization programmes (Kelly, 2012). Early childhood interventions, such as Sure Start, have also been shown to possess the potential to generate greater savings than investments made in later life (Meadows, 2011). Reducing the availability of alcohol and banning alcohol advertising are highly cost-effective strategies in influencing consumption and its negative consequences (Anderson *et al.*, 2009). These kinds of investments may not yield returns for many years, however.

A major criticism of economic evaluation is that it gives primacy to efficiency over equity in decision making. This continues to be a source of some debate in the public health field where 'levelling up' of those in the poorest health is advocated if health inequalities are to be reduced (Whitehead, 1992). In policy terms the goals of equity and those of efficiency are difficult to reconcile: policies tend to improve fairness while decreasing efficiency or improve efficiency while increasing health inequalities (Sassi *et al.*, 2001). Efficiency matters, however, because resources are scarce and those used in one way cannot be used elsewhere.

Although there is often pressure to evaluate, the cost of evaluation may itself be prohibitive. 'Natural experiments' can sometimes offer a relatively low-cost alternative. They allow the impact of differences in exposure on outcomes to be analysed at a population level with the aim of making causal inferences (Craig *et al.*, 2011). Twin, adoption and migration studies are classic examples of natural experiments. In the public health field, natural experiments include a variety of studies that have focused on legislative and other policy changes directly and indirectly related to health. Studies in England (see, for example, Sims *et al.*, 2010) and Scotland (see Pell *et al.*, 2008) have explored the impact of the legislative ban on smoking in public places on hospitalization for acute coronary events, for example. Natural experiments have also been used extensively to study the impact of price on alcohol consumption (Anderson, *et al.*, 2009). These studies have shown that increasing the price of alcohol is a highly cost-effective strategy. A study in Finland found that a 33 per cent cut in tax in 2004 was followed by an increase in alcohol consumption and an increase in alcohol-related mortality in men and women within two years (Ludbrook, 2009). Similar findings have been found in other countries, and have provided the evidence-base for calls to introduce a minimum price per unit of alcohol. A before-and-after approach has also been used to study the impact on participation levels in physical activity of holding the Olympic Games. A systematic review of these studies concluded that there was little evidence to support claims for an 'Olympic effect' (Mahtani *et al.*, 2013). Although not without their problems, natural experiments provide opportunities for scientific evaluation in circumstances where exposed and unexposed population groups can be compared using sufficiently large samples to detect outcomes of interest, and accurate data from routinely collected sources on exposure, outcomes and possible confounding variables are available (Craig *et al.*, 2011).

More specialized forms of evaluation have also developed in recent years. Health impact assessment (HIA) for example, is an approach specifically designed to estimate 'the effects of a specified action on the health of a defined population' (Scott-Samuel, 1998: 704) and draws on approaches used in environmental impact assessment. HIA also seeks to understand the impact in terms of its distribution within the population to see who might be affected most and least. One of the first HIAs to be carried out involved the European Union's Common Agricultural Policy (Dahlgren *et al.*, 1996). Since then the methodology has been applied to a wide range of policies such as those relating to transport, food production, air quality, urban development and mental health. Advocated by the WHO, it has been used extensively in Europe following regulatory requirements (Fehr *et al.*, 2012). It is a particularly relevant decision-making tool in public health because it seeks to predict the consequences of various plans and proposals and thus has the potential to avoid various harms.

Notwithstanding the array of methodologies, evidence from evaluation is often seen as insufficiently robust for decision-making. While the scientific research community continues to view RCTs as the 'gold standard' for making causal inferences, in policy circles 'stories' often exert a powerful influence on policymakers (Roberts *et al.*, 2012). Stories can provide a straightforward and easily understood example of impact with little of the complexity, uncertainty or caveats that tend to accompany scientific evidence. No matter how strong the evidence from RCTs, it may still be rejected, overlooked, or suppressed if it does not align with either planned interventions or the dominant political view (Stevens, 2011: 237). The debate relating to the minimum pricing of alcohol illustrates how evidence arising from evaluation is shaped in various ways for political purposes.

Conclusion

Although evaluation has become characterized by methodological pluralism in recent years, debate about various approaches is likely to continue. Pressure to produce evidence of 'what works' (and perhaps 'how' it works), will expand the increasingly complex empirical evidence-base. However, the extent to which new evidence is required to inform policy makers about how to address most of the **global health** issues is debatable. Ultimately, political will to act on the available evidence is required if health, particularly among those most disadvantaged, is to be improved.

EVIDENCE

Context

The notion of using the 'best available evidence' as a basis for decision-making emerged in the medical and **health** care fields during the 1970s, alongside growing concerns about the quality of care and the effectiveness of interventions (Grol and Wensing, 2004). Since then, the idea of evidence-based **policy** and practice has permeated many other fields including social welfare, criminal justice, **education**, sport development and public health. The rhetoric of evidence-based policy and practice signals a shift away from a reliance on everyday observation and experience towards **evaluation** and the use of 'objective' and 'robust' empirical research data. Increasingly, however, this rhetoric has become interwoven with notions of cost and 'value for money'. This has led some observers to conclude that an emphasis on evidence really reflects a continuing political desire to ration resources, as well as regulate the professions through requiring greater transparency and accountability in decision-making (Rycroft Malone, 2006). As a consequence, debates surrounding the generation and use of evidence tend to be politically charged, particularly in public health, and require careful scrutiny.

Defining evidence

Definitions of evidence within public health are sparse. The main academic field within which debates about the meaning of evidence have taken place has been philosophy. In a court of law, however, evidence tends to be defined in terms of 'facts' – observations, communications, materials and so on – believed to be pertinent to a case. Judicial systems use processes of argumentation involving the weighing-up of accumulated evidence in order to arrive at judgements. A similar process is used in the field of evidence-based policy and practice. Evidence-based **medicine**, for example, is defined as 'the conscientious, explicit and judicious use of current best evidence in making decisions about the care of individual patients' (Sackett *et al.*, 1996: 71). Evidence does not, in other words, 'speak for itself' but requires intelligent interpretation (Roberts, 2009). The process of weighing-up and interpreting evidence is made complex because of disagreement about what counts as evidence, a matter which tends to vary across disciplinary and professional fields. In **epidemiology**, for example, Porta defines evidence as 'scientific knowledge' (2008: 87). This implies that evidence – data, the researcher's interpretations and conclusions – produced through the scientific method is necessarily credible. It also implies that scientific evidence has an 'intrinsic authority', particularly when supported by statistics that lend an 'appearance of certainty and legitimacy that seems beyond challenge' (Neylan, 2008: 17).

Porta's definition conflates evidence with scientific knowledge. Philosophers, however, tend to view evidence as preceding knowledge. According to this view, 'knowledge requires justification, and justification is a matter of having sufficient evidence for one's beliefs' (Joyce, 2004: 296). The corollary to this is that evidence is judged according to its ability to explain phenomena. This implies that evidence is more adequately conceptualized as a multifaceted and pliable concept, its status being provisional as well as a matter of degree. Although it has become commonplace to talk in terms of the *best* evidence, Dopson (2006) argues that there is no such thing. This in turn opens up possibilities for different forms of evidence to be drawn on in the development of knowledge.

The significance of evidence for public health

Until relatively recently, the scientific view of evidence has been the predominant influence on evidence-based public health. Killoran (2010: 459) argues, however, that the goals of public health are different from those of medicine and health care, as reflected in the following definition of evidence-based public health: 'the process involved in providing the best available evidence to influence decisions about the effectiveness of policies and interventions aimed at improving health and reducing inequalities'. Governments in many countries have placed an increasing emphasis on generating evidence of the effectiveness and cost-effectiveness of public health interventions through evaluation as well as using evidence to inform policy and professional practice.

The issue of *quality* of evidence – including what counts as evidence – has become a preoccupation in evidence-based thinking in the public health field. The notion of a hierarchy of evidence provides a tool for grading different forms of evidence (relating specifically to cause and effect relationships) on the basis of (largely epidemiological) study designs. Some scientific consensus has emerged about the relative strengths of different types of studies designed to test the effectiveness of interventions. Rankings reflect this consensus in as much as those study designs judged to be better able to control various forms of bias and confounding that threaten a study's internal validity are placed at the top of the hierarchy. Systematic reviews and meta-analyses, and RCTs are, therefore, located at the top of the hierarchy, followed by various forms of observational studies, with expert opinion and lay knowledge at the bottom (Greenhalgh, 2010).

Decisions are rarely made on the basis of evidence from a single study, no matter how strong the study design. Hence processes for synthesizing research findings have been developed. Systematic review is a standardized method that involves identifying, selecting and critically appraising all published studies on a specified topic or question. The end product – the systematic review itself – presents a synthesis of the current state of knowledge about a subject. If the review is based on results from RCTs, a meta-analysis is included, combining results from all the studies that have been located and reviewed. The end result is the derivation of a pooled statistic, viewed as producing 'unbiased conclusions if performed appropriately' (Leandro, 2005: 2). Of course, systematic reviews and meta-analyses can only be as sound as the studies on which they are based, hence the use of strict inclusion criteria relating to study quality. Studies that are under-powered (having insufficiently large samples) normally would be excluded. Because systematic reviews often combine a large number of individual RCTs they sit at the top of the hierarchy. Systematic reviews, however, may suffer from publications bias, that is to say, the tendency for positive (rather than negative) results of effect to be published.

Cochrane (1984) took the view that the RCT should be the starting point for generating evidence of effectiveness because of its potential to reduce bias. The use of RCTs in evidence-based public health is, however, problematic for a number of pragmatic, financial and ethical reasons. There are also conceptual and theoretical issues to consider. Can the social world – the populations and communities whose health is the focus of improvement – be meaningfully studied using an RCT or does this design reduce the complex, dynamic and interconnected nature of social life to the extent where it ceases to reflect the reality of people's everyday lives? Kelly argues that a simple application of the hierarchy of evidence would be inappropriate for assessing public health evidence because:

> Public health actions frequently consist of long causal chains from the intervention and outcome, involving individual behaviour in complex social **settings**. In these long causal chains multi-factorial processes are at work with many intervening variables exercising a moderating or mediating effect.
>
> (Kelly, 2012: 111)

This causal complexity poses a particular problem for public health programmes and projects directed at the wider **determinants** of health and reducing health **inequalities**. Not only might there be limited evidence available to inform the development of projects with specific communities and goals in mind, the kind of evidence required may well differ from that traditionally used in public health (Dunne *et al.*, 2012). In this regard, appraising evidence in terms of its *local* relevance is paramount in **health promotion** and public health, conflicting with the claim of generalizability that is the hallmark of scientific evidence (Potvin *et al.*, 2011).

Several developments have sought to increase policymakers' and practitioners' access to evidence. In the UK, NICE, which expanded its role to include public health in 2005, has produced evidence appraisals of the effectiveness and cost-effectiveness of predominantly surgical procedures, medical devices and drugs. One of the main uses to which systematic reviews have been put is the development of guidelines. Kelly and Moore (2012) describe a guideline as an evidence-based protocol that provides optimal approaches to a particular issue. NICE, for example, produces national guidelines to standardize practice on the basis of evidence. A further development in the early 1990s was the Cochrane Collaboration, an international network of independent, not-for-profit organizations, which prepares, disseminates and promotes the use of evidence about health care and public health interventions (www.cochrane.org). The *Cochrane Database of Systematic Reviews* contains systematic assessments of evidence of the effects of interventions, prepared and updated by collaborating authors working in a Cochrane Collaborative Review Group. In a similar vein, the Campbell Collaboration (C2) was established in 2000 to prepare and disseminate systematic reviews in education, crime and justice and social welfare (www.campbellcollaboration.org).

Some have argued for an expanded approach to evidence to include social science research and evaluation methods as well as expert opinion and lay knowledge (Exworthy, 2011; Popay and Williams, 1998; Rychetnik *et al.*, 2004). These views reflect a growing emphasis on the inclusion of qualitative research findings as evidence. Berridge (2010) argues that historical evidence can also be used to inform policy, and act as a counter to the 'folk history' that is often used in justifying policy decisions. Analysing historical developments (what might be termed a retrospective natural experiment) has the potential to lead to a better understanding of contemporary phenomena without the necessity of having to generate new evidence. The potential value of historical analyses may be difficult to realize in public health, however, for a variety of reasons, not least of which is the dominance of the scientific paradigm. Yet there are some signs of a shift in thinking regarding the potential value of other forms of evidence. Synthesis of qualitative studies has emerged as a new methodology, for example. This might reflect, at least in part, policymakers' interests in learning from the experiences of service users (Ring *et al.*, 2011). The Cochrane Collaboration Qualitative and Implementation Methods Group focuses on methods and processes for the synthesis of qualitative research as well as how qualitative research might be integrated with evidence from systematic reviews of effects. Appraising the quality of qualitative research continues to be a matter of some debate, however, making it difficult to decide what studies to include. Narrative reviews – an increasingly common feature of many health-related journals – are systematic overviews of topics that draw on qualitative, quantitative and theoretical studies. They might also include 'grey literature', a type of literature that has become more common in recent years. The Luxembourg definition of grey literature has found its way into the public health field in terms of 'that which is produced on all levels of governmental, academics, business and industry in print and electronic formats, but which is not controlled by commercial publishers' (Hopewell *et al.*, 2008: 2). This includes research reports, conference abstracts, personal correspondence and so on. While potentially useful, these forms of evidence also raise questions about how to judge their quality. Nevertheless, Korjonen and Ford (2013) argue that grey literature constitutes an important source of evidence for public health practitioners.

Increasingly, the focus of research attention has shifted towards understanding how policymakers and practitioners use evidence – what has been called, the knowledge transfer, translation or utilization process. However, the path from evidence to policy or practice is rarely linear or straightforward. On the basis of their review of research in a range of policy areas, Nutley *et al.*, (2002: i) concluded thus: '[the view that] evidence is created by experts and drawn on as necessary by policy makers and practitioners – fail as either accurate descriptions or effective prescriptions'. Policy-making is an inherently political process shaped by ideological and economic factors. The public health field is replete with examples of how governments have tended to re-negotiate their relationship with scientific evidence depending on their perception of, for example, the prevailing views of the public. In the UK, the government's drug policy was criticized by its own adviser for ignoring scientific evidence and overestimating the dangers of ecstasy (Humphreys and Piot, 2012). The governments of most countries ignored the wealth of evidence linking cigarette smoking with lung cancer and other diseases over several decades prior to the introduction of the legislation banning smoking in public places. In the USA, the Obama administration lifted the ban on federal funding for needle exchange schemes to prevent HIV transmission, citing scientific evidence as its justification for action (Humphreys and Piot, 2012). Governments have also introduced policies that might be viewed as politically expedient rather than evidence-based. In the UK, Changing Childbirth involved a fundamental change in the provision of maternity care, a national policy for which there was no evidence (Black, 2001). Policy decisions that are taken and implemented in the absence of evidence might amount to experimentation (Katikireddi *et al.*, 2011). In the USA, the Bush administration set an ozone standard irrespective of the scientific evidence (Grifo *et al.*, 2012). In the UK, in spite of the extensive evidence-base on social inequalities in health there is little evidence that this has influenced policies to reduce such inequalities (Orton *et al.*, 2011; Petticrew *et al.*, 2009). Political concerns about the sedentariness of children and young people are expressed despite the growth in sport and physical activity participation in recent years (Coalter, 2013: 3). These examples illustrate how policymakers use evidence selectively and with particular (political) purposes in mind.

In the medical field, direct attempts by governments to change health professionals' practice using evidence-based clinical guidelines – so-called top-down approaches – have been relatively unsuccessful. Research has shown that health professionals (including doctors and others with a strong scientific training), give greater weight to personal experience or eminent colleagues' opinions rather than the 'best scientific evidence' (Dopson, 2005). This leads Dopson to conclude that it is 'notoriously difficult to implement research evidence in the face of strong professional views and complex organizational contexts' (Dopson, 2006: 85). Furthermore, because there are degrees of uncertainty attached to health-related evidence, practitioners have the 'space' within which to reach their preferred view. In discussing the value of mammography **screening**, Parascandola (2003) argues that in a climate of uncertainty scientists' values influence their interpretations of evidence. The contested character of evidence means that it can be interpreted, re-interpreted, rejected, used selectively and challenged. Evidence utilization is therefore better viewed as a dynamic and political process, in which science and values are often interwoven. The shift in terminology towards 'evidence-informed' or 'evidence-enhanced' rather than 'evidence-based' is perhaps more congruent with the everyday reality of policy-making and practice. Overall, using evidence on its own as a basis for shifting prevailing views is unlikely to be successful.

Conclusion

Finding, generating, understanding and using evidence have become core dimensions of public health policy and practice and pose considerable challenges, not least of which is the time and skills necessary to engage with these processes. Increased access to information via the Internet has, in a number of ways, contributed to the complexity of these processes. Sifting and selecting that which might be of most relevance and value to any particular public health issue can become overwhelming. Yet in core areas, there remains a dearth of good quality, diverse studies to inform public health action, particularly that which is pertinent at a local level.

GLOBAL HEALTH AND GLOBALIZATION

Context

Taking a global perspective on **health** reveals complex and shifting patterns of disease worldwide, alongside stark social **inequalities** in health. In many of the poorest countries, health problems are deeply entrenched despite decades of foreign aid and action through the MDGs on hunger, disease, illiteracy, environmental degradation and discrimination against women. Infectious and chronic degenerative diseases increasingly co-exist in all countries, with the latter making an increasing contribution to mortality in low- and middle-income countries, primarily through increases in CVD (Magnusson, 2009). All countries remain vulnerable to the threat of pandemics from, for example, influenza. Given this context, a system of global collaboration and authoritative leadership has been called for since the 'global health crisis ... is not primarily one of disease but of governance' (Kickbusch and Seck, 2007: 162). Yet, the development of a global infrastructure remains elusive. Increasingly national governments have assimilated health issues into their security, foreign and development policies (see, for example, DH, 2011; Norwegian Ministry of Foreign Affairs, 2012) perhaps signalling a retreat to a 'fortress' mentality in which countries seek to protect themselves without due regard to their interconnectedness with the rest of the world (Collin and Lee, 2007). Integrating a global perspective into public health has become increasingly important since it has the potential to shed light on how and why health problems endure.

Defining global health and globalization

In the public health field, there has been a notable shift in language in recent years from 'international health' to 'global health' (Brown *et al.*, 2006). Yet it is only in the last few years that there has been any systematic consideration of the distinct conceptual value of the term 'global health'. International health (and the earlier term 'hygiene and tropical **medicine**') was (and still is) used to refer to health work in developing countries (Koplan *et al.*, 2009) and was (and still is) often associated with so-called 'foreign aid'. 'International' in this context tends to indicate a one-directional process, aid flowing from richer to poorer countries through agreed protocols to assist the latter in coping with their own health and development problems. The sociological concept 'globalization' refers to 'the spread of interdependencies between countries' (Roberts, 2009: 112). 'Global health' thus suggests a more complex set of connections (interdependencies) that transcend nation states. These connections – in relation to trade and the movement of goods and people, for example – are not new. Globalization is, however, generally thought to have accelerated and intensified during the twentieth century insofar as global connectedness has become multidirectional, multifaceted, dynamic and complex, such that it has become difficult for anyone to fully comprehend or control the global world. In effect, globalization exposes all societies and economies to a world system (Schrecker *et al.*, 2008) and, as the recent global financial crisis illustrates, what happens in one country has significant implications for other countries, often rapidly so.

Most definitions of global health, however, have not been underpinned by an appreciation of globalization. They tend to either conflate global health with public health (Fried *et al.*, 2010) or offer a broad descriptive definition that refers to geographical reach, level of co-operation, range of disciplines and values such as equity (Koplan *et al.*, 2009). The advantage of framing 'global health' with reference to globalization is that it directs attention to the mechanisms that generate global health problems – the global **determinants of health** – as well as shedding light on the various possibilities for their resolution.

The significance of global health and globalization for public health

Because it involves interdependencies that have economic, political, human and cultural dimensions, globalization has considerable significance for understanding health. Deepening interdependencies between low- and high-income countries have resulted from trade liberalization (particularly through deregulation), which has increased the complexity of public health problems for poorer countries (Blouin *et al.*, 2009; Walt, 1998). Trade liberalization has enabled tobacco companies, for example, to expand their global market into low- and middle-income countries, where an estimated 82 per cent of the world's smokers reside (Collin and Lee, 2007). Of the six million smoking-related deaths in 2011, 80 per cent were in low- and middle-income countries (Erikson *et al.*, 2012). The USA (the fourth largest tobacco producer) threatened countries such as South Korea and Thailand with retaliatory trade sanctions if they did not open up their economies to competition (Collin and Lee, 2007). This example illustrates how trade agreements can undermine national autonomy in relation to public **policy** (Pollock and Price, 2003). Following the ratification of the WHO Framework Convention on Tobacco Control (FCTC) (the first global public health treaty negotiated by the WHO, the objective of which is to reduce global tobacco consumption), plans to develop land that had been used for tobacco farming for crops such as bamboo were met with resistance among Asian and African farmers. Given that tobacco generates considerable revenue for governments, unless there is political resolve to support alternative land usage developments (even where these are profitable) it seems likely that little will change (Kirby, 2012).

Globalization has implications for nation states, increasing the pressure on them and other global policy actors – such as the UN, the IMF and the G20 – to co-operate (Buse *et al.*, 2005; Gostin and Mok, 2009). There is, however, no global governance structure to lead and facilitate collaboration. In this regard, the WHO, as a specialist agency of the UN, has occupied an ambiguous and at times controversial position in the last decade or more. It is perhaps the only organization that has the necessary authority to lead a global alliance (Kickbusch and Seck, 2007). Two recent developments suggest this might be the case. First, the WHO was responsible for developing a set of 'global rules' in the form of the International Health Regulations 2005 (IHR). The IHR is an international legal instrument that requires the 194 member states to report public health events in an effort to strengthen global public health security. It also requires countries to improve their public health surveillance and response systems (www.who.int/ihr/en/). Second is the FCTC (discussed above), which came into force in 2005. Unlike the IHR, however, the FCTC has no binding obligations on countries. Nonetheless, the FCTC has been a catalyst for mobilizing support from member states and other international organizations such as the World Bank, because it linked tobacco control to other policy arenas such as human rights (Collin and Lee, 2007).

Within the international public health field (including a number of non-governmental organizations such as Oxfam) there has been extensive criticism of a number of global institutions such as the World Bank, the IMF and the G20, not only on the grounds that they work to protect the interests of high-income countries but also because they advocate market solutions that neglect matters of social justice. The WHO has also become embroiled in debates about its neutrality and its (in)ability, for example, to advocate social equity (Lee, 2010). There are new sites of resistance, however, that are confronting powerful vested interests. Global political ideologies, such as the anti-globalization movement, have presented themselves as an alternative to market globalism (Steger and Wilson, 2012). This social movement has a value-base that aligns with those who argue for health as an international human right and that health inequalities are preventable, unfair and unjust. On this view, developments in human rights law and practice could be a vehicle for improving institutional and state accountability to communities (Gostin *et al.*, 2011). Other civil society movements have also emerged such as CorpWatch (www.corpwatch.org/index.php), which has challenged transnational corporations in relation to their human rights and social justice practices. CorpWatch exposed the poor working conditions in Nike factories in Vietnam, forcing them to change some of their corporate policies. The People's Health Movement set up 'WHO Watch' to mobilize people to critique the work of the WHO. The recent proposal by the current Director General of the WHO to extend the inclusion of the private sector in the financing and governance of the WHO (Colvin, 2011) drew criticism from Medicus Mundi International (a network of private not-for-profit organizations). Vigilance towards the WHO, it appears, is necessary if the best interests of low-income countries are to be protected. Given that sufficient knowledge exists to prevent most of the enduring health problems in low-income countries, the remaining struggle centres on values and ideas (Lee, 2010). The same struggle is likely to limit the extent to which the recommendations in the report from the CSDH (2008) are implemented.

Global health policy is further complicated by the entry of new independent and powerful – symbolically and economically – actors, such as the Bill and Melinda Gates Foundation (Ollila, 2005). The Foundation distributed 1,094 grants totalling $8.95 billion dollars between 1998 and 2007 (McCoy *et al.*, 2009). Not only does the distribution of grants shape global health priorities, the Foundation also proactively shapes policy through its representation on the governing structures of many global health **partnerships**. The Foundation's involvement in the field of malaria control has drawn criticism from the WHO on the grounds that it was crowding out some scientists' views. There has also been criticism concerning the Foundation's emphasis on new technologies and the neglect of issues such as maternal health. These developments are problematic not solely because they have limited transparency and accountability but because they tend to fragment complex problems into specific 'downstream' health issues, treating the symptoms rather than the root causes.

A particularly pertinent issue in many low- and middle-income countries has been access to an adequate system of **primary health care** (Samb *et al.*, 2010). An especially controversial aspect of aid programme support has been the widespread adoption of user fees for health care services – payment at the point of service for drugs, diagnostic investigations, consultation fees, for example – which rarely benefit the poor, including pregnant women, because they prevent them accessing care when they need it (Meessen *et al.*, 2011). Equally problematic is delayed and partial access. Drug resistance can be the outcome if people can only afford part of a drug treatment, particularly when drugs are over-prescribed (Whitehead *et al.*, 2001). Given the revenue generated through user fees their abandonment is unlikely. Some countries, however, have sought to mitigate their effects for the poor and vulnerable (Bigdeli and Ir, 2010). A related issue is the capacity and capability of the workforce given the extensive migration of qualified clinicians from low- to high-income countries in recent years, with countries such as the UK eager to meet their own skills shortages (Collin and Lee, 2007).

Conclusion

If health is to be improved and inequalities narrowed, strong global leadership is required. The WHO has been identified in some quarters as fulfilling this role (Kickbusch *et al.*, 2007). Norway, for example, has stated that it will seek to support WHO as a leading normative organization for promoting global health (Norwegian Ministry of Foreign Affairs, 2011: 23) within the context of a reformed UN system. Others argue that the WHO's role needs redefinition and the UN should lead a global health panel (Mackey and Liang, 2013). But the UN has also been criticized as supporting market mechanisms that have proved harmful to the health of some of the poorest nations. Whether or not the WHO or the UN can lead with authority, credibility and diplomacy in this crowded and complex policy arena remains to be seen. The best that may be possible is the assemblage of a loose collection of temporary alliances emerging out of some mutual recognition of self-interest. New global health players, such as the BRIC countries (Brazil, Russia, India and China), however, may play an increasingly important role, bringing an alternative perspective to collaboration, rooted in the values and models of their domestic programmes (Global Health Strategies Initiatives, 2012). The increasing plurality of organizations acting in the global health arena continue to add to its complexity.

HEALTH

Context

Efforts to improve population health take place in a context of complex and shifting patterns of disease and illness. Chronic degenerative diseases such as CVD and cancers have become major causes of mortality and morbidity in high-income countries. However, many low- and middle-income countries have also experienced rises in the prevalence of these diseases in recent years, where they co-exist alongside endemic infectious diseases. Since the 1970s, a number of new diseases have emerged – estimated at one or more per year (WHO, 2007). Recent examples include SARS (Severe Acute Respiratory Syndrome – a potentially fatal respiratory infection caused by a virus that appeared in China in 2002) and H1N1 influenza ('swine' flu), which became a pandemic in 2009. At the same time, some diseases are re-emerging where social and economic living conditions are poor – TB and cholera, for example. Other diseases show an upward trajectory, emerging as major challenges to public health: obesity, injuries and mental illness, for example. There are also global threats to health from the consequences of human activity, such as **climate change**, bio-terrorism and nuclear accidents. Japan's Fukushima Daiichi nuclear plant disaster in 2011, where the combined effect of an earthquake and tsunami led to the devastation of the plant, illustrates the short-, medium- and long-term health consequences for individuals and their environments of such phenomena.

Notwithstanding this global picture of real and potential threats to health, overall life expectancy at birth has improved considerably over the past century. Average life expectancy at birth across all 34 of the Organization for Economic Co-operation and Development (OECD) countries in 2009 was 79.5 years, an increase of 11 years since 1960 (OECD, 2011b). The difference between the life expectancy of men and women has also narrowed during the last 30 years in most countries and is predicted to disappear by 2030 in England, when both sexes could live to their late 80s (Mayhew and Smith, 2012). These averages, however, obscure a much more complex pattern of inequalities in health both between and within countries. Social divisions in terms of class, income, ethnicity and gender give rise to differences in life expectancy of some magnitude. In England, for example, geographic analysis of life expectancy shows a clear north-south divide, with higher life expectancy in the south, specifically in Kensington and Chelsea, one of the most affluent areas of London, where men have a life expectancy of 85.1 years and women 89.8 years (Office for National Statistics (ONS), 2011). At a local level, however, life expectancy can vary within the space of a few miles: in Glasgow male life expectancy varies across the city from 54 to 82 years (CSDH, 2008). There are also signs that recent gains in life expectancy can, under certain social, economic and political conditions, be reversed, as relatively recent events in Russia illustrate (Cockerham, 2000). At a population, group and individual level, health, illness and disease fluctuate and co-exist; health, it seems, cannot be taken for granted.

Defining health

The pursuit of health has become a highly valued social practice (Crawford, 2006). Health, however, seems to defy straightforward description, having multiple, contested meanings. It is increasingly linked to the word 'well-being', also a contested concept. The UK government recently decided to develop a measure of well-being that could be used to guide and evaluate policy choices (Wallace and Schmuecker, 2012). However, given that health and well-being tend to be conflated with happiness, mental health and individual psychology (Atkinson, 2011) as well as life satisfaction, there is scope for generating further conceptual confusion. A consequence of placing greater emphasis on well-being in official definitions – particularly in terms of measurement – is that 'health' may become more narrowly defined.

Formal definitions of health can serve several purposes. Because they are developed by institutions that have a vested interest in health, definitions tend to be framed in terms that express particular values and beliefs, emphasizing those facets that institutions choose to prioritize. In 1948, the WHO published its constitution, a central aspect of which was the definition of health as 'a state of complete physical, social and mental well-being and not merely the absence of disease or infirmity', adding that 'the enjoyment of the highest attainable standard of health is one of the fundamental rights of every human being' (WHO, 2006: 1). These two principles reflect those of the UN of which the WHO is a specialized agency. The emergence of the UN (1945) and the WHO (1946) in the post-war period reflects the strong degree of consensus among world leaders at that time about the need to work together for world peace and social progress, of which human rights – including the right to health – were considered a fundamental part. The principles embodied in the constitutions of both organizations reflect these aspirations and ideals.

The WHO definition was the first formal definition to move away from the medical notion of health as an absence of disease. It articulated a positive, expansive, multidimensional view of health and, by including the idea of 'well-being' it extended the definition upwards (Roberts, 2009). It was not until the publication of the *Ottawa*

Charter (WHO, 1986) that the original definition was supplemented with two statements: first, that health was a resource and a means to a good productive life rather than an end in itself; and second, that health was generated (and eroded) in the settings of everyday life. The definition of health as a resource – as embodied biopsychosocial capital that individuals and organizations can invest in – emphasizes the idea of resilience and coping. Eriksson and Lindstrom (2008) argue that this idea reflects core ideas in Antonovsky's salutogenesis theory (1996). Although the idea of health as a resource has gained some currency, it has had little influence in guiding policy and practice (Williamson and Carr, 2009).

The WHO definition has been criticized for being unrealistic and unachievable (Lupton, 1995). Others have argued that it is not 'fit for purpose' in a context of high chronic disease prevalence, in which few would achieve 'complete' health (Huber *et al.*, 2011). Such criticism has prompted the development of new definitions. Huber *et al.*, for example, define health as 'the ability to adapt and self manage' (2011: 236). This definition reflects the notion of resilience found in the *Ottawa Charter* while at the same time emphasizing individual responsibility for health. Representatives of the International Union for Health Promotion rebutted this reformulation in the following terms: 'health is created when individuals, families, and communities are afforded the income, education, and power to control their lives; and their needs and rights are supported by systems, environments, and policies that are enabling and conducive to better health' (Shilton *et al.*, 2011). As these reformulations illustrate, all definitions share one thing in common: they are underpinned by values.

The significance of health for public health

It is only in the relatively recent past that research has explored lay understandings of health (rather than illness and disease). Much of this work has taken place in Europe in general and the UK more specifically. Less is known about how people think about health beyond these geographical areas, particularly among some of the indigenous populations of the world. Research on lay understandings has also been less common among men (Robertson, 2006). The academic literature on lay perspectives on health uses various terms, such as 'understandings', 'knowledge', and 'beliefs' to reflect the different degrees of validity that lay views are accorded. Encounters between professionals and lay people can be difficult when differing conceptualizations collide. Historically, this has tended to be seen as 'expert' professionals' knowledge being superior to lay beliefs. However, the user involvement movement of the past few decades has begun to challenge this orthodoxy, at least in theory if not in practice. Lay views of health, however, are not distinct from nor unrelated to professional or official views. In many countries, medical ideas in particular have diffused through a variety of processes, including the media, and have become part of the everyday lexicon of the general public. In fact, both professionals' and lay 'world views' comprise a complex mix of official and personal values, beliefs and facts. Given this complexity, Shaw (2002) questions the validity and utility of the 'laity' concept itself. This suggests that, in analytic terms, 'professional' and 'lay' may be something of a false dichotomy. Nonetheless, those involved in the health field – who tend to think and feel that health is a value that ought to be protected, promoted and prioritized over and above other values – may encounter differing perspectives and values. This includes working with others for whom 'health is not necessarily a pressing and overriding value consciously considered on a daily basis' (Bury, 2005: 8).

Research on lay views of health has explored three interrelated areas: what health means to people, how people understand the causes of health and illness, and how people explain inequalities in health. The first large-scale study of what health means to people included 9000 people in Great Britain (England, Scotland and Wales)(Cox *et al.*, 1987). The study included two questions that asked people to think about health in relation to someone they thought was healthy as well as in relation to themselves. On the basis of their responses a number of different conceptualizations of health were identified: the absence of illness; being able to cope physically and mentally; fitness; energy; psychosocial well-being; behaviour; and, a reserve (Blaxter, 1990). These ideas contain notions of health as an attribute (bodily processes), health as relational (social or psychosocial influences that create health) and health as 'doing' (Blaxter, 1990; Bury, 2005). Health is thus a multidimensional concept. Furthermore, how health was understood varied in relation to age, gender and social class. Older women, for example, tended to articulate views that expressed psychosocial dimensions of health, while younger women were more likely to value social relationships, particularly with children and family more widely. Younger men were inclined to emphasize health behaviours and the physical dimension of health. Other research has shown that people in lower socio-economic groups are more likely to see health and illness in terms of whether or not they are sufficiently well to go to work (Calnan, 1987). Not only do views on health reflect continuity and change over an individual's life course, they also reflect the commonplace cultural values and beliefs of people's differing social positions.

Blaxter's work reveals the idea of health as a reserve, similar to the idea of health as a resource expressed in the *Ottawa Charter*. In other words, health is viewed as capital that can be depleted over time or in relation to certain actions such as smoking, as well as invested in, for example through social interaction with friends. This illustrates the point that health, illness and disease are not necessarily viewed as distinct or static categories. Those who live with a chronic disease (such as diabetes) or disability, for example, may still see health as a possibility. In these situations being healthy tends to be viewed as a present-centred phenomenon specifically related to how each person feels on a particular day (Bury, 2005). Health is thus best viewed as a dynamic concept, shifting in relation to the moment-to-moment feelings associated with people's everyday lives.

The idea of 'lay epidemiology' has been developed to explore how people explain good or poor health (Davison *et al.*, 1991). This is significant for those working in public health because how people view the world, particularly their expectations of it, will guide their actions (de Swann, 2001): if people understand the causes of health in a particular way, this will influence, to varying degrees, their attitudes and actions. Lay views tend to accommodate official ideas about the causes of health, illness and disease. Research on CHD for example, concluded that people integrate ideas about behavioural risk factors with other cultural ideas, such as luck and destiny (Davison *et al.*, 1991). Research in the field of mental health, however, indicates that some 'official' ideas about the causes of health may be more readily embraced than others. The idea of mental illness residing in the body – in terms of brain chemistry, levels of neurotransmitters, and so on – dominant in psychiatry for many years, is commonly expressed in lay views. Yet sociological studies on depression suggest that life events involving loss and threat have a substantial impact on the development of the illness in the presence of other factors such as a lack of a confiding relationship and low economic status (Brown, 1984). Viewing mental illness as connected to social relations seems to have penetrated lay understandings to a lesser degree. This may reflect the way in which mental health tends to attract negative judgements, especially in the form of blame, from which families and sufferers wish to distance themselves (Bury, 2005). A parallel can be draw from the field of social inequalities in health, which also seems to have permeated people's views to a limited degree (Daghofer, 2011). This may reflect people's reluctance to identify themselves in terms of inequality (Blaxter, 1997). Although lay people tend to emphasize personal responsibility for health, in the eyes of some, policies, governments and environments remain important (Herzlich, 1973; Hughner and Kleine, 2004). Such complexity reflects the dialectical way in which ideas about health are mediated in different cultural contexts (Bury, 2005). It also reflects the ways in which people accommodate ideas they find disconcerting into some kind of rational world view through which they attempt to make sense of health and illness in their everyday lives (Davison *et al.*, 1991).

Conclusion

Health continues to be a matter of considerable public concern (Crawford, 1980). In public health, the pressure to measure health outcomes, particularly as a means of gauging improvements in health, reflects this interest. Nonetheless, the difficulties inherent in measuring health as a positive concept or state means that 'negative' measures of health – such as death, disease, illness and behaviours – continue to be the predominant way of assessing population health. The extensive research on lay concepts of health and illness, however, suggests the general public view health in more complex terms. As Blaxter (2010: 162) points out, 'neither in lay perceptions, nor as manifested in their actual experience, are health and illness simply logical opposites'. Lay perceptions of how disease is caused and how health is manifested have a number of implications for policy and practice. Significantly, it may be short-sighted to assume that professionals' views are necessarily more authentic and valid than lay views. It also seems likely that debates about improving health and well-being will increase in complexity and raise new ethical issues. New technologies, in particular, are likely to be a significant part of the developing picture, with their promise to enhance normality and delay disease, infirmity and death.

HEALTH EDUCATION

Context

In one form or another, health education has had a long association with public health. It is, however, an ambiguous term associated as it is with **health promotion, health literacy** and **social marketing**. The emergence of health promotion in particular, alongside the re-emphasis on **behaviour change** over the past 30 years, has contributed to creating a complex milieu in which health education continues to be debated. Some have viewed the proliferation of terms as a 're-branding' of health education in an effort to revitalize an orthodox field. In England, however, health education (in one form or another) appears likely to remain part of public health not least because of the continuing **policy** emphasis on 'informed' healthy choices (Secretary of State for Health, 2010). The tendency for health education to be presented as a 'safe', straight-forward and value-neutral activity hides the more complex character of its assumptions and intentions.

Defining health education

Central to defining health education have been attempts to identify an 'essence' in order to differentiate it from (while linking it to) health promotion. Drawing on ideas from the philosophy of **education** and notions of learning and autonomy, Tones and Tilford (2001: 30) define health education as 'any intentional activity that is designed to achieve health or illness-related learning, that is, some relatively permanent change in an individual's capability or disposition'. They go on to argue that learning might involve a shift in aptitude, values, beliefs, attitudes or behaviour, emphasizing the voluntaristic character of health education. Tones and Tilford's definition has endured alongside a number of theoretical typologies that describe different ways of conceptu-alizing health education (Beattie, 1991; French and Adams, 1986; Tones, 1986). Reflecting wider theoretical debates of the time, Tones (2002b) argued that the purpose of health *education* is to empower individuals and communities. The 'new health education' (reproducing the idea of the 'new public health') is presented as radical and as having the potential to be the 'driving force' of health promotion (Green, 2008: 451). Defining the 'essence' of health education in terms of voluntarism and empower-ment implies a diversity of outcomes that include the possibility of people acting intentionally in ways that others might view as 'unhealthy'.

The significance of health education for public health

At its simplest, health education has taken the form of disseminating health-related information to persuade (or sometimes shock) the public to act with due regard to their own health and that of others. Historically, children and mothers have been a particular target of information campaigns. In England during the 1960s and 70s, mass publicity campaigns and national programmes such as the 'Look After Yourself!' scheme were the mainstay of governmental efforts to persuade people towards healthy choices (Rodmell and Watt, 1986). More recently, population-level campaigns in a number of countries have targeted smoking, drug **prevention**, sexual health, '5-a-day' healthy eating and physical activity. Common to these types of initiatives is a tendency to present **lifestyle** as a matter of individual choice and personal responsibility with little if any reference to the differential access to resources or contextual constraints that render the notion of individual 'choice' problematic (Naidoo, 1986). This form of health education (persuasion using information presented as 'facts') can lead to victim-blaming: an ideology that blames individuals for their poor health and urges them to take more responsibility, while at the same time deflecting attention away from the social **determinants** of health and health behaviour (Crawford, 1977). This 'radical critique' of health education (Rodmell and Watt, 1986) has given rise to considerable theoretical debate within the field. Some have seen the critique as primarily directed at the narrow, medical and behaviourist form of health education practice that had become commonplace at that time rather than an attack on health education more generally. However, the emerging field of health promotion, centred as it was on a critique of individualism, is viewed in some quarters as having eclipsed health education in any form.

The relationship between information, knowledge and behaviour is far from straightforward, however. Knowing about the health **risks** associated with smoking and excessive alcohol consumption, for example, does not necessarily lead to the adoption of healthier lifestyles. Furthermore, sustaining **behaviour change** has also been shown to be problematic, particularly among some groups. A growing appreciation of the limits to health education has shifted attention towards trying to better understand health behaviour. A plethora of psychologically-based models have been developed and applied in the health field: the theory of reasoned action (Azjen and Fishbein, 1980), the health belief model (Rosenstock, 1974) and stage-based models such as the TTM (Prochaska and Diclemente, 1983). These models have some appeal, not least because psychological variables might appear more amenable to change than socio-demographic variables (Armitage and Connor, 2000). Such models, however, have promised much but delivered little in terms of understanding how to shift health behaviours in the desired direction. They have also been criticized on the same grounds as health education, namely for a narrow behaviourist focus that underplays the influence of context. Bandura's social cognitive theory based on the concept of self-efficacy – 'a belief in one's capabilities to organize and execute the courses of action required to produce given levels of attainments' (Bandura, 1998: 624) – is something of a departure in that it seeks to address 'the sociostructural determinants of health as well as the personal determinants' (623).

Empowerment continues to be a central organizing concept for health education and health promotion and is particularly relevant to understanding **inequalities** in health and how they might be addressed. In health education, Freire (1972) has been a particularly influential theorist, perhaps because he viewed knowledge and understanding as central to emancipation. His method of critical consciousness raising among 'the oppressed' involved developing an appreciation of the root causes of people's subjugation, as well as reflecting on actions – at an individual, group and societal level – needed to bring about change. In the Freirian process, 'power' is viewed as an aspect of all human relations; people's interests are bound up with those of others, with some groups possessing greater degrees of power to act, protect and preserve their interests. It follows from this that power relations can be understood at different, although interconnected levels: as a feature of interactions between people as well as operating in systematic ways through society (Ribbens McCarthy and Edwards, 2011). Power can also be used to maintain the status quo; governments and other powerful elites can decide not to take action in the face of public pressure or accumulating evidence, for example.

In the health education literature the terms self-empowerment and **community** empowerment are used to convey the different levels at which greater control over decisions and actions affecting health might work. Several ideas have been used to theorize the basis of individual and group-based empowerment, including the concept of self-efficacy. More recently Sen's capability approach has emphasized 'assets' as the foundation of 'positive capabilities' that can be used to 'identify problems and activate solutions' (Morgan and Ziglio, 2007: 17). A critical perspective would suggest that people's social position (in relation to class, ethnicity and gender, for example) gives rise to differing degrees of power and control and it is this that needs to be equalized through political action (Rissel, 1994; Friedli, 2013). Thus, no matter how assertive people perceive themselves to be, or how well-equipped in terms of knowledge, personal skills and so on – individual capabilities and assets – poverty alleviation, for example, requires a political solution. All in all, if health and ill-health are shaped by socio-economic and political structures then attempts to change personal behaviour through empowerment are essentially misconceived (Tesh, 1988). Individual-level conceptualizations of empowerment thus miss the point in that processes of empowerment seek to *redistribute* power, increasing the capacity of those with less power to change things alongside a diminution in the power of others.

In many countries, health education continues to be part of the school curriculum, reflecting a degree of consensus that schools have a responsibility to ensure that children and young people are well-informed, not least because of many parents' disinclination to talk to their children about issues such as sex and relationships (Wilson *et al.*, 2010). In England, personal, social and health education (PSHE) has occupied a somewhat uncertain position over the years as a statutory or non-statutory curriculum subject. Given the pressure on schools to increase their performance in relation to core subject areas (such as mathematics and English), PSHE has been viewed as less of a priority, particularly in the secondary school **setting**, receiving scarce resources, including limited time and few teachers with the confidence and expertise to deliver the subject well (Formby and Wolstenholme, 2012; Macdonald, 2009). The effectiveness of PSHE and the extent to which it is evidence-based have also been called into question (Hale *et al.*, 2011). Debates about effectiveness, however, raise questions about the aims and purposes of PSHE. Ostensibly the aim is to support the personal development and learning of each child in relation to health and well-being, but questions about effectiveness suggest that there is an expectation that PSHE will impact on choices about lifestyles.

Sex and relationships education continues to be viewed as problematic in many countries. Concerns have been expressed about its propensity to encourage earlier sexual activity, while others argue that it is likely to discourage or delay sexual activity as well as enable young people to practice safe sex when the time comes. In the USA, the former view has manifested itself in 'abstinence only' approaches – driven in large part by neo-conservative federal policies and funding – rather than comprehensive sex and relationships education (Collins *et al.*, 2002). Research has shown that teenagers who receive comprehensive sex education have a lower risk of pregnancy compared to those who receive abstinence only or no sex and relationships education. Furthermore, research has shown that comprehensive sex education was not associated with an increased risk of sexual activity (Kohler *et al.*, 2008). Neither is there any research that suggests that abstinence only programmes delay sexual activity (Collins *et al.*, 2002). However, enhanced sex education programmes are also limited in the extent to which they serve to reduce conceptions or terminations, a finding that is perhaps unsurprising given the strong association of early pregnancy with socio-economic determinants (Henderson *et al.*, 2006). Comprehensive sex education is more likely to be effective – in the sense of supporting young people to make their own choices safely and without coercion – if the wider determinants of early sexual (and unsafe) activity are also addressed.

School-based health education, however, takes place within a complex arena characterized by shifting power relations between policymakers, school governors, parents and teachers, a context in which ideological arguments tend to prevail sometimes to the detriment of children and young people's health and well-being. Although health education based on a model of critical pedagogy might serve children and young people's best interests it is unlikely to be implemented in practice in schools, given its emphasis on Freire's (1972) ideas of critical consciousness raising and empowerment. Varying conceptualizations of health education underpin these discussions, however. Some have argued for health educators to act as advocates in the policy process, sensitizing the public to the arguments of policymakers, not just in scientific and technical terms but also in relation to values, including reflection on their own value position (Breton *et al.*, 2007; Green, 2008). The extent to which those with a role in health education want to embrace a more politically contentious model of practice remains to be seen, however. Passive, information-driven approaches may well continue to be the mainstay of health education – despite their limited impact on behaviour – because they constitute a palatable and ostensibly politically 'neutral' approach.

Conclusion

Thinking critically about health education involves reflecting on why specific models and concepts emerge in particular political contexts as well as whose interests are being served by their promulgation (Friedli, 2013). In policy and practice, a key tension centres on the goals of health education. These can vary along a spectrum from being instrumental and focused on behaviour, through to approaches that give primacy to voluntarism and empowerment. Public health policy in many countries, however, continues to emphasize health education as a route to behaviour change. Such approaches are more likely to be successful among those living in the most advantaged circumstances. Elsewhere, success is more likely if they are supported by other broader policies for creating supportive environments (Benzeval *et al.*, 1995).

HEALTH LITERACY

Context

The concept of **health** literacy surfaced in the early 1970s in the **health education** field. Since then, it has been applied widely in health care **settings** in the USA, where low levels of health literacy have been associated with poor health, lower usage of prescribed medications and preventive health services, and higher likelihood of being admitted to hospital (Institute of Medicine, 2004). The usage of health literacy beyond the USA has been more limited, however. There are, nonetheless, signs that interest is expanding in Europe. In part, this reflects a growing recognition that people are increasingly confronted with diverse forms of health-related information via a range of media, including persuasive marketing information extolling the health-related benefits of various products. In addition, health services regularly communicate with patients about their care and treatment via invitations to participate in **screening**, through explaining prescribed medication regimes, as well as communicating **risk** information (Raynor, 2012). There has also been a trend in countries such as the UK to engage patients in the management and care of their own conditions (Coulter and Ellins, 2007). Health literacy is seen as relevant to helping people navigate this complex terrain. The extent to which health literacy has relevance beyond clinical settings is however, debatable. In the public health field, some have also questioned whether there is anything new and useful in the concept that has not already been captured by terms such as health education and empowerment (Tones, 2002a; Wills, 2009).

Defining health literacy

Definitions of health literacy have been extensively debated in recent years but no universally agreed definition has emerged (Wills, 2009). A recent systematic review of the field identified 17 definitions and 12 conceptual models (Sørensen *et al.*, 2012; Sørensen and Brand, 2013). This situation is perhaps unsurprising given debates within the field of literacy about the meaning and forms of different 'literacies' (financial literacy, nutritional literacy, computer literacy, emotional literacy and so on) and their constituent social and cognitive skills (Nutbeam, 2009). Recognizing different literacy domains – such as health literacy – implies that generic literacy skills are necessary but insufficient to develop understanding of specific subject matter; in other words, domain-specific content and skills are also essential. According to this view, a person may be literate but not necessarily health literate.

Most definitions of health literacy refer to people's access to, and comprehension of information sufficient to enable them to act in relation to their health. The US Institute of Medicine (2004: 32), for example, defines health literacy as 'the degree to which individuals have the capacity to obtain, process and understand basic health information and services needed to make appropriate health decisions'. Here, use of the phrase 'to make appropriate health decisions' suggests that health literacy primarily relates to patient compliance. The distinction between medical and public health literacy has been at the centre of definitional debates. Peerson and Saunders (2009) use the term 'medical literacy' to refer to comprehension of health care-related inform-ation and argue that it should be differentiated from 'health literacy' (keeping well in everyday life) as a distinct form of literacy. Bennett *et al.* (2009), for example, propose a definition of public health literacy that shifts the focus away from the individual level and gives primacy to the social, political and environmental **determinants** of health.

Nutbeam (2000) has been particularly instrumental in elaborating the concept of health literacy within the public health field. Drawing on Freebody and Luke's (1990) classification of literacy, he presents a three-fold typology of health literacy based on what it is that literacy enables people *to do*. According to this framework, functional health literacy refers to having the reading and writing skills to be able to understand factual information about health, similar to the definition proposed by the US Institute of Medicine cited above. Interactive health literacy concerns the development of personal skills – such as problem solving and decision-making, as well as higher order cognitive skills – said to enable individuals to act on their knowledge and under-standing of information and apply it to new health-related situations. Critical health literacy, on the other hand, refers to advanced cognitive, analytic and social skills sufficient to exert greater control over health-related situations. This form of health literacy is particularly in keeping with the *Ottawa Charter*'s emancipatory aims, which focus on empowering people to increase control over their lives (WHO, 1986). It also chimes with Freire's idea of **education** as critical consciousness-raising, the purpose of which is to achieve social and political change. Fundamentally, the idea of a 'critical' health literacy implies a sceptical stance towards information and **evidence** and the use of literacy skills in uncovering assumptions, challenging authority and, potentially, engaging in social and political action. In other words, although health literacy is an individual capability, it can be directed towards **community** and population-level ends. In this regard, Nutbeam (2000) argues that all three forms of health literacy are, by degrees, related to empowerment.

The WHO definition reflects Nutbeam's emphasis on literacy skills – not only reading, writing, and numeracy but also critical appraisal and decision-making skills: 'health literacy represents the cognitive and social skills which determine the motivation and ability of individuals to gain access to, understand and use information in ways which promote and maintain good health' (Nutbeam, 2000: 264). Nutbeam (2009) argues that health literacy is the outcome of health education, as well as education more generally, rather than synonymous with it.

The Institute of Medicine's (2004) and the WHO's (Nutbeam, 2008) definitions are the two most frequently cited (Sørensen *et al.*, 2012). Based on a content analysis of different definitions of health literacy, Sørensen *et al.* define health literacy as

> linked to literacy and entails people's knowledge, motivation and competences to access, understand, appraise and apply health information in order to make judgements and take decisions in everyday life concerning healthcare, disease prevention and health promotion to maintain or improve quality of life during the life course.
>
> (Sørensen *et al.*, 2012: 3)

A key aim in producing this definition was to provide an agreed platform for the development of valid measures of health literacy. It reflects the core ideas in the definitions of Nutbeam and the Institute of Medicine, thereby integrating the medical and public health domains. Comprehensive as the definition is, it may be difficult to operationalize, however. Others have tried to delineate and define the sub-types of health literacy more precisely (see for example Sykes *et al.* (2013) in relation to critical literacy). Given the impetus to develop valid measures of health literacy it seems likely that debates relating to definitions will continue.

The significance of health literacy for public health

Nutbeam (2009) argues that health literacy can be measured in much the same way that literacy is measured in schools: in other words, as a measure of performance. The TOFHLA (Test of Functional Health Literacy in Adults) – relating to reading fluency – and the REALM (Rapid Estimate of Adult Literacy in Medicine) – relating to vocabulary – are two instruments widely used in the USA to measure health literacy. Both instruments measure an individual's reading comprehension in a medical setting; in other words, they measure functional health literacy (Baker, 2006). The Health Activities Literacy Scale (HALS) also developed in the USA, is a more comprehensive measure but takes 30–40 minutes to complete, an issue that might influence the test's acceptability to patients. No existing test measures comprehension of spoken health-related information, important in clinical encounters (Baker, 2006). The European Health Literacy Project 2009–2012 developed a new instrument based on the definition cited above (Sørensen *et al.*, 2012) to collect population-level data on health literacy in eight countries. The 47-item questionnaire uses a 4-point self-report scale to measure perceptions of difficulty associated with different health tasks (HLS-EU Consortium, 2012). This is the first instrument to have operationalized health literacy as a composite construct.

A number of studies in different population groups have shown that low levels of functional health literacy are a feature of high-income countries, where a third to a half of people experience difficulty understanding their health care to the extent that it has implications for their health (Raynor, 2012). In the UK, for example, Bostock and Steptoe (2012) found that approximately a third of adults aged 52 or more had difficulty reading basic health information. In Canada, 55 per cent of adults (16–65 years) were found to have less than adequate health literacy skills (Rootman and Gordon-El-Bihety, 2008) and in the USA, some 90 million adults lacked basic health literacy (Carmona, 2006). Low health literacy in the USA has been associated with a higher risk of developing diabetes mellitus, heart failure and asthma, as well as of developing complications from these conditions (Chinn, 2011; Rowlands, 2012). Strategies to strengthen patients' health literacy have a number of beneficial outcomes, including improving patient safety, reducing use (and costs) of health services and improving self-care (Coulter and Ellins, 2007). Coulter and Ellins (2007) argue that health literacy is central to patient engagement and, if not addressed, has the potential to widen health **inequalities**. Significantly, however, low levels of health literacy reflect low levels of basic literacy. In England, approximately 16 per cent of adults (5.2 million people) are 'functionally illiterate', that is, have literacy levels below that expected of an 11-year old (Jama and Dugdale, 2012).

Various studies have found that women, older people, and those from a lower socio-economic or minority ethnic group are more likely to have low health literacy (HLS-EU Consortium, 2012; Kickbusch and Maag, 2008). Visually and/or hearing impaired people have also been shown to have relatively low levels of knowledge about diseases such as cancer (Powell *et al.*, 2008). Thus, health literacy – like literacy itself – is patterned according to various forms of social disadvantage. Chinn (2011) argues that critical health literacy is an asset distributed in social networks as a form of **social capital**. Some social networks may be better endowed with health information assets than others, giving advantages to those involved. Those with a higher level of education and economic advantage are better positioned not only to access but also to understand and respond to information about their health. Differences in levels of health literacy may therefore reflect differences in class position or educational attainment, in other words, they are a symptom of deeper structural inequalities.

Although Nutbeam (2000) articulated a broad, composite view of heath literacy, relatively little attention beyond the academic field has been given to critical health literacy. The CSDH (2008: 189) argued that 'The understanding of the social determinants of health among the general public needs to be improved as a new part of health literacy.' The CSDH claimed that this form of health literacy was an important element in strategies to reduce health inequalities. Lay understandings of the causes of poor health tend not to be articulated in terms of social inequalities, especially among those who are most likely to experience social disadvantage (Blaxter,

1997). More recent research suggests this might be changing. Davidson *et al.*'s (2006) qualitative research showed that people living in disadvantaged circumstances articulated a range of views that indicate how inequalities adversely affected their health and well-being.

The CSDH (2008) also identifies the responsibility of public and private organizations to communicate information in ways that make it comprehensible. Health care systems in many developed countries are difficult to navigate and made more complex by health professionals through the language and terminology used in clinical encounters (Rudd, 2010). Power relations, including controlling access to information in various ways, have been extensively researched in health care. The conclusion tends to be that clinicians and other health care professionals have made little progress towards more empowering, mediating or enabling models of practice (Anderson and Funnell, 2005; Nugus *et al.*, 2010) as advocated in the *Ottawa Charter*. Raynor (2012) argues that strengthening health literacy (of any type) has the potential to give rise to actions that diverge from the advice given by health care professionals. 'Decision-aids' have been introduced into health care contexts to help people participate in decisions by weighing up harms, benefits and uncertainties relating to treatment and screening. A recent review found that while such 'aids' can improve people's knowledge of options and involvement in decisions, they have a variable effect on their actual choices (Stacey *et al.*, 2012). This underscores the limits to knowledge (or health literacy) in effecting health-related decisions (Peerson and Saunders, 2009).

Conclusion

In a relatively short period of time, health literacy has achieved widespread political currency. In consumer-oriented societies the volume of health-related information of variable quality creates pressure for improved knowledge and skills if such material is to be critically appraised and used as a basis for decision making. Navigating an increasingly complex health care system also demands similar competence. Being 'health literate' is thus promoted as an important matter of personal responsibility. The expansion of the concept to include critical health literacy extends the notion to the political realm and challenges established systems of governance (Chinn, 2011). This conceptualization is thus relevant to raising the profile of inequalities in health and arguing for action on the social determinants of health (Mogford *et al.*, 2010). Recognizing the differences between the various forms of health literacy is therefore important if public health action is to move away from solely individually-oriented approaches. As Wills (2009: 4) points out 'Being able to read a food label is one thing, understanding why a Macdonalds [sic] is so cheap, filling and ubiquitous is another'. Integrating critical health literacy into practice is likely to be challenging, however.

HEALTH NEEDS

Context

Addressing **health** and health care needs has always been fundamental to the purpose of public health. In recent years this has manifested itself in terms of efforts to confront the wider **determinants of health** – meeting the need for food, shelter, employment, affection, protection, equality, and so on. When people have unequal access to these and other prerequisites for health, a variety of needs are generated to which the **welfare state** has been designed to respond. In recent times, however, pressures on welfare systems have become considerable, particularly since the global financial crisis of 2008 and the period of sustained financial austerity that has ensued in very many countries. With its focus on creating the conditions to support health, however, public health has the potential to reduce needs and demand for welfare services. A focus on **prevention** is likely therefore to be especially attractive to governments.

Defining health needs

The concept of 'need' is difficult to pin down. A variety of disciplines – philosophy, economics, social policy, **ethics**, as well as public health and health care – have sought to clarify and define the concept. Disagreement remains, however. New terms such as 'capabilities' (Nussbaum, 2011), as well as the increasing influence of economic concepts relating to 'priorities' and 'affordability', have increased the complexity of the definitional terrain.

A key dimension of contention centres on the extent to which needs can be objectively defined, becoming in the process undeniable. If viewed in these terms, then people should have a constitutional right to have their needs met as a matter of social justice. The discourse relating to the wider **determinants of health** and social **inequalities** in health has been increasingly couched in such terms in recent years. Doyal and Gough's (1991) theory of human need is particularly pertinent to public health given its societal (population-level) perspective based on an understanding of human beings as interdependent and therefore unable to meet all their needs themselves, its focus on prerequisites and its relevance to understanding inequalities. According to this theory, needs are defined in terms of 'a particular category of goals which are believed to be universalisable' (Gough, 2003: 8): that is to say, those that are in everyone's interests for all to achieve, as distinct from individual personal preferences. The theory is based on the twin goals of avoidance of serious harm and social participation, the achievement of which are dependent on a hierarchy of needs: societal preconditions (such as political rights); universal satisfier characteristics (such as food, water and shelter); and, basic needs (physical health, cognitive capacity). This theoretical position presents needs in instrumental terms in that they enable people to reach specified goals. Although concerned more broadly with what it means to be a human being, Doyal and Gough's theoretical framework has much in common with Dahlgren and Whitehead's (1991) model of health determinants, as well as ideas articulated in the *Ottawa Charter* relating to the prerequisites for health. Viewed from the perspective of public health, it reflects a view of need consistent with the wider determinants of health and helps make the distinction between *health* needs and *health care* needs. It also provides a framework for understanding the generation of social inequalities in health.

An alternative view is that needs are socially constructed and related to social and cultural norms that shift over time and **place**. This opens up the possibility for needs to be judged according to whether or not they are legitimate. Hence, whether or not something is evaluated as a need is contingent on the prevailing views of dominant groups in contemporary society – especially policymakers. Robertson (1998) argues that this puts needs squarely in the political domain and underscores their essentially contested character. Much of the political (ideological) discourse underpinning arguments for financial austerity measures since 2008 reflects judgements about whether or not people are in 'real need' and/or 'deserving' of support. In such a context the language of need tends to be replaced by the more restricted concept of priorities (Foreman, 1996).

Both the objective and relativist views – health needs as identifiable and universal or as socially constructed – are central to understanding health needs. The extensive empirical **evidence** on the determinants of health is well-established; health flourishes under particular circumstances. Obfuscating the evidence, directly denying it, or asserting that the consequences that flow from the evidence cannot be afforded reflects political expediency.

The significance of health needs for public health

Although prevention holds out the promise of reducing demand for services, in most high-income countries there have been few signs of a major shift in effort away from reactive services towards addressing the wider determinants of health. This means that services continue to play a key role in supporting people during times of hardship. The concept of 'need' has been the accepted basis on which public services have been provided ever since the establishment of welfare states (Percy-Smith, 1996). In recent decades, however, public services have come under sustained attack in many countries and the question of how needs, particularly health needs, should be met has become one of the most highly contested issues in public policy. What characterizes the contemporary landscape is the increasingly complex mix of provision through the market, the voluntary and **community** sector, informal support from friends and family members as well as the state. The point to note here is that access to services is not necessarily straightforward, particularly for disadvantaged groups. Inequalities in access can exacerbate more fundamental inequalities in health.

Bradshaw's (1972, 1994) fourfold typology of needs can be used to illustrate how needs are managed within, for example, the health care system. He differentiates between normative, felt, expressed and comparative need. Normative need is that which is defined by experts, often on the basis of some 'standard'. Although experts differ in terms of their professional opinion and standards shift over time, in the health care field normative need remains the primary basis for defining need. It has become commonplace in health care for normative judgements to be made in terms of a person's 'capacity to benefit' from an intervention (Culyer, 1998: 79). This judgement implies that effective interventions (those that can lead to health gain) are available. Increasingly, cost-effectiveness **evaluations** that compare health gains to costs are used to prioritize resources in order to maximize benefits relative to costs (Donaldson and Mooney, 1991). Here need is defined in terms of 'care that is required to bring about the maximum possible health improvement within given resource constraints' (Allin *et al.*, 2010: 466). The incorporation of an economic perspective shifts the focus away from assessed needs, which may well remain unmet.

Felt need is that which is defined by lay people based on their perceptions and is often equated with wants or personal preferences. The increasing commodification of health and health care has not only blurred the boundaries between needs and wants, but also created demands for all manner of products and interventions. A *felt* need tends to manifest itself as an *expressed* need when a person takes action and seeks a service. Some felt needs, however, may not be expressed for a variety of reasons, including people's beliefs relating to the availability, effectiveness and fairness of services. The needs of people with mental health issues or who are homeless, for example, may well remain unmet due to stigma. Expressed need tends to be viewed as 'demand' by economists in particular, with GPs being seen as key gatekeepers in regulating demand. A point to note here is that GPs also generate demand. Health needs may be medicalized, for example, in that doctors judge needs in relation to what services they can provide, rather than more broadly in relation to the wider deter- minants of health. Furthermore, regardless of the severity or character of needs, the referring behaviour of doctors and the availability of local and regional services (the latter in turn being dependent on the priorities of politicians and the resources they have made available) influence whether or not needs are addressed. Referral rates, for example, tend to reflect the characteristics of doctors rather than the health of populations. Similarly, hospital admission rates reflect the supply of hospital beds rather than severity of need (Wright *et al.*, 1998). The geographical variation in the quality and quantity of health care services continues to be a factor influencing people's access to services. Hart's (1971) inverse care law remains pertinent to understanding the poorer access to health care in areas of **deprivation** where needs are likely to be greater than elsewhere. Bradshaw's construct of comparative need refers to the aim of providing equivalent care to people with similar characteristics. If there is a shortfall, then some individuals are, comparatively, in need. In England, equity audits have been used to reveal how fairly services are distributed relative to the health needs of different groups and identify gaps in provision (Low and Low, 2006).

Out of this complexity a variety of unmet needs emerge, representing the burden of illness and disease in the community. Health needs assessment (HNA) has developed as a population-based methodology for objectively assessing the nature and extent of health needs in a specific area. Cavanagh and Chadwick (2005: 3), for example, define HNA as 'a systematic method for reviewing health issues facing a population, leading to agreed priorities and resource allocation that will improve health and reduce inequalities'. Its emergence reflects a desire to develop a rational basis for planning health and related services. Most HNAs use mixed methods, combining existing statistical, epidemiological and documentary sources with direct observations in the community, consultation with key informants (such as providers of services) as well as with members of the community. The aim is to build a picture of health needs, the determinants of health, as well as the existing pattern of provision for supporting needs. Although advocated as a way of addressing equity, economic perspectives tend to permeate planning processes.

Rapid appraisal (RA) and rapid participatory appraisal (RPA) are particular types of HNAs that have been used predominantly in low- and middle-income countries for several decades. What differentiates these approaches from HNAs is the greater involvement of local people in the identification of local problems as well as in decision-making about what to prioritize and what actions to take (Foreman, 1996). Professionals tend to have a role in collating relevant data as well as a support role in helping lay people make sense of information, facilitating the decision-making process. The commitment in RA and RPA is towards empowerment and community development. As the names suggests, the aim is to work quickly and reduce costs. A strength of the approach is that it can add insights from the community, including those relating to the needs of disadvantaged groups about what matters, which may well differ from professionally-oriented perceptions. It can also reveal the extent to which solutions reside beyond the immediate locality (Brown *et al.*, 2006).

In England, an annual Joint Strategic Needs Assessment (JSNA) has been a statutory requirement for the local authority since 2007, the resulting document to be used to inform the commissioning of local services to address identified needs. Relevant needs are defined as those capable of being met by the local authority's exercise of functions (DH, 2013). To support the JSNA, areas have access to locally relevant data relating to population characteristics (age and sex structure, black and minority ethnic population, child poverty, pensioners living alone, long term unemployed and so on), prevalence of health-related conditions (such as obese children) and behaviours (for example, binge drinking among adults), health service activity (such as hospital admissions) and epidemiological information (death rates by cause) (see for example, www.localhealth.gov). Consultation with patients, services users and the wider community should also be carried out and included in the JSNA.

As with HNAs, the JSNA provides a basis for local decision-making. However, it remains to be seen how it will be used and with what consequences. Making sense of detailed and complex information of the type described above is likely to pose challenges for those less familiar with this way of working. Furthermore, translating information into a coherent and integrated health and well-being strategy, as required, is also likely to prove difficult. It may be particularly challenging given how difficult it is to connect health and well-being to the wider determinants of health in other than theoretical terms. Although investing in new services to meet needs may be straight-forward, the historical pattern of services is likely to make disinvestment decisions particularly difficult. Fundamentally, however, the JSNA – in common with HNAs more generally – provides a tool for priority-setting and resource allocation. In other words it is likely to be deployed as an economic tool for rationing because 'capacity to benefit' will always exceed resources.

Conclusion

Assessing local health needs remains an important part of public health practice, ostensibly providing a rational basis for planning and commissioning services. If comprehensively carried out, it has the potential to include local views on needs as well as uncover unmet needs. The challenge for local policymakers, however, is in translating information about health needs into coherent plans for action, particularly given the inevitable economic constraints. Perhaps more fundamentally, health needs assessments provide an opportunity to re-think the customary emphasis on meeting needs through service provision rather than attending to the conditions of everyday life wherein needs are generated. Housing policy, and the provision of social housing in particular, provides an example of how health needs might be better met through a focus on the fundamental causes of poor health (Link and Phelan, 1995).

HEALTH PROMOTION AND THE 'NEW PUBLIC HEALTH'

Context

Ideas surface in particular contexts. Such is the case with the emergence and development of **health** promotion, an idea popularized during the 1980s through the work of the WHO. In 1984, the WHO's European Regional Office established a new programme in 'health promotion', a vision clarified in a later publication – *The Concepts and Principles of Health Promotion* (Health Promotion, 1986). This document described health promotion as representing 'a unifying concept for those who recognize the need for *change* in the ways *and* conditions of living in order to promote health' (WHO, 2009: 29). In 1986, the first international conference on health promotion was held in Ottawa, where the *Charter for Health Promotion* was launched, with the subtitle 'the move towards a new public health'. These specific events were manifestations of a longer-term process of development at the WHO, which earlier had given rise to the *Alma-Ata Declaration* (1978) and Health for All by the Year 2000. The influences shaping this process extended beyond the WHO, however. The Canadian *Lalonde Report* (Lalonde, 1974) is often cited as providing the main impetus for the creation of a new programme in health promotion, through its critique of the role of health care in improving population health alongside a refocusing on the role of the environment and individual **lifestyle** (Raeburn and Rootman, 1989). Broader global events during the 1970s and 1980s were also influential and included the recognition of new and entrenched health problems in low-, middle- and high-income countries; growing recognition of **inequalities** in health between and within countries; a global economic crisis; disillusionment with the power, costs and limited effectiveness of **medicine**; and a questioning of the **ethics** and effectiveness of **health education** approaches to changing behaviour. The women's movement and the green movement were also sources of influence that shaped the thinking of key actors at the WHO (Kickbusch, 2007). However, it seems that the birth of the health promotion programme was a painful one, particularly in the form of tensions between the technical and activist groups within public health at the WHO, as well as the medical and non-medical paradigms (Berridge *et al.*, 2006: 30). These tensions have endured. As many have observed, health promotion, as well as the new public health, continue to be contested concepts.

Defining health promotion and the new public health

According to Kickbusch – who led the WHO's global health promotion programme, which included responsibility for drafting the *Ottawa Charter* – health promotion was 'not a new and separate discipline, but a necessary and timely reconsideration of public health' (Kickbusch, 1986: 3). Thus, the intention was to revitalize, reorientate and 'modernize' public health (Ashton, 2007), shifting the dominant paradigm away from its reliance on therapeutic, medical interventions towards action on the **determinants** of health (Ashton and Seymour, 1988; Breslow, 1999). The journal *Health Promotion* (latterly *Health Promotion International*) was established to 'reflect and contribute to new developments in public health' (Kickbusch, 1986: 4). However, an unintended consequence of the addition of this new terminology to the established fields of health **education** and the (old) public health has been considerable debate about boundaries, definitions and meanings. One starting point for making sense of these issues is to understand the concept and principles – and not merely the definition – of health promotion from the perspective of the originators at the WHO. The definition they proposed emphasized health promotion as a process – that is to say, a field of human action – the aim of which was to change the power relations that lead to poor health for some and better health for others by 'enabling people to increase control over, and to improve their health' (WHO, 1986: 1). Nearly a decade later, the *Bangkok Charter* (WHO, 2005a: 1) defined health promotion as a process of 'enabling people to increase control over their health and its determinants'. Thus, people's health was linked directly to the prerequisites for health. Five action areas were identified in the *Ottawa Charter* that sought change at macro (building healthy public **policy**), meso (creating supportive environments for health; reorienting health services) and individual and group (strengthening **community** action for health; developing personal skills) levels. Health was thus presented in ecological terms; that is to say, it was related to, and interdependent with, the social, political and economic environment, mediated through macro, meso and micro levels. The redefinition of health in the *Ottawa Charter* as a 'resource for everyday life, not the objective of living' (WHO, 1986: 1) also repositioned the purpose and scope of health promotion.

Although the WHO has continued to seek a consensus about the meaning and purposes of health promotion and its related concepts (Smith *et al.*, 2006) debate continues regarding whether health promotion is a subset of public health, the other way round, or, if in fact they are overlapping categories (Scott-Samuel and Springett, 2007). Academic and professional tensions have continued to beleaguer debates, which tend to overlook the original motive to 'revitalize' public health. Those working within health education have also sought to clarify its relationship with health promotion given that, initially at least, the latter term displaced the former overnight as health education units were re-named health promotion units in England. In the health education field there has been a tendency to emphasize the empowering consequences of health education in ways that support health promotion goals (Tones, 1996). According to this analysis, health promotion is health education plus healthy public policy (Green and Tones, 2010). However, definitions of health promotion and health education vary by country (see for example Taub *et al.*, 2009). Health promotion has also been reframed in terms of **social marketing** and as health improvement at various times and in different contexts. In England, it seems that health improvement has been used as a more 'neutral' term, devoid as it is of the ideological and emancipatory underpinnings that characterize health promotion. In setting out its own view of the public health field, the UK Faculty of Public Health identifies three domains of public health practice: health improvement, health protection and improving services, and makes no reference to health promotion. Some have argued that it does not matter if the term 'health promotion' has been abandoned as long as the underpinning way of thinking influences policy and practice within and beyond the health sector (Wills *et al.*, 2008). This chimes with Ashton's argument (2007) that health promotion is fundamentally about ways of working.

The significance of health promotion and the new public health for public health

How far, then, has the rhetoric of health promotion influenced public health policy and practice, fields which themselves might be described as being in a state of flux?

Inevitably, people interpret ideas in the everyday contexts of their working lives. This has given rise to health promotion definitions, concepts and principles being more or less visible in the policy documentation of different nation states. That said, the Nordic countries have tended to integrate health promotion ideology into policy in various ways. A Norwegian government document on achieving good health for all, for example, defines health promotion as 'the sum total of society's organized efforts to maintain, improve and promote the population's health by weakening factors that entail a health risk and strengthening factors that contribute to better health' (Klepp, 2010: 6). This resembles the commonly cited definition of public health in the Acheson report (1988: 4), viz 'the science and art of preventing disease, prolonging life and promoting health by the organized efforts of society'. These perspectives are emblematic of the convergence of fields as the WHO initially intended.

The social democratic **welfare state** that is a feature of Nordic countries espouses equity, universalism and redistribution of resources as core values (Povlsen *et al.*, 2011). Health promotion concepts and values are more easily integrated into public health and welfare policy in contexts where they go with the grain of the dominant political ideology. In Sweden, for example, health targets have been set in relation to the determinants of health rather than health behaviours and, more generally, public health has been integrated with general welfare policy (Pettersson, 2007; Vallgårda, 2007). The advantage of this form of policy development is that it allows health to be addressed – rather than side-stepped – as an essentially political issue and through several policy streams. These examples also illustrate the possibilities for healthy public policy (health in all policies) as articulated in the *Ottawa Charter* and by Milio (1981). Policy development, however, takes form as an aspect of the elected government. In Norway, for example, there have been shifts in emphasis between structural and more individually oriented measures over time. Since 2003, however, and the election of a socialist government there has been a renewed emphasis on universal structural measures (Fosse, 2009). These national differences, as well as shifts over time, illustrate the influence of prevailing ideologies on how health issues are understood and responses constructed. In this regard, Raphael (2013a: 95) concludes 'that it is the political economy – or form of welfare state – of a nation rather than its explicit commitments to health promotion concepts – that shape provision of the prerequisites of health'.

In many ways, the emergence of health promotion was a direct challenge to public health practice because it proposed a shift in 'mind-set and professional ethos' (Kickbusch, 2003: 384). Health promotion involved enabling all people to achieve their full health potential through mediating and **advocacy**, as well as through developing alliances across organizations, professions, disciplines and sectors. Health promotion also raised broader questions about the development of an appropriately skilled and knowledgeable workforce who could respond to the vision set out in the *Ottawa Charter*. Notwithstanding the ways in which these issues played out in different national contexts, an enduring theme has been debate about the position of health promotion as a discipline, discourse and profession vis-à-vis public health. Kickbusch (2007) lamented what she saw as the uncoupling of the subtitle to the *Ottawa Charter* ('the move towards a new public health') from the concept of health promotion on the grounds that it gave rise to schisms that ran counter to the interdisciplinary and collaborative rhetoric of health promotion while militating against the development of a multidisciplinary, multiprofessional, intersectoral field of action as intended. Thus, two divergent groups emerged, provocatively referred to by Ashton as 'health promotion apartheid' (2007: 233). In countries such as England, a 'new' cadre of health promotion specialists emerged from the health education units located within the National Health Service (NHS) (Ewles, 1996). After an initial expansion, and through a series of organizational changes, these have merged into public health departments, a pattern repeated in Canada and Australia (Wills *et al.*, 2008). Although the concept of health promotion was based on a notion of professional and disciplinary integration, the relative power of the public health profession as a branch of medicine meant that it was, to varying degrees, able to resist change.

In England, however, the then government actively supported the development of new senior professional roles in public health (open to candidates from a range of disciplines) as a means of progressing the development of multidisciplinary public health (Evans, 2003). The first Directors of Public Health were appointed in 2002, a development that was both controversial and radical (Evans and Knight, 2006). The health promotion profession, together with like-minded colleagues in public health, is said to have been highly influential in the development of multidisciplinary public health (Evans and Knight, 2006; Orme *et al.*, 2007). The consequences of this radical development are difficult to unravel but some have concluded that health promotion ideology had become marginalized rather than mainstreamed (Wills *et al.*, 2008) through 'hegemonic absorption' (Scott-Samuel and Springett, 2007: 211). These boundary tensions (Evans, 2003) continue to unfold against a background of increasingly complex organizational restructuring in many countries, which is a reminder that all professions, even those with greater degrees of autonomy, are constrained by the broader political context. Furthermore, implementing health promotion in practice – through advocacy, empowerment and so on – challenges professionals to examine their own values, competence and skills and demands considerable reflexivity, as well as the time and inclination to do so (Andrews, 1999, 2006).

Debates have continued to polarize around the centrality of medical *or* non-medical knowledge, skills and expertize, the importance of population *or* individually based approaches, the use of scientific and technological interventions *or* social and political approaches and so on. The history of public health, however, reveals the problems of such dichotomous thinking. The science and technology of sanitary engineering in the mid-nineteenth century was important in providing the necessary infrastructure for improving specific aspects of the environment but left untouched the root causes of the societal conditions in which the labouring classes lived and that exposed them to multiple risks (Ross, 1991). This example illustrates the multilevel character of public health problems as well as the necessity for multilevel responses.

Conclusion

The emergence of health promotion has much in common with the development of a 'new social movement'. The health promotion framework developed and promulgated by the WHO was unequivocally ideological, directly challenging the status quo. The intention was to improve health *and* health equity. The framework articulated a clear set of values: empowerment, participation, equity, social justice, inclusivity and so on. It also challenged the ostensibly 'objective' scientific basis of much conventional public health work. This vision remains relevant to contemporary public health policy and practice. In recent years, however, the WHO's role has been constrained in various ways. As a specialist agency of the UN it occupies a specific position within a bureaucracy of powerful global institutions that include the World Bank and the IMF. Nonetheless, a number of groups, organizations and practitioners have adopted the ideas espoused in the framework. These ideas have also given rise to new social movements, such as the People's Health Movement, which emerged in 2000, the stated aim of which was to work for better health for all in a better world. Ostensibly less constrained than the WHO, such networks may provide considerable momentum in promoting the values and aspirations of the health promotion movement.

INEQUALITIES IN HEALTH

Context

At a population level, there have been remarkable improvements in **health** over several decades. The estimated life expectancy at birth of the world's population has been increasing since 1950, initially with gains in all regions (Leon, 2011). Stark differences emerge, however, when data are disaggregated and comparisons made between and within countries. In 2010, between-country differences in life expectancy for example, varied from 32.5 for males in Haiti (43.6 years for women) to 80 years for men in Iceland (84.4 years for women) (Salomon *et al.*, 2012). Within high-, middle- and low-income countries differences in life expectancy can also be stark (Braveman and Tarimo, 2002). In Scotland, for example, life expectancy varies from 54 years in Calton (a deprived area of Glasgow) to 82 years in Lenzie (an affluent part of the same city some 12 km away) (Marmot, 2010). The Westminster area of London has the highest gap in male life expectancy in England at 16.9 years (Cheshire, 2012; London Health Observatory, 2012). A consistent finding in high-income countries is that despite well-developed welfare systems (which include high per capita health care expenditure) differences in life expectancy have persisted and, in countries such as England, widened in recent years.

In the UK, the Black Report (Black *et al.*, 1988; Department of Health and Social Security [DHSS], 1980) on inequalities in health is widely seen as having 're-discovered' differences in mortality across social groups, which have subsequently been documented in a number of countries (see, for example, Mackenbach *et al.*, 2008). The Black Report revealed the patterning of health in relation to social (occupational) class. Since then, the subject of health inequalities has undergone a process of politicization in several countries insofar as the findings from academic research have been, to varying degrees, debated in the public sphere and become an issue for politicians to address. Consistently documented as they have been over many years, health inequalities raise fundamental questions regarding the enduring effect of socio-economic position on health (as well as other social divisions such as gender and ethnicity) as well as the role of **policy** in narrowing such entrenched differences. This is contested territory, however, at a variety of levels.

Defining inequalities in health

Three terms – disparities, inequalities and inequities – have been used, often inter-changeably, to describe the patterns of health between and within countries, terminology shifting in relation to time, context and geography. In some political contexts (the UK in the 1980s, for example) 'geographic variations', 'differences' and 'disparities' were the terms used, while 'disparities' continues to be favoured in the USA. The term 'inequalities in health' has become more commonplace internationally in recent years, although the WHO has tended to prefer the phrase 'health inequities' (the distinction centring on notions of equality and justice).

Graham (2007: 4) discusses three different approaches to describing and under-standing health inequalities: health differences between individuals in a population; health differences between population groups; and health differences between groups occupying unequal positions in society. Taking the individual as the unit of analysis has been strongly criticized on the grounds that it fails to reveal the ways in which health is patterned across different social groups (Braveman, 2006). The second perspective explicitly does this by describing health in relation to social groups: in relation to age, sex, income quintile, area **deprivation** score and so on. This approach reveals differ-ences in health across social groups without linking them to inequalities relating to people's unequal social position. The use of ostensibly more neutral terminology de-politicizes the social patterning of health because it avoids explicit reference to differences as being 'unequal' (inequality) or 'unfair' (inequity). The third perspective, however, explicitly links health to social position within a social hierarchy (whether related to gender, ethnicity, social class or some other social division) and refers to health differences as 'social inequalities in health'. It draws directly on the sociological concept of stratification – socially structured inequalities – that give rise to a social hierarchy of relations, such as class divisions (Roberts, 2009). Position in the class structure is especially significant for understanding health inequalities (as well as other inequalities, such as income), not least because it influences life chances and shapes **lifestyles**, as well as conditioning many important life choices (Goldthorpe, 2010). According to this third perspective, 'a health disparity/inequality is a particular type of difference in health ... it is a difference in which disadvantaged social groups ... system-atically experience worse health or greater health **risks** than more advantaged groups' (Braveman, 2006: 167). Structural **determinants** (wider, social determinants) of health and well-being, such as the **education** system, labour market and welfare system, are mediated by people's social positions (socio-economic and gender, for example) through pathways associated with housing, neighbourhood, behaviour and so on (Graham and Kelly, 2004; Graham et al., 2006).

For some, the term 'health inequalities' is descriptive rather than evaluative – revealing patterns as 'differences, variations, and disparities in the health achievements and risk factors of individuals and groups ... that need not imply moral judgement' (Kawachi et al., 2002: 647). However, the WHO, as well as the public health field more widely, increasingly view socially structured health inequalities (rather than individual or group-based differences) as profoundly unfair and unjust (CSDH, 2008; Marmot, 2010; Raphael, 2013a). Accordingly, the social patterning of health is viewed as an ethical issue wherein health inequalities *are* health inequities. Whitehead and Dahlgren (2006: 4) argue that 'essentially, all systematic differences in health between different socio-economic groups within a country can be considered unfair and therefore classed as inequities'.

Deciding the extent to which something is unfair and morally unjust is far from straightforward, however. Carter-Pokras and Baquet (2002) point out that if health is viewed as a matter of individual responsibility, then health disparities or health inequalities will not necessarily be viewed as health inequities and as unfair. On the other hand, social inequalities in health refers to systematic differences in health between socio-economic (and other) groups, which are generated and maintained by social arrangements that are themselves unjust (Graham, 2007) and which 'offend common notions of fairness' (Whitehead and Dahlgren, 2006: 3). This line of argument involves moving from empirical descriptive observations to explicit normative judgements based on particular values that relate the social production of health differences to their supposed inevitability and unfairness. Thus, the WHO has increasingly and explicitly linked the pursuit of equity in health to the pursuit of social justice – a fair society (Marmot, 2010) – in which there is an 'absence of systematic disparities in health or in the major social determinants of health between groups who have different levels of underlying social advantage/disadvantage' (Braveman and Gruskin, 2003: 254).

These types of argument, to varying degrees, draw on Rawls' theory of distributive justice (1971) and Sen's (2004) capability approach. Although different in a number of important respects, both premise their arguments on the degree to which social structures ensure people's access to the resources (Rawls' 'primary social goods') and opportunities (Sen's 'capabilities') needed to enjoy good health throughout life. Perhaps because Sen refers specifically to health in a way that is explicitly absent from Rawls' approach, his arguments have been drawn on in international debates relating to human development and the need to evaluate societies not so much in terms of GDP but rather in terms of the degree to which they equalize people's substantive freedoms and capabilities (Graham, 2007). Both arguments focus on the basic structures of societies and the mechanisms that give rise to social inequalities. Thus, justice is undermined 'if society's main economic, social and political institutions require sacrifices from the worse off groups purely for the benefit of the better off groups' (Peter, 2001: 165). From this it follows that social inequalities violate the principle of moral equality and are therefore unjust. Peter (2001) argues that Rawls' theory provides a compatible framework for analysing the social determinants of health as well as pursing ethically-oriented **advocacy** in order to address health inequalities at the level of the social structure and as a matter of social justice.

Using definitions that differentiate patterns of health from judgements about fairness (that is, differentiating between *inequality* and *inequity*) may be preferable because it avoids making assumptions regarding what is or is not fair. While there is some consensus that social inequalities in health are a feature of all modern societies, there remains considerable disagreement whether or not such inequalities are unfair or even modifiable through state action. The maintenance of the class system in neo-liberal societies, for example, would be viewed as necessary by some, regardless of the health consequences (Kawachi *et al.*, 2002).

The significance of inequalities for public health

The burgeoning international **evidence** relating to the social distribution of health inequalities is complex and controversial. Using the official classification of the Registrar General's Social Classes (RGSC) (based on occupation), the Black Report (DHSS, 1980) documented a social *gradient* in mortality: that is to say, differences in mortality stretched right across the six social classes in a step-wise or linear fashion, with those at the top of the hierarchy (Class I professional occupations) having lower mortality and better life expectancy than those below them (II intermediate occupations; IIIn non-manual skilled occupations; IIIm manual skilled occupations; IV partly skilled occupations; V unskilled occupations). Thus, although those in the poorest circumstances had the poorest health, they represented one pole of a broader social gradient. The gradient in health has been extensively documented in a number of countries using level of income, level of education, occupation and area deprivation. Moreover, although differences in life expectancy provide the clearest evidence of the social patterning of health, a similar picture emerges in relation to infant mortality and birth weight, long-standing illness and disability, and self-reported health (Diderichsen *et al.*, 2012). Use of the term 'health inequalities' in the plural also illustrates the multiple ways in which both social inequalities and different dimensions of health are related (Graham, 2007).

In the UK, mounting criticism of the RGSC classification led to its replacement in 1998 with the National Statistics Socio-Economic Classification (NS-SEC), used for the first time in the 2001 UK Census. The classification measures the employment relations and conditions of occupations on the grounds that these are 'central to showing the structure of socio-economic positions in modern society and helping to explain variations in social behaviour and other social phenomena' (ONS, 2010b: 3). The eight-class version covers the whole adult population, including those who have never worked or who are long-term unemployed (Class 8). A similar classification has been produced for comparative European research. The NS-SEC has been used in the Marmot Report (2010) and elsewhere to reveal the social gradient in health in relation to socio-economic position. Some countries (Norway and the USA, for example) use level of education as the main measure of socio-economic position. Whatever the approach, a social gradient consistently emerges.

Social class has an economic basis, relating to people's position in the labour market. Level of economic resources has long been associated with health and quality of life. In this respect the history of public health is anchored in the transformation of England during the Industrial Revolution (*c.* 1750–1860) and the resulting living conditions (Szreter, 1997). The development of laissez-faire (industrial) capitalism during this period gave rise to a division of labour that created a social hierarchy in the form of the class system. New classes reflected not only new occupations but also new forms of wealth and power that become increasingly concentrated among those at the top of the social hierarchy. The impact of these developments on health was, however, different across social divisions. Those with limited income experienced poorer living and working conditions, exposing them to a variety of risks and hardships, an outcome of which was a lower life expectancy compared to the owners of factories and mills. More recently, the health consequences of social, political and economic upheaval have been documented in the post-Soviet countries, which experienced a six-year fall in life expectancy between 1990 and 1994 during the break-up of the USSR, with working class men particularly affected (Leon, 2011).

A rich seam of work has explored the relationship between socio-economic position and health using level of income, both in absolute and relative (income inequality) terms. This literature is especially complex and controversial, particularly in relation to the potential policy implications of linking widening health inequalities with widening income inequalities. The relevance of a country's economic resources (national income in terms of GDP per capita) to health has been extensively explored. Research since the 1970s has revealed that life expectancy increases rapidly in poorer countries during the early phases of **economic development** (Preston, 2007; Wilkinson and Pickett, 2010). Increasing GDP per capita by relatively small amounts has the potential to lift substantial proportions of people out of poverty, supporting a decline in childhood mortality and increasing life expectancy (Gordon, 2010). This point is also relevant to high-income countries where poverty, particularly persistent poverty, is associated with poorer health (Benzeval and Judge, 2001) and reflects the emphasis that Black (DHSS, 1980), Acheson (1998) and Marmot (2010) placed on the alleviation of poverty, especially child poverty. However, increases in life expectancy begin to tail off (at about $5,000 per capita in 2006) and eventually plateau with 'diminishing returns' from increasing per capita income (Preston, 2007: 488). This suggests that the relationship between economic development and life expectancy is less straightforward for those countries aligned along the plateau, many of which (but not all) are high-income countries such as Norway, the USA and Japan (see Wilkinson and Pickett, 2010: 7).

Although GDP is generally viewed as a good indicator of living standards in a country it provides no basis for understanding how economic resources are used (Preston, 2007). Varying life expectancy at a given level of national income per capita may, at least in part, reflect differences in how resources are used within a country. Costa Rica and Cuba have life expectancies that exceed what might be predicted from their GDP per capita. National policies influence the distribution of resources in particular ways at specific points in time and in response to a wide variety of events and circumstances. Policy decisions have differential consequences for sections of the population, some decisions tending towards equalizing social inequalities (and hence health inequalities) while others advantage those already in the best health, widening social and health inequalities further. Goldthorpe (2010) notes that unless the basic structures of inequality are altered, any changes are likely to be ephemeral and easily reversed.

The link between absolute income and health also holds for individuals within countries (Bloom and Canning, 2007), including the so-called 'egalitarian' Nordic countries (Huijts *et al.*, 2010). This means that at any given level of income (for example, in relation to quintiles) an individual's health status is the same, regardless of the income of others in the population (Kawachi *et al.*, 2002). Longitudinal studies indicate that long-term income (rather than income at any one point in time) is particularly significant for health (Benzeval and Judge, 2001). Studies that focus on income tend to suggest a materialist/structuralist explanation for the social gradient in health – the preferred explanation in the Black Report. A materialist perspective can explain how differences across socio-economic classes remain against a background of improvements in population health over time. Even though the health of those in the lowest socio-economic position improves, reaching that of those in the highest socio-economic position, in the intervening period the latter have moved further ahead (Blane, 1985). This is consistent with contemporary research indicating that the widening of health inequalities in recent years has primarily been driven by improvements among those already in the best health (Marmot, 2001).

Materialist/structuralist explanations tend to refer to standards of living and emphasize access to tangible resources such as food, housing, amenities and services, as well as a car, a telephone and so on (Kawachi *et al.*, 2002). Access to these resources is mediated through people's socio-economic position. Increasing income gives people more options for providing a standard of living commensurate with that needed for a healthy life (Link and Phelan, 1995). A healthy life depends on income in relation to needs, which are likely to be greatest among those in the lowest socio-economic position. Their vulnerability is particularly threatened by limited capacity to work (Deaton, 2002). Materialist/structuralist explanations also provide a way of linking inequalities in educational achievement to social inequalities in health. The accrual of wealth among those in higher socio-economic positions provides opportunities for using resources (paying school fees, private tuition and moving to an area with the best schools, for example) to further the educational achievements of their children, increasing their chances of obtaining a good university education and higher lifetime earnings, as well as more satisfying and secure employment (Major, 2011).

The relationship between income *inequality* (relative income reflected in income distribution within a country) and health has also been extensively explored by economists, epidemiologists and sociologists. Their findings tend, however, to be somewhat inconsistent and controversial, attributable, at least in part, to differences in methodology (Wilkinson and Pickett, 2006) as well as poor quality income data in some studies (Judge *et al.*, 2001). The publication of *The Spirit Level* (Wilkinson and Pickett, 2010) created considerable debate, not only in relation to the interpretation of the patterns of health inequalities documented but also in respect of a number of methodological and statistical issues (see, for example, Noble, 2011, for an exposition of the criticisms). Nonetheless, a recent paper concluded that approximately 90 per cent of over 200 studies have found some support for the relationship between income inequality and health (De Maio, 2012). Wilkinson and Pickett measured social inequality using income inequality (utilizing the ratio of the income of the top 20 per cent to the bottom 20 per cent) in a number of high-income countries and explored its relationship to health (life expectancy and mental illness for example) as well as a range of other social problems (such as teenage births and violence). They concluded that countries with smaller income inequalities tended to have better health and social outcomes. The significance of this relationship is important given that income inequality has widened in a number of countries since the late 1970s, primarily driven by faster growth in the top 10 per cent richest households compared to the bottom 10 per cent (OECD, 2011a). Salaries among top earners have risen particularly rapidly.

There has been considerable debate about how to interpret the described gradients in health and other social problems in relation to income inequality. Building on previous work (Brunner, 1997; Chandola *et al.*, 2006; Wilkinson and Pickett, 2006), Wilkinson and Pickett (2010) advanced a psychosocial explanation linking income inequality to low social status. Drawing on evidence from a range of disciplines (biology, animal behaviour, as well as **epidemiology**) they argued that psychosocial factors (for example, uncontrolled threats to self-esteem, feelings of inferiority) mediated a variety of biological consequences via neuroendocrine stress responses over the **lifecourse**. Thus, socio-economic position (an attribute of which is income inequality) was linked to stratification in terms of status. For some sociologists, this oversimplifies a much more complex conceptual understanding of social inequality in relation to class, the preferred indicator of which is occupation (market situation) and it is this that confers status rather than income (Goldthorpe, 2010). Because social class represents a position in the system of economic production and distribution it tends to give rise to class culture and common lifestyles (Roberts, 2012). This means that status rankings are likely to reflect class inequalities that have an institutional basis. Nonetheless, in recent years there has been debate among sociologists that trends towards greater consumption and forms of lifestyle that attract prestige may have led to status becoming more important (Roberts, 2009). In highly commodified societies, such as the USA, status might be more significant than elsewhere (Bartley, 2012a).

Although materialist and psychosocial explanations are sometimes seen as competing, they can be related: social structure influences psychosocial processes as it does access to material resources. Having a home, for example, has both a 'material interpretation and a psychosocial one' (Kawachi et al., 2002: 649). Links can also be made to health behaviours, particularly in respect of smoking and physical inactivity (Marmot, 2001). These (and other) health behaviours also show a social gradient, emphasizing the relevance of context in understanding the differing ways in which people respond to their circumstances. Behavioural and cultural factors such as smoking can be seen as indicators of other differences between the social classes (Blane, 1985; Abel, 2008). Thus, social class provides a way of integrating these differing explanations.

Much less is known about the social patterning of health in relation to other kinds of social division (such as ethnicity, disability, gender, sexuality) or how different dimensions of disadvantage interact and cumulatively shape the chance of living a healthy life (Graham and Kelly, 2004). Ethnic inequalities have been explored extensively in New Zealand and Australia and found to be stark. Comparisons of men and women in relation to life expectancy and various causes of mortality also reveal marked differences. In recent years, the tendency has been to view these differences less in biological terms and more as socially constructed and culturally transmitted, although this also remains controversial.

How health inequalities are explained has considerable implications for the framing of policy. In theory, if health inequalities are to be narrowed then a faster rate of improvement among the more disadvantaged groups is required; in other words, there needs to be a reversal of the trend seen over the last 30 or more years. There needs to be, in other words, a 'levelling up' so that the health of all social groups moves towards that of those in the highest (Whitehead and Dahlgren, 2006). Directing attention to the unequal distribution of health determinants has been advocated (Graham and Kelly, 2004). At a global level, national strategies reflect differing ideological commitments to addressing a social gradient across the whole population rather than a problem of a smaller minority with the greatest needs, which has been found to differ even among the Nordic countries (Vallgårda, 2010). Although there may be greater awareness among policymakers of the extent of health inequalities, their complexity seems to give rise to strategies that continue to target those most in need (Baum et al., 2013).

In England, the Black, Acheson and Marmot Reports each made a number of recommendations relating to social inequalities in health. In the case of the Black Report, they were dismissed as economically unrealistic and ideologically unpalatable to the incoming Conservative government. Reducing inequalities evidently requires political will rather than any technological or scientific innovation (Gordon, 2010). Determinants associated with childhood development in general, and education in particular, both of which relate to parental social position, are especially important (Diderichsen *et al.*, 2012). Whether or not income should be redistributed to reduce income inequality is hotly contested.

A number of countries (The Netherlands, Sweden, Finland and England, for example) have implemented policies aimed at narrowing health inequalities. In the case of England, the Labour government (1997–2010) set out to implement many of the recommendations of the Acheson Report through a variety of strategies, including the introduction of a minimum wage, increased benefits, increased spending on education, as well as specific programmes directed at areas of deprivation (Mackenbach, 2011a). However, despite concerted action, health inequalities persisted during this period (Font *et al.*, 2011; Mackenbach, 2011a). Difficult as it is to measure the effect of such multifaceted strategies, taking a longer-term view might be more instructive given the likely time-lag in effects (Bambra, 2012). Nonetheless, there is some consensus that in spite of the duration and the intensity of Labour's strategy it did little to alter inequalities in health. Policies, of course, can also widen inequalities as well as narrow them (Lorenc *et al.*, 2013).

Conclusion

Social inequalities in health have been documented in several countries. They have also been shown to persist over time, widening in recent years in many high-income countries. The policy responses of governments to the global financial crisis has, furthermore, brought new challenges in relation to reducing inequalities. By 2015, the UK government, for example, plans to spend a lower proportion of its GDP than any other major European country, the consequence of which will be a reduction in public services and welfare benefits (Dorling, 2012). These trends are likely to widen inequalities at a faster rate than in the previous decade (Barr *et al.*, 2012). Indeed, it seems that countries with large inequalities (such as England) are less likely to invest in collective goods (Mackenbach *et al.*, 2013), relying instead on behaviour change interventions. Given the evidence indicating that social inequalities in health have structural origins, this is likely to be a public health policy that widens rather than narrows health inequalities.

LIFECOURSE PERSPECTIVES

Context

Lifecourse perspectives have become increasingly common in public health in recent years. In part, this reflects the growing influence of lifecourse **epidemiology** as well as the social and behavioural sciences in understanding patterns of **health** and disease. Both the CSDH (2008) and the Marmot Review (2010) based much of their analysis of social **inequalities** in health on a lifecourse perspective, prioritizing early childhood as a key entry point for policymakers. Notwithstanding the conceptual and methodological complexities of lifecourse studies, there is an increasing appreciation of the value of studying health and its social distribution over the entire life span (Bartley, 2012b). While lifecourse studies reveal generational continuities in disadvantage and its consequences, they also provide a way of exploring resilience against the odds.

Defining a lifecourse perspective

Taking a lifecourse perspective means focusing on social biography, thereby shifting the emphasis away from the traditional adult **lifestyle** model of disease **risk**. Although definitions vary across disciplines, there is much common ground. All take as their starting point a developmental position – that is, health and well-being are under development from the time of conception through all the major life stages: prenatal life, infancy, childhood, youth, early, middle and late adulthood. The process of moving through these stages tends to be regarded not as driven simply by biology but, rather, as unfolding within a social context that involves major status passages marked by 'life events', such as going to school, entering the employment market, marriage, becoming a parent, and retirement (Roberts, 2009). Within the general field of lifecourse studies emphasis varies in the extent to which biological, psychological or social processes and outcomes are the focus of attention. Lifecourse **epidemiology** has tended to focus on biological processes and disease outcomes. In recent years it has broadened its scope to include a range of psychosocial processes and health-related outcomes. What a lifecourse perspective offers, however, is the potential for integrating biological, psychological and social models of health as well as explaining the interaction between these factors in the development of health and disease (Ben-Shlomo and Kuh, 2002). This broader perspective is encapsulated in Gilman's (2012: 2124) view of lifecourse epidemiology as seeking to understand 'the extent to which long-term health and well-being are influenced by factors very early on in the life course ... [and] the mechanisms accounting for these influences'. In other words, it seeks to understand, for example, why smaller babies tend to have shorter lives, by examining how physical and social exposures and experiences during gestation, childhood, adolescence, young adulthood and later adult life independently, cumulatively and interactively influence health (Porta, 2008). Nonetheless, lifecourse influences on developmental trajectories are, in part, complex because they can give rise to processes that raise health risks as well as protect against them. That said, studies indicate that risks – as well as protective factors – tend to cluster among some groups.

Recent work has sought to differentiate the lifecourse concept further. Graham *et al.* (2010), for example, used the concept of 'socioeconomic lifecourse' (**education** and current socio-economic circumstances, for example) and 'domestic lifecourse' (such as age of becoming a mother, current cohabitation situation) to understand the social patterning of cigarette smoking. This more nuanced approach to studying the lifecourse reflects its multidimensional character.

The significance of a lifecourse perspective for public health

Over several decades, a number of countries (the UK, New Zealand, the USA and the Nordic countries in particular) have invested in long-term follow-up studies of children. Together, these have considerably advanced understanding of risk and protective factors across the lifespan. Developments in computing and statistics in recent decades have also given rise to improved capacity and capability to analyse large and complex datasets in terms of continuities and change, by linking data from one part of the lifecourse to another. The British Birth Cohort Studies (carried out in 1946, 1958, 1970, 2000) alongside the UK Life Study (2012) have been especially influential, based as they are on large representative samples of the population with long-term follow-up. The 1958 Birth Cohort Study, for example, included approximately 17,500 infants born in one week and followed-up at ages 7, 11, 16, 23, 33, 42 and 46 years of age. Data on family background, health, cognitive and behavioural development, educational achievement, employment and family formation have been collected. The repetition of birth cohort studies also allows comparison between different cohorts (for example, 1958 with 1970), allowing the effects of age, period and cohort to be disentangled (Chandola and Marmot, 2004). Repeated cross-sectional surveys (on different cohorts of people rather than the same people) cannot provide the same insights. Researchers can apply for free access to the birth cohort data through the UK data archive.

In some countries, such as Norway, record linkage studies offer a cost-effective and more efficient way of conducting follow-up studies. This approach is dependent on having a unique identifying system – as is the case in Norway – that gives a personal identification number to each person. This enables information contained in different health records (as well as other kinds, such as education records) to be brought together and related. Privacy, confidentiality and civil liberty issues have precluded many countries from introducing a unique identifier system.

The 'critical periods' model has been prominent in lifecourse studies. It is of potential value in public health because it focuses attention on where in the lifespan policymakers might effectively direct their attention. In biological terms, a critical period refers to the susceptibility of tissues and organs to harmful influences, such as sub-optimal nutrition, the consumption of alcohol during pregnancy or exposure to chemicals found in everyday items. Typically, critical periods are those during which organ systems are developing through processes of rapid cell division and differentiation during prenatal life. Exposure during a developmental 'window' (of limited duration) can have lasting biological effects on anatomical structures and metabolic systems (sometimes referred to as biological programming) but the consequences may only become apparent many years later. Outside this window, there is no increased risk through exposure. The pioneering work of Barker (1998) on the foetal origins of disease – now more commonly referred to as the developmental origins model – has been influential in this regard. His retrospective epidemiological approach showed that death from heart disease in later life was more likely among those who were smaller at birth and one year, a pattern that has been found in many countries (Ben-Shlomo and Kuh, 2002). Poor prenatal growth has also been linked to the development of non-insulin dependent diabetes and hypertension in later life (Chandola and Marmot, 2004). Analysis of data from the Dutch famine (1944–45) found that maternal undernutrition during gestation, especially early gestation, increased the risk of glucose intolerance, coronary heart disease and disturbed blood coagulation in later life (Roseboom *et al.*, 2006).

The concept of critical periods has been extended to children's development during the postnatal period, particularly in relation to brain development. The brain has considerable developmental plasticity (capacity to change and develop in response to sensory stimulation and learning) postnatally. This means that from birth up until the age of about two, children's brain development remains particularly susceptible to a broad range of harms. Moreover, their development becomes increasingly interdependent with others in their expanding social world. Appropriate stimulation, care and support have the potential to create the conditions for optimal development. This explains how 'children's physical, emotional and cognitive capabilities [are] inseparable from what is popularly known as "growing up"' (Graham, 2007: 145). Bronfenbrenner's (1986) ecological (multi-level) model of child development provides a point of reference for understanding the lifelong significance of processes of interaction throughout the whole of childhood. Lifecourse studies have tended to focus on the prenatal environment, early infancy and childhood. More recently, adolescence as a major period of transition and identity formation, has been the focus of attention in studies that have sought to understand how health-related behaviours such as physical activity might track into adulthood and contribute to adult health inequalities (Due *et al.*, 2011).

Although terminology varies, Ben-Shlomo and Kuh (2002) argue that the term 'sensitive' (rather than critical) period is preferable to use when referring to behavioural development. They argue that a sensitive period is more open-ended than a critical period; there is a time period during which exposure can have a strong effect but beyond that weaker effects are still possible. To some extent the developmental origins model gets round these issues because it includes the idea of accumulated risk over the entire lifecourse. Some studies have shown, for example, that the association between insulin resistance and low birth weight only holds for those who become obese in childhood or adulthood. This implies biological systems may be compromised by earlier events but that the consequences vary depending on other exposures (Chandola and Marmot, 2004). Theoretical models that seek to explain the pathways that link exposures to various outcomes are likely to become more sophisticated as new **evidence** emerges. Central to lifecourse studies, however, is the analytic process of linking exposures, events and experiences to specific outcomes in a temporal sequence. This approach enables clustering of risks or protective factors among some groups and chains of risks to be explored, where one adverse exposure or experience leads to another. A lifecourse approach has been used to explain social inequalities in health in terms of socially patterned experiences and exposures at different stages of the life span (Ben-Shlomo and Kuh, 2002). The point here is that social and economic policies can influence how people move through different life stages, a matter that is of particular significance during 'socially critical periods' (Bartley *et al.*, 1997: 1195). This provides a way of understanding how social phenomena might become 'embodied', that is to say, incorporated into the biology of people. The dynamic and complex character of biological and social interactions as children progress through the lifespan, as well as their capacity for adaptation to events and experiences, however, poses considerable theoretical and methodological challenges for lifecourse studies.

In public health, childhood and adolescence have become recognized as formative periods during which developmental health unfolds with long-term consequences. It is well-established that a poor start in life significantly limits the extent to which children can realize their potential (Graham and Power, 2004). The interdependence of children with their parents for love, care and attention, directs attention to the family environment. Parenting capacity is, however, interdependent with parental income, the family home and neighbourhood, as well as parents' own health and well-being, all of which are important to children's healthy development (Bartley, 2012b). Stress during childhood has been linked to susceptibility to future stress, possibly through influencing biological processes relating to the stress response (Adam and Kumari, 2009). Lifecourse studies also indicate that the most developmentally supportive environment for children is a stable household with two parents, both of whom are in paid work (McMunn *et al.*, 2012). The policy implications of these findings point towards supporting parents at home and in work through flexible working arrangements and parental leave, among other things. Currently, for those in full-time employment, working hours are longer in the UK than any other European country (Bartley, 2012b). How adolescence is negotiated has also been shown to have longer-term consequences for adult mental health. Both early and delayed entry into adult roles seem to have implications for mental health. At every stage of the lifespan, however, positive relationships with friends and family have a central place in developing resilience and various capabilities. Success in **education** has benefits that stretch throughout the lifespan and well into older age. Although the mechanisms are unclear, those with a higher level of education are less likely to experience Alzheimer's disease than those with a lower level (Bartley, 2012b).

Conclusion

Lifecourse studies represents a dynamic and changing field. Such studies are providing rich data of direct relevance to public health in general and public health policy in particular. The ecological and multilevel perspective on which such studies are based opens up a range of policy options for both how to create the conditions to support healthy development as well as when and how to intervene to prevent harm (Graham, 2002). While early family support and intervention remain of particular importance, the lifelong relevance of succeeding at education and having a network of good friends are an especially significant part of the picture.

LIFESTYLE

Context

'Lifestyle' has become the preferred way of talking about how people live their lives, not just in the public health field but in many disciplinary and professional arenas. In public health, lifestyle is identified as a major **determinant** of **health** and is frequently targeted for intervention. In relation to physical activity, for example, efforts are directed at those with 'sedentary lifestyles' in order to increase their activity. Yet, until relatively recently, people's ways of life were customary and somewhat inevitable, circumscribed by their income, their family circumstances and how they earned their livings (Roberts, 2009). They had, in other words, little *choice* in how they lived their lives. Choosing how to live has become possible in consumer societies where there is considerable scope for spending money on non-essentials. The relatively recent emergence of the term 'lifestyle' reflects this shift in society, inferring as it does freedom to choose one's 'style of life'. 'Choice' is, therefore, central to discussions relating to lifestyle. In the public health field, 'lifestyle choice' tends to be somewhat uncritically invoked as a way of explaining people's behaviour. A more critically informed perspective on lifestyle suggests a more cautious approach to the term is required if it is to be of value in understanding patterns of behaviour.

Defining lifestyle

In the public health field, lifestyle has been conceptualized, operationalized and defined in two contrasting ways. The 'lifestyle model of disease' emerged in the latter half of the twentieth century as a consequence of the increasing role played by **epidemiology** in public health (Hansen and Easthope, 2007). Large-scale cohort studies such as the Framingham study (initiated in 1948 in a small town in Massachusetts, USA) identified several (lifestyle) behaviours that were associated with an elevated **risk** of cardio-vascular disease. Smoking, lack of exercise and over-eating (specifically saturated fat) were established as 'risk factors' and CVD was defined as a 'lifestyle disease'. The premise of the lifestyle model is that diseases are the result of unhealthy clusters of behaviours and disease **prevention** requires **behaviour change** (or lifestyle modification). Definitions based on this model tend to emphasize individual behaviours or habits viewed as *intentionally* chosen by individuals. A particular feature of public health **policy** in a number of countries in recent years has been an emphasis on lifestyle diseases and risk factor modification.

There has, nevertheless, been a sustained critique of the lifestyle model of disease in recent years, based upon three interrelated issues. The most fundamental of these relates to the causal mechanism implied by the lifestyle model of disease. Most diseases are caused by a web of interrelated proximal and distal factors, illustrated particularly well in the case of CVD. Reducing **causality** to a single aetiological agent, such as lifestyle, or a specific behavioural aspect of lifestyle, oversimplifies complex phenomena (Vallgårda, 2011). The lifestyle model of disease is, therefore, reductionist in that specific behaviours (risk factors) are viewed in isolation from other relevant factors; that is to say, there is no linking of distal with proximal factors. The model also offers little by way of understanding how lifestyles are developed and maintained. Critics argue that 'choice' is more complex than implied by an individually oriented and reductionist approach to lifestyle. The emphasis in public health on lifestyle at the expense of other factors has given rise to the term 'lifestylism', used to refer to the 'pathologizing' of common forms of social behaviour, such as sedentary behaviour and smoking (Rodmell and Watt, 1986: 4).

Drawing on these criticisms, an alternative perspective on lifestyle has emerged in recent years. Informed by a sociological understanding of human action, this perspective focuses on the interplay between social circumstances and behaviours, moving beyond individual lifestyle risk factors. Cockerham (2000: 1314) for example, defines health lifestyles in terms of 'collective patterns of health-related behaviour based on choices from options available to people according to their life chances'.

Defining lifestyle in terms of 'collective patterns' shifts the focus away from individuals towards groups based on wider social divisions – such as social class. In this vein, Abel *et al.* (2000: 63) propose the following definition: 'health lifestyles comprise interacting patterns of health-related behaviours, orientations, and resources adapted by groups of individuals in response to their social, cultural and economic environment'. The development of more critically and theoretically informed definitions of lifestyle such as those cited above, provides a more adequate basis for understanding how (un)healthy lifestyles are developed and maintained, as well as providing some insight into why they are so difficult to change.

The significance of lifestyle for public health

Health and lifestyle surveys are routinely used to chart lifestyle patterns in populations and population sub-groups. The Health Survey for England is an example of such a survey, carried out annually and involving the collection of data at a household level on general health, smoking, drinking alcohol, height, weight, blood pressure, use of health services and medication, as well as socio-demographic information. Such surveys reveal that health-related behaviour varies according to social position (Calnan and Williams, 1991). Those in more disadvantaged circumstances, for example, are more likely to smoke, have a poorer diet, be less physically active during leisure time, be less likely to use preventive health care services and more likely to have unplanned and earlier pregnancies (Benzeval *et al.*, 1995). Indeed, there is a tendency for these behaviours to cluster among social groups (Buck and Frosini, 2012; Coulter, 1987). A gradient in lifestyle behaviours was found in the Whitehall studies (of the British Civil Service) where those in lower grades of employment were more likely to smoke, be overweight and physically inactive, as well as have higher blood pressure. The gradient in lifestyles relating to particular forms of behaviour has been used as the basis for explaining the poorer health of those in lower grades (and social groups more generally). The Whitehall study found, however, that differences in lifestyles across employment grades explained approximately one-third of the increased risk of death from CVD (Davey Smith *et al.*, 1990). **Evidence** from these and other studies indicates that while differences in lifestyles remain important, they provide only part of the explanation for the social gradient in health. The findings also raise questions about how these differences in patterns of lifestyle are developed and why those in higher socio-economic positions are more likely to change their lifestyles in a healthy direction.

Drawing on the work of sociologists such as Weber and Bourdieu, Cockerham (2000) has explored these questions and developed a more complex and contextually-oriented conceptualization of lifestyle. From a Weberian perspective, life conduct (life choices that people have in their selection of lifestyles – that is to say, self-directed behaviour) and life chances (the probability of realizing choices) make up the two interrelated dimensions of lifestyle. According to this view, the likelihood of realizing choices is anchored in structural conditions such as social class, gender, age and ethnicity. In short, lifestyles are life choices shaped by life chances and it is this that gives rise to the observed collective patterns of behaviours that are described as 'lifestyle'. The collective dimension of lifestyle choices is captured in the concept group habitus – systems of durable, transposable dispositions shared with others (Bourdieu,

1984; Elias, 1991). Thus, class cultures, for example, influence social practices, such as food habits, and these habits in turn, help reproduce class culture. Group norms and interpersonal dynamics more or less 'force' the choice to eat in particular ways, drink alcohol or smoke, for example, a particular group habitus tending to channel behaviour routinely down prescribed paths. The greater propensity of young working class males to engage in higher risk behaviours compared to their middle-class counterparts is a further illustration of this process. Beyond class, nationality, gender and ethnicity also influence lifestyle formation (Cockerham, 2005). Thinking in terms of collective patterns of behaviour also provides a mechanism for understanding how health is unequally produced (Abel and Frohlich, 2012).Viewing lifestyles as meaningful social practices associated with the constraints and opportunities of a particular social location provides a potentially more adequate way of conceptualizing the notion of choice. Graham (1989) suggests that patterns of behaviour are likely to involve 'health compromises' rather than 'choices' especially for those in more disadvantaged circumstances. Cockerham (2000) provides examples of the way in which social location patterns lifestyles with reference to alcohol consumption and the development of CVD in Russia. For men, meeting with friends has traditionally involved drinking strong vodka over a short period of time accompanied by small snacks. The expectation is that each man will drink as much as the others in the group regardless of the desire to do otherwise. Changes since the fall of communism have given rise to a convergence in levels of drinking between men and women in Russia, alcohol consumption having become much more common among women (Hinote *et al.*, 2009). Hinote *et al.* conclude that a change in political ideology has meant that women were 'more able to embrace these behavioural practices, if they wish to do so' (1259).

There is little to suggest that this more complex and critically informed perspective on lifestyle and lifestyle choice has informed public health policy and practice. The restricted form of the terms (based on individual, personal responsibility, and disease risk) has found its way into **social marketing**. Here, the concept lifestyle is used to imply a particular identity, reflected in the kinds of things people buy, the activities they are involved in and the tastes they have. These constitute so-called 'lifestyle groups' based on patterns of consumption. Clusters of behaviours form the basis upon which different lifestyle groups are constructed, each conveying a particular kind of identity. The extent to which these lifestyle groups can be considered robust and valid categories independently of social markers such as social class has, nevertheless been keenly debated. Although lifestyles are patterned – particularly in relation to age and life-stage – they are also fluid in that 'some are lived only on holiday, at weekends or on nights out' (Roberts, 2009: 149).

Although policymakers have recognized the need to confront the wider determinants of health if **inequalities** are to be narrowed, specific policies and strategies have tended to be formulated in terms of targeting individual lifestyles and behaviours. This tendency has been termed 'lifestyle drift' and viewed as one of the main explanations for the limited progress made on narrowing health inequalities (Baum, 2011; Popay *et al.*, 2010). Lifestyle has become embedded in public health policy and practice discourses in many countries. For practitioners, emphasizing choice and personal responsibility can give rise to feelings of inadequacy, helplessness and failure among those who are the target of their behaviour change efforts. Regardless of practitioners' personal and professional 'philosophies of practice', however, it may be difficult to work against the grain of dominant ideologies (Rodmell and Watt, 1986).

Conclusion

The widely referred to *Ottawa Charter* (1986) argued that the aim of **health promotion** is to 'make the healthy choice the easy choice' through policies that remove obstacles to healthy living. In England more recently, a reformulation of this idea has been expressed in a number of government documents in which healthy lifestyles are discussed alongside notions of personal responsibility and individual free choice, with a more limited role for the state beyond providing health information (DH, 2004; Secretary of State for Health, 2010). Drawing on a number of well-established sociological ideas can, however, lead to a more fine-grained appreciation of how 'processes shape the lifecourses and biographies of individuals' (Williams, 2003: 140), an aspect of which is lifestyle formation and reproduction. In particular, a more sociologically informed perspective can help us understand how 'lifestyle choices are also ways that individuals can exercise some semblance of agency when many events and forces seem beyond their control' (Hinote *et al.*, 2009: 1261). Recognizing the interplay between individuals and social context over time thus leads to a more realistic appreciation of how lifestyles emerge and are sustained.

MEDICINE

Context

Medicine has become a major system of knowledge and practice in contemporary society. It is not surprising, therefore, that medical ideas have become 'institutionalized and embodied in law and administration' (Blaxter, 2010: 11). Contemporary medicine is practiced within a system of health care involving varying degrees of organizational complexity in different countries. The rise of modern medicine reflects the influence of science and technology, as well as the complex array of contemporary illnesses and diseases with which it is concerned. It also reflects the considerable power of the medical profession. Although medicine as a profession continues to receive considerable respect, it has come under increasing criticism in recent years. Within public health, criticisms have centred on medicine's 'downstream' approach to **health** and disease and neglect of the wider social **determinants** of health; the limited effectiveness of many treatments; the disempowering character of clinical encounters; and the financial costs of medicine. Questions continue to be raised about the value and place of medicine in contemporary society.

Defining medicine

The term 'medicine' is derived from the Latin *ars medicina*, meaning the art of healing. In prehistoric times, healing was entwined with spiritual and mystical belief systems. Over time, however, different systems of medicine have developed in various parts of the world: Chinese, Babylonian and Roman forms of medicine and Ayurvedic medicine in the Indian subcontinent, for example. These different systems were each rooted in particular cultural beliefs that framed the causes of illness and disease and the ways that health could be restored (Kleinman and Mendelsohn, 1978). The shift towards a rational and empirical approach to health and disease is believed to have begun during the sixth century BC (Sigerist, 1961) but was propelled towards the modern form during the enlightenment (seventeenth and eighteenth centuries). Greek medicine is believed to be the foundation from which Western scientific medicine has developed. Modern, Western medicine as a system of ideas and practices, as well as a profession, developed rapidly during the nineteenth century, predominantly as a consequence of developments in science. The work of early bacteriologists, such as Koch, and their interest in discovering the causes of infectious diseases, was influential in shaping views of disease. This brief historical sketch illustrates some of the key characteristics of medicine as it has come to be practiced in the twenty-first century. Definitions of medicine are sparse, however, and tend to relate to the many and varied specialisms. In broad terms however, medicine is viewed as the science and practice of diagnosis, treatment and **prevention** of diseases. The medical model, discussed below, provides a more detailed framework for exploring the character of modern medicine.

The significance of medicine for public health

Popular academic reference to the 'medical model' is rooted in the pre-eminence of medicine in the modern world. It is used to describe the dominant approach to health in Western societies. Blaxter (2010) refers to the *bio*medical model to reflect the influence of the biological sciences – its methods and principles – on the development of medicine. As an 'ideal type', the (bio)medical model comprises several interrelated ideas: (i) the philosophical concept of mind-body dualism, (that the mind and the body – the mental and the material – can be treated separately); (ii) health as the absence of 'disease'; (iii) *ill*-health as a deviation from 'normal' (in terms of biological variables such as blood pressure); (iv) diseases having theoretically identifiable causes, referred to as the doctrine of specific aetiology; and (v) each disease having its own distinct set of universal features. The (bio)medical model is viewed as reductionist in that it reduces explanations for disease to pathology – abnormalities residing in the cells, tissues, organs and systems of the body. Medical practice (and reasoning) – evident during clinical encounters between doctor and patient – centres on diagnosis on the basis of signs and symptoms and treatment. In this manner, medicine is viewed as adopting a mechanical metaphor (Nettleton, 1995), viewing the body as a machine that, although 'broken', can be 'fixed'. Such conceptual models are representations of phenomena, which inevitably over-simplify reality. Unsurprisingly, the (bio)medical model has come under increasing scrutiny and criticism since the 1960s both from within and outside the medical profession. As Roberts (2009: 166) observes, 'nowadays the model is acknowledged by all concerned to be a parody of current medical thought and practice'.

One of the central criticisms of medicine, however, relates to the way in which medical ideas – such as those relating to diagnosis – are imported into an analysis of social problems. The term medicalization – the process of framing social phenomena as medical issues – emerged at some point in the 1970s as a critique of medicine, originally from within psychiatry but was developed subsequently by sociologists. Zola

(1972: 495) argued that 'if anything can be shown in some way to affect the workings of the body and to a lesser extent the mind, then it can be labelled … "a medical problem"'. Defining a problem as 'medical' results, it is claimed, in the *creation* of patients (Blaxter, 2010; Crawford, 1980). The encroachment of medicine into more and more aspects of everyday life not hitherto deemed 'medical' – childbirth, menstrual discomfort and the menopause – has been discussed extensively, particularly among feminists. Various forms of 'deviance' – madness, alcoholism, homosexuality – have also been 'medicalized' only, in the case of the latter, to be subsequently de-medicalized (in 1973) when it was no longer viewed as a clinical mental disorder. Gambling 'addiction', on the other hand, has recently become the subject of medical attention with the development of new guidelines for **screening** and treatment (Bowden-Jones and Smith, 2012). Pharmacological developments have accelerated the process of medicalization in recent years, making 'treatments' available for unhappiness, male sexual difficulties, chronic fatigue and childhood hyperactivity. This has particularly been the case since the emergence of the Human Genome Project in 2000, promising advances in genomics and the transformation of medicine through the development of personalized medicines – that is to say, medicines tailored to the 'prediction, diagnosis and treatment of the individual' (Tutton, 2012: 1721). However, few such pharmacological developments have materialized to date.

Medicalization has largely been constructed as a negative phenomenon – one that tends to result in interference in people's lives, eroding their capacity to care for themselves and others (Illich, 1975). To this extent, medicalization is said to serve the particular interests of powerful groups by exercising social control over others (Zola, 1972). In the case of HIV/AIDS, for example, routine screening offers a way of detecting HIV status and providing medication. Detection of pre-disease states can, however, be viewed as extending medical surveillance into the lives of apparently healthy people. A similar point can be made in relation to lowering the cut-off points for cardiovascular **risk** factors (blood pressure and serum cholesterol) that can lead to large numbers of people designated as in need of medical treatment (Le Fanu, 2012). The process of medicalization can also lead to iatrogenesis – literally, 'doctor-generated' adverse effects of medical interventions (Porta, 2008: 121). While medicine is not the only profession that gives rise to adverse consequences, Bunker (2001) estimated that there were between 75,000 and 150,000 iatrogenic deaths in the USA annually, including those that resulted from medical error. Others, however, have argued that there have been real clinical and symbolic benefits of medicalization. Defining a condition as appropriate for medical attention opens up opportunities for the alleviation of symptoms. Notwithstanding the difficulties faced by health professionals in 'detecting' and responding appropriately to women in a violent relationship, recent developments in the UK have publicized the health consequences of domestic violence for women and their children, contributing to the reduction in stigma and blame that has been attached to it. In other cases, such as chronic fatigue syndrome, patients can benefit from a diagnosis simply because it helps them make sense of unpleasant experiences and offers possibilities for managing and living with the condition. In reality, medicalization is likely to have both positive and negative consequences. The critical question is whose interests are served by medicalizing phenomena?

Medicine has become increasingly complex in recent decades. While scientific and technological developments have expanded the number of 'conditions' that can be detected and treated, broader socio-cultural processes are equally significant. Blaxter (2010) points out that as well as being dependent on doctors, 'patients' can also drive medicalization – in the case of plastic surgery, for example. There are, nevertheless, several developments that appear to run counter to medicalizing trends. For example, members of the public can be less passive and more critical in clinical encounters (Williams and Calnan, 1996) partly as a consequence of the dramatic growth in information technologies such as the Internet (Greenhalgh and Wessley, 2004). Such democratizing tendencies – including an increasing emphasis on the involvement of service users in health **policy** and practice (Branfield and Beresford, 2006) – are relevant to understanding how clinical encounters might be changing. In addition, new developments, such as an increasing use of complementary therapies, reflect varying degrees of disenchantment with modern medicine. One aspect of this trend is the (re)emergence of self-care. Recent evidence suggests that for GPs at least, these and other factors combine to limit their powers of discretion (Cheraghi-Sohi and Calnan, 2013). Research has shown that the reporting of diverse aspects of biomedicine relevant to everyday life in various media has become more mixed in recent years (Hallin *et al.*, 2013).

As well as the (bio)medical model, the medical *profession* itself has come under increased scrutiny. Professions have always been characterized by their relative autonomy. The medical profession continues to exert authority and power over others – patients as well as other professional groups such as nurses and other allied professions – in matters relating to health. In spite of developments that have sought to regulate and control the medical profession in recent years, its members continue to exercise control over the organization and terms of their work (Gabe *et al.*, 2004), although there are some signs that this is changing.

From a public health perspective, significant questions have been raised about the role of medicine in relation to improvements in population health. McKeown (1976) questioned the orthodoxy that increases in life expectancy since the mid-nineteenth century were due to medical therapeutic interventions. His analysis of the declines in death rate in Britain due to different types of infectious diseases (air-borne; water/food borne; contagion; other) led him to conclude that improving nutrition as a result of better living standards (including increased earnings for those in employment) was the most likely explanation for the patterns he observed. McKeown also demonstrated that, with the exception of smallpox and diphtheria, the substantial declines in mortality occurred well before the time at which either effective immunization procedures or therapies (antibiotics, for example) were available. However, McKeown's analysis created considerable controversy. Szreter (1988), for example, questioned McKeown's analysis in relation to the decline in mortality during 1850–1914, not so much in terms of his overall conclusion but rather in terms of the way he gave primacy to nutrition above improvements in sanitation. Szreter argues that an aspect of rapid industrialization during this period was chaotic urban congestion and that this was considerably ameliorated by public health intervention. As he points out, although the employed were better off they still lived in squalor. Szreter focuses upon the politically and ideologically motivated actions of groups (including medical officers of health and other doctors) who collectively brought about a number of strategic public health developments, such as the London sewerage system.

Trying to separate the effects of medical care for an entire population from those of other determinants of health is fraught with difficulty but similar analyses have been carried out in other countries. Mackenbach (1996) analysed the contribution of medicine to mortality decline in the Netherlands between 1875 and 1970. He estimated that between 5 and 18.5 per cent of the total decline could be attributed to health care. Wolleswinkel-van den Bosch *et al.* (1998) also concluded that medical care and technology had been particularly important after the introduction of antibiotics in the Netherlands after 1945. Focusing on data from the USA, Bunker (2001) concluded that 5–5.5 years of the 30-year increase in life expectancy since 1900 and half of the 7–7.5-year increase since 1950 could be attributed to clinical interventions. This led him to conclude that medicine was a major determinant of life expectancy in the USA.

While the contribution of medicine continues to be debated, conditions in various countries at different times suggest that medicine can have considerable impact when other prerequisites have been met (Frankel, 2001). Furthermore, it seems self-evident that some medical interventions (such as removal of cataracts) can, at relatively low cost, significantly improve quality of life. Nevertheless, in spite of large increases in expenditure on health care, there remain high levels of ill-health in most populations, as well as new and emerging health problems.

Drawing on the sociological critiques of medicine, many working in public health have become critical of medicine and medicalization, particularly on the grounds that it separates 'conditions' from the social systems that have given rise to them (Roberts, 2009). Isolating the body from the person and the person from the wider social, cultural and biographic determinants of health not only leads to a very partial understanding of health but also to a tendency to deploy a narrow range of interventions. A recent example is the case of HIV/AIDS where the social causes (poverty, lack of **education** and power among women, access to free and reliable contraception and so on) have been displaced by a focus on antiretroviral medication. As Barbour (2011) argues, in such cases the public health issue becomes 'reframed' in terms of ensuring equal access to medication rather than focusing on the social determinants of HIV/AIDS.

Conclusion

In the early decades of the twenty-first century, medicine and the organization of health care with which it is entwined, are undergoing considerable re-examination in many countries as a consequence of both economic and political imperatives. In England, doctors and other health care professionals are increasingly likely to become employees of private sector organizations as an expanded mixed economy of health care provision emerges (see, for example, the Health and Social Care legislation in the UK). Diversification of job roles is likely to accelerate within modern medicine as duties formerly the sole preserve of doctors continue to be reallocated, particularly as doctors become further involved in management and administration. Whether or not these developments create opportunities for reorienting health care towards a **health promotion** model of practice (WHO, 1986) remains to be seen.

OFFICIAL STATISTICS

Context

Official statistics, in one form or another, constitute the bedrock of public health. Indeed, the public health movement of mid-nineteenth century England gathered considerable momentum and force on the basis of the officially documented patterns of mortality associated with the cholera epidemics in London. Since then, governments in many countries have invested considerable resources in expanding systems for the collection, analysis and dissemination of data relating to population **health** and illness, the economy and many aspects of social life. While of considerable value to a variety of constituent groups beyond governments, official statistics can be highly contentious. Politicians, academics and the media regularly debate the veracity and interpretation of the latest government figures. The emergence of independent 'fact-checking' websites such as Fullfact (http://fullfact.org), which focuses attention on statistics and statements released by politicians and the media, reflects a demand from various groups for 'believable' facts. Understanding these issues requires a critical appreciation of the processes through which official statistics are produced as well as the uses and misuses to which they are put. At best they constitute a rich resource for public health policy-makers, practitioners and researchers. At worst, they can be used to obfuscate and camouflage the reality they are meant to clarify.

Defining official statistics

Official statistics in the form of quantitative data are often referred to as national statistics. Consequently, government statistics departments in many countries are named the bureau or office of national statistics. Both terms signal the source and ownership of the statistics, namely the government. Reflecting this key feature, Kerrison and Macfarlane (2000: 2) define official statistics as those that are 'collected, commissioned or published by the central government departments and agencies, local government and NHS [or other health service]'. Although structures vary from country to country, together these departments and agencies make up a government's statistical service. These data collection activities reflect the state's 'financial and legislative power' to collect information about its population (Levitas and Guy, 1996: 2). Not only does the term 'official statistics' sound authoritative, it also lends an air of authenticity to statistical information produced by a government; in other words, it suggests government statistics are credible and provide a sound basis for planning, forecasting, policy-making and so forth.

Governments produce an extensive array of official statistics. Core areas of work include vital (civil) registration systems for recording live births, deaths (including cause of death) and marriages (and subsequent changes to marital status); the census (providing information about the population and its social, economic and demographic characteristics); and a large number of population-based surveys based on nationally representative samples. Increasingly, statistical outputs are also derived from various kinds of routinely collected administrative data from publicly funded services, agencies and programmes. Annual crime statistics based on reported crimes and quarterly returns on unemployment from claimant returns, for example, are the by-products of these administrative processes.

In recent years, a number of global institutions such as the WHO, the OECD and the UN, as well as Eurostat (the statistical office of the EU) regularly produce statistics on a country-by-country basis. Statistics published by these organizations tend to come under the umbrella of official statistics because they draw on national statistics provided by governments. The British Household Panel Survey for example, contributes to the European Household Survey (Roberts, 2009). Under EU law, member states are required to collect and provide specific statistics to enable the production of European-wide statistical outputs. Approximately 80 per cent of official statistics collected by the UK government's statistical service is required by EU law (Travis, 2013).

The significance of official statistics for public health

Countries vary in the robustness and comprehensiveness of their statistical services. The UK Statistical Service is generally viewed favourably in relation to other similar comparator countries, as well as having some particular strengths in longitudinal studies and access to microdata (records containing individual-level information) (Holt, 2008). Online access to datasets and the increasingly sophisticated use of web-based tools to analyse and present data at a variety of geographic levels have increased the potential value of official statistics in studying trends and informing local strategies. Although health care data are important for revealing patterns of service usage and outcomes ensuing therefrom, the statistics produced by most, if not all government departments are of considerable relevance to public health, relating as they do to the wider **determinants** of health and social **inequalities**. For researchers, in particular, they constitute a cheap and often largely under-explored resource.

Documenting public health phenomena in order to make them visible relies on official statistics. Governments, for example, use their statistics to highlight issues and justify the need for **policy** attention. The US government is unusual among high-income countries in not reporting health statistics by social class, preferring instead to present analyses in terms of race and gender (Kawachi *et al.*, 2005). Recent proposals in England to withdraw from data collection in key areas of public health – smoking, teenage pregnancies and drinking – as well as reconfigure the current format of the census (Travis, 2013) have provoked considerable debate. Without up-to-date statistics, issues become less visible, more contentious and easier to ignore. Withdrawing from data collection in sensitive policy areas on the basis that they are the inevitable consequence of financial austerity also obscures what might be the politically motivated character of such decisions. In England, the cost of the 2011 Census – approximately £480 million, £1 per person, per year of the 12-year planning and operational cycle – has been judged as 'good value for money' and comparable to that of many other countries (ONS, 2012). In the broad scheme of austerity measures, the savings are likely to be negligible.

Campaign groups in particular use official statistics to draw attention to issues and build their case for change as part of their **advocacy** role. Women's groups, for example, have long campaigned for the right to have domestic violence recognized as a public issue. In many countries, however, it is only in the relatively recent past that official statistics have been collected, making it possible to document the extent of domestic violence. Since 2004/5, the Crime Survey for England and Wales has included questions on domestic violence. This survey is a particularly valuable source of data because it covers crimes not reported to, or not recorded by the police and therefore better represents people's experiences of crime. In the case of domestic violence, this is particularly important because it is not recognized as an official specific criminal offence and does not appear as a separate category in crime statistics. By providing prevalence estimates, surveys of this kind have uncovered the extent of domestic violence. Access to survey data as well as to police records has allowed the patterns of domestic violence to be explored in more detail, such as its significant increase during sporting events such as the World Cup (Brimicombe and Café, 2012). The WHO (2005b) multi-country study of women and domestic violence has contributed to documenting how widespread domestic violence is and how far-reaching its impacts on the health and well-being of women and their children.

But judging whether a phenomenon constitutes an issue in need of attention extends beyond the presentation of statistical data. This has become abundantly clear in relation to social inequalities in health. Mortality statistics have been used extensively to document the social gradient in health for men and women, as well as reveal the stark differences in life expectancy across social classes. Researchers have consistently documented this pattern across time and **place**. Considerable debate remains about the interpretation, however. In other words, official statistics can be used to provide the platform for theoretical speculation; they cannot be used to prove an explanation.

Official statistics also have a potential role to play in policy development. In reality, however, such statistics have been used primarily to monitor policies rather than inform new policy choices and designs (Holt, 2008). Policy monitoring in the form of 'performance management' using key indicators and targets has become common in many countries. In England, it has become the predominant means of identifying under-performing public services (Hood, 2006). Administrative data relating to hospital waiting lists – a contentious issue with a high political profile – have been used to monitor and judge the performance of hospitals, and the adequacy of resourcing health services in general. Surveys are also used to fulfil a monitoring role. The annual Active People Survey commissioned by Sport England, for example, tracks trends in sport participation as a way of monitoring its aim to increase participation. The data also form the basis for tracking the impact of the 2012 Olympic Games on sport participation. At a global level, the United Nations Children's Fund (UNICEF) and the WHO publish annual mortality statistics by country to monitor progress towards the MDGs (Boerma and Stansfield, 2007). However, systems of civil registration continue to be absent in many parts of the world, particularly those where mortality is high. The WHO (2013) estimates that approximately two-thirds (38 million) of 57 million annual deaths and almost half the world's children go unregistered. Many countries do not have the necessary laws or infrastructure to make it obligatory to register births and deaths. Judging progress on the MDGs has been difficult because of limited access to high quality data.

Official statistics can also play a role in surveillance and forecasting. 'Public health intelligence' is a term used to describe the collection, interrogation, synthesis, interpretation and presentation of statistics (and other forms of data) in order to clarify their public health significance. A recent development in England has been the expansion of online systems relating to small area data (such as at the local authority level) in relation to, for example, health profiles and alcohol profiles, a trend apparent in other countries such as Norway (see for example www.norgeshelse.no). In England, the government has established national public health knowledge and intelligence teams to focus on specific health priorities, such as obesity and mental health. Together, these systems provide a wealth of locally relevant data to support the identification of **health needs** and formulation of local health strategies. Statistical modelling is a particular form of public health intelligence that has increasingly been used for planning and allocating resources. This approach has been employed to generate prevalence estimates of HIV/AIDS and mortality projections in many African countries (AbouZahr *et al.*, 2007). More recently, ONS statistics relating to alcohol-related liver deaths have been utilized to project deaths and potential lives saved if **evidence**-based policies were implemented (Sheron *et al.*, 2011).

Notwithstanding these uses of official statistics, a number of concerns relating to their quality and comprehensiveness remain. In most countries with well-developed statistical services – supported by a legally-binding code of practice – official statistics are collected to a high technical standard, with continuity in many measures over several years allowing trends to be documented. However, all official statistics (as all data derived from human processes) have limitations. In surveys, for example, developing valid, reliable and acceptable frameworks for categorizing phenomena is challenging. In spite of pressure from a number of groups, this explains why the 2011 Census in England (as in most other countries) did not include a question on sexual orientation (ONS, 2010a). Problems of categorization are particularly relevant to administrative statistics because they are collected for specific (administrative) purposes. Secondary analysis of such statistics is hampered by their incompleteness (missing data/not recorded), inaccuracy of records, as well as the absence of key socio-demographic information relating to disability, sexual orientation, postcode and so on.

The transparent production of official statistics potentially provides a mechanism by which the public can hold the government of the day to account for how it has used resources. It is thus 'at the heart of the democratic contract between the public and its elected government' (Holt, 2008: 327). That said, considerable disquiet among researchers and the public more broadly about the credibility of official statistics endures. The independence of a government's statistical service – in terms of structure and process – has been the subject of considerable debate. Norway's central statistical office has operated independently of its government since 1876 (www://ssb.no). By contrast, a new, independent agency – the UK Statistics Authority – was established in 2008, reporting directly to Parliament rather than to ministers, a move that was designed to restore public confidence in the statistical system (House of Commons Public Administration Select Committee, 2013). A recent survey by Ipsos Mori (2013) concluded, however, that low levels of confidence in politicians and their use of statistics remains; seven per cent of respondents thought politicians used statistics accurately when talking about policies. Among the 27 member states of the EU, public trust is lowest in Britain, illustrating a gap between the quality of statistics produced by the government and public confidence (Holt, 2008). A particular issue in Britain relates to the public's awareness of 'political spin'. Several recent examples illustrate that ministers have used government statistics selectively and ambiguously. In 2013, the UK Prime Minister, David Cameron, claimed in a party political broadcast that the Government was reducing the nation's debt, when it was actually rising (Mason, 2013). (He later received a rebuke from the UK Statistics Authority for confusing accumulated debt with annual public sector borrowing.) Regardless of changes to the system, political manipulation of official statistics persists. The introduction of measures of well-being into the Integrated Household Survey in 2011 in England was a direct consequence of prime ministerial influence, which may seem, on the face of it, innocuous. The construction of a 'well-being index' has drawn criticism, however, on the grounds that it conceptualizes happiness and well-being in individual, subjective terms, bound up with personal choices, rather than social circumstances (Tomlinson and Kelly, 2013). In other words, it reflects a particular ideology with specific implications for policy.

There are also a number of subtle ways of influencing the statistical system. In relation to government surveys, 'troublesome' questions can be removed or modified, new ones added and different ways of categorizing people or phenomena based on different definitions introduced. Broad patterns of statistics can also be used to frame issues in particular ways to justify ideologically-informed policy choices, often picked up and fanned by the media to create a 'moral panic'. The ageing of the population has been used to justify raising the pension age as well as reforms to public sector pensions (Marshall, 2011). An Ipsos MORI (2013) poll in the UK, found that people think the population is much older than it is, estimating 36 per cent of the population to be over 65 compared to the official estimate of 16 per cent. Why the general public's perceptions are misaligned with official statistics on this and other issues is likely to relate to a lack of trust in the government, current issues of concern among the population, as well as 'moral panics' created by the media.

All these issues reflect the tendency at every level of government to accentuate success and soften failure, particularly because statistical outputs are one means by which the performance of public servants might be judged (Holt, 2008). In other words, they are a fact of political life and evident in countries beyond the UK. The Argentine government, for example, was accused of massaging statistics, leading *The Economist* to remove Argentine inflation figures from its website (Radical Statistics, 2013). Two further points can be made here. First, statistics are commonly presented as immutable 'facts' rather than the outcome of a social process. Second, they are valuable *and* limited, and always require intelligent interpretation. The political process as played out in the media, however, often militates against the considered use of official statistics.

Conclusion

The debate relating to official statistics is likely to become more rather than less contentious in at least two areas. The collection of data from private sector suppliers of public services for monitoring and **evaluation** purposes remains controversial. Given the penetration of the private sector into the public realm in many countries this is a particularly pressing issue. The protection of commercial interests has been used to justify suppression of data (Holt 2008). Second, there is the issue of privacy. Legislation in the UK (in 2006) relating to a national identity card scheme was repealed in 2011 amid concerns of excessive government surveillance. Schemes such as those used in some Nordic countries based on a 'unique identifier' have the potential to link all records together. Of greater significance, perhaps, is intrusion from the commercial sector. Large amounts of data are recorded automatically in connection with credit card use, internet access, electronic tickets, traffic surveillance and so on; people leave an increasingly complex and large electronic 'footprint'. The significance of all these developments in terms of who has access to which forms of data about whom remains to be seen.

PARTNERSHIPS AND PARTNERSHIP WORKING

Context

Various forms of 'working together' have been advocated in the public health field since the 1980s. A number of global institutions, such as the WHO (1986, 1999, 2005a) and the UN Millennium Project (2005), have highlighted the importance of co-ordinated, co-operative and sustained strategies – across sectors, professions and disciplines, as well as with the **community** – for improving the prerequisites for **health** and reducing health **inequalities**. They argue that the complexity of modern societies and the wide range of **determinants** of health require concerted, collaborative action. In the UK, the idea of 'partnership', as well as the related notion of 'joined-up government', emerged as one of the defining features of the **policy** rhetoric of the Labour government from its election in 1997. The intuitive appeal of partnership working – that it is unequivocally a 'good thing' – has meant that it has endured as the preferred policy instrument across a range of domains, in a number of countries beyond the UK (Canada and Australia, for example). **Advocacy** of partnerships (as a way of working) has, nevertheless, outstripped empirical **evidence** of its effectiveness in bringing about particular policy goals, although the theoretical advantages of working together for mutual benefit have been well rehearsed (Dowling *et al.*, 2004). Nonetheless, working in partnership continues to be promoted as a way of addressing complex issues, such as improving health and well-being and reducing social inequalities in health.

Defining partnerships and partnership working

The term 'partnership' appears extensively in policy and related documents, yet there is little consensus regarding its definition. In fact, several different terms are used to describe co-ordinated working arrangements: developing alliances, intersectoral collaboration, multi-agency working, joined-up working, service integration, and networking, for example (Purcal *et al.*, 2011). These terms all refer to new forms of inter-organizational working based on horizontal (rather than vertical) forms of relationships and which emphasize collaboration, reciprocity and mutual benefit. Yet there is still much ambiguity about the term partnership, partly generated by its unrestrained application to diverse organizational relationships.

Many definitions tend to focus on the technical and managerial aspects of partnership working. The Audit Commission, for example, defines partnership working as a form of

> joint working arrangement where partners are otherwise independent bodies co-operating to achieve a common goal; this may involve the creation of new organizational structures or processes to plan and implement a joint programme, as well as sharing relevant information, **risks** and rewards.
>
> (1998: 8 (emphasis added))

Definitions of alliance-building and intersectoral collaboration similarly tend to emphasize organizational, managerial and technical dimensions of working together on agreed goals, as well as the presumed benefits that accrue therefrom. Much effort and time has been given to establishing partnership structures and systems – what Hunter and Perkins (2012: 50) refer to as 'over-engineering partnerships' – disregarding more substantive issues such as aims, purposes and mechanisms of policy implementation. Increasingly, however, a more critical perspective on partnerships has been evident in the academic literature, drawing attention to the social relational aspects of partnerships and the power struggles that reside therein (Diamond, 2006; Pollitt, 2003). Derkzen *et al.* (2008: 464), for example, view partnerships as 'sites of political organization, characterized by inequality and difference, in which power is an important constitutive element'. Viewing partnerships as constituted by mutually-oriented interdependent people (in other words, as existing in and through people, not independently of them) has, in particular, the potential to shed light on the difficulties of partnership dynamics.

Joined-up working, particularly applied to the idea of joined-up government, is a related term that has also been applied (somewhat ambiguously) to new ways of working. Pollitt (2003: 35) defines joint working as the 'aspiration to achieve horizontally and vertically co-ordinated thinking and action' across departments of government. This idea has been applied to all levels of government: local, regional, national and global. Implicit in this terminology is the aim of working together in order to limit situations in which different policies and strategies undermine each other. In the health field, Milio (1981, 1988) uses the term 'health in all policies' to illustrate that focusing on the health implications of all policies developed by different government departments has the potential to maximize their health benefits. Transport policies that promote road building at the expense of public transport and cycle lanes, are likely to undermine the efforts of health and sport policies seeking to promote active travel, for example. Working in a joined-up way also has the potential to raise awareness of the health consequences of policy decisions and organizational practices in different sectors, as well as bring about service integration at the policy, strategy and service level (Pollitt, 2003). Most efforts towards joint working, however, have been evident at a local and regional level, with central government having largely failed to follow its own rhetoric (Boyce and Hunter, 2009).

The significance of partnerships and partnership working for public health

Partnership has been advocated as the solution to a multitude of health and social welfare problems. In particular, it has been promoted as the *only* way to address 'wicked issues', that is to say, complex policy problems, which themselves are difficult to delineate, falling between the responsibilities of agencies and for which there are no straightforward or easily agreed solutions (Rummery, 2009). In England, a large number of partnerships between local authorities, health services and the voluntary sector have been established in the last two decades, the aim of which has been to address a variety of entrenched public health problems relating to disadvantaged communities. These locally developed and implemented partnerships were primarily concerned with bringing about service integration, eradicating duplication and creating new services to meet identified needs. Collaborating across different policy, service and practice domains has the potential to create a variety of synergies that would not only lead to the creation of innovative solutions to complex problems but also improve the quality, efficiency and effectiveness of services. HAZs, healthy living centres, Sure Start local programmes, healthy schools programmes and the New Deal for Communities were examples of local partnership programmes designed to improve – among many other things – health and well-being. Working in partnership with the community was also a central feature of these programmes. The development of local strategic partnerships (LSPs) in most English local authority areas followed on from these diverse programmes and became the focus for addressing health inequalities through targets in local area agreements (Perkins *et al.*, 2010). Partnership structures continue to develop in England, following a change of government in the UK in 2010 (health and well-being boards and clinical commissioning groups effectively replacing LSPs). However, collaboration between public, private and voluntary and community sector organizations remains a core, mandated feature of arrangements. One outcome of this process of partnership formation is an increase in the complexity of local governance arrangements (a mix of organizational and **place**-based). These arrangements are, furthermore, fluid, limiting the possibilities for developing trust, viewed widely as the bedrock of effective collaboration. Establishing lines of accountability in this context can also be difficult (Marks *et al.*, 2010). Developing some form of shared understanding of health is also likely to be challenging when collaboration across diverse groups and agencies is required (Cameron *et al.*, 2008).

Partnership-based programmes and structures have been extensively researched in relation to their processes and outcomes. In terms of the former, there is substantial evidence that partnership working is time-consuming and difficult (Purcal *et al.*, 2011), particularly in relation to participation, collective decision-making and leadership (Hunter and Perkins, 2012). Differing values give rise to persistent conflicts that tend to fragment and polarize rather than integrate policy and practice (Davies, 2009). This can lead to 'silo mentality' (focusing on the needs and demands of a person's organization) behind a 'veneer' of partnership working (Hunter and Perkins, 2012: 49), and give rise to suspicion and rivalry among partners (Carlisle, 2010). Integrating voluntary and community sector organizations into partnerships can be particularly difficult when they are viewed by others as not only troublesome but as junior members who have to earn their place in the partnership (Sinclair, 2011). Although partnerships tend to be presented as non-hierarchical, the reality of working within a partnership suggests that various forms of hierarchy emerge over time. Furthermore, there is little evidence to suggest that partnerships have any direct effect on health (Smith *et al.*, 2009b). A recent systematic review concluded that there was no 'reliable evidence that interagency collaboration, compared to standard services, necessarily leads to health improvement' (Hayes *et al.*, 2012: 2). Perhaps the most that partnerships can do is increase the profile of public health and health inequalities across a range of sectors, as research has suggested (Smith *et al.*, 2009a).

Evaluation of partnerships is, however, fraught with difficulties, particularly in relation to attributing the consequences of partnership working to specific health outcomes. Furthermore, no matter how well-organized, focused and resourced partnership are, they may be limited in the extent to which they can act on the wider determinants of health and reduce local social inequalities in health. Yet, local authorities have a number of powers to 'place-shape' (that is to say to influence the character of local environments) but rarely appear to use them (Dorling, 2010)

In England, the extensive restructuring of the public health system has at its core a variety of partnership structures. The extent to which these collaborative arrangements can work effectively alongside the extension of processes of competitive tendering remains to be seen, however. Competitive contracts have been found to undermine collaborative work and trust (Milbourne, 2009). It seems likely, furthermore, that public–private partnerships will increase in the future. The Global Alliance for Vaccines and Immunization (GAVI), which promotes the immunization of all the world's children is described as a public–private global public health partnership. It includes governments, the WHO, UNICEF, the Bill and Melinda Gates Foundation, non-governmental organizations, research institutes and vaccine manufacturers. In England, the Public Health Responsibility Deal was launched in 2011 as a partnership of public sector, academic, voluntary sector and commercial sector organizations, the aim of which is to agree practical approaches to address a range of public health issues including those relating to food, alcohol and physical activity. The formation of voluntary partnerships to make pledges is a mechanism that has been used elsewhere in Europe (Bryden *et al.*, 2013). The approach has been the subject of extensive criticism, primarily on the basis that it provides a mechanism for commercial organizations to influence policy in ways that serve their own interests. The involvement of the alcohol industry has, in particular, drawn comment, given its recent efforts to prevent the introduction of minimum pricing legislation in spite of evidence that this can bring about population-level benefits in patterns of drinking. Voluntary public–private partnerships are, however, more likely to be effective if they involve sanctions for non-participation or non-compliance with objectives (Bryden *et al.*, 2013). This illustrates a further development and application of the term 'partnership'.

Conclusion

There is some consensus that governments have viewed partnerships as a panacea for a broad range of deeply entrenched public health and other related problems. As a mechanism for addressing local health issues, partnership continues to be attractive to policymakers conveying as the term does some mutual benefit from collaboration that obscures the power dynamics inherent in such arrangements. Nevertheless, as Dickinson and Glasby (2010: 815) argue, it is 'not that [partnerships] cannot work, but more that they often do not work' for well-documented reasons that include their over-ambitious aims. Moreover, their effectiveness might be enhanced if less attention was given to their structure and more to their purpose, and if the purpose was to solve a specific problem within a limited duration (Hunter and Perkins, 2012). On the other hand, partnerships may not necessarily be an appropriate way to address some issues. Narrowing social inequalities in health, for example, requires a structural, rather than a local partnership solution. The tendency has been, however, for these types of so called 'wicked problems' to be managed rather than solved (Rittel and Webber, 1973). It seems that in public health, partnerships have become the predominant form of managing them.

PLACE

Context

The geographical patterning of **health** and health **inequalities** has been well-documented ever since mortality records began being systematically compiled. Differences in life expectancy, for example, can be stark between as well as within countries. In England, the 'north-south divide' has been used to refer to the substantial excess mortality from all causes in the north of the country, a pattern that has endured over several decades (Hacking *et al.*, 2011). Geographical variation over relatively small distances – between the east and west of a city for example – has also been described in many countries. It is only in the relatively recent past, however, that researchers have turned their attention to studying how 'place' – particularly in the form of local neighbourhoods – shapes health. To some degree this refocusing on the context reflects renewed interest in the wider **determinants of health**. In public health **policy** terms, the contemporary focus on place reflects a political emphasis on locally-based strategies for addressing local **health needs** and problems. In England, this policy emphasis has endured over several decades in spite of limited **evidence** of its effectiveness in either improving health or reducing health **inequalities**.

Defining place

Although seemingly straightforward, place is a particularly slippery concept to tie down, and definitions tend to be lacking in the public health literature. Rather, place tends to be presented axiomatically as geographic space or area. This tendency is illustrated in the use of administrative areas (electoral wards or local authority boundaries, for example) to identify areas of **deprivation** and for targeting resources. Areas have also been more arbitrarily identified on the basis of perceived needs and problems as happened in the case of some Sure Start local programmes in England. Researchers have increasingly recognized, however, the limitations of defining place in terms of a bounded geographic area equated, metaphorically, to a 'black box' (Macintyre *et al.*, 2002). Of particular note is the conflation of place (what a location is and means for people) with space (where a location is as a specific geographic position), a critical distinction made in recent years by geographers studying the spatial patterning of health (Tunstall *et al.*, 2004). A neighbourhood for example, may well be defined in administrative or geographic (space) terms. As a *place* to live, however, a neighbourhood is likely to carry a variety of emotionally-charged meanings for residents as well as offer access, by degrees, to a range of health-related social and material resources. This conceptual differentiation between space and place opens up possibilities for defining place as a more complex and socially constructed idea.

In public health, nevertheless, the predominant approach to defining place has been in spatial terms. In part, this reflects the influence of **epidemiology** and the use of multi-level statistical modelling in studying patterns of health and disease. A common approach has been to conceptualize place in terms of two dimensions that make measurement of specific variables possible: a compositional dimension that relates to the people living and working in an area (the 'composition' of the population), and a contextual dimension that relates to the characteristics of the environment. The assumption underpinning this approach is that the effects of context on health can be separated out from those of the characteristics of the people living there (Tunstall *et al.*, 2004). Dichotomizing place in this way not only presents a static view of people and places but also neglects the 'mutually reinforcing and reciprocal relationship between people and place' (Cummins *et al.*, 2007: 1835).

The development of a more nuanced definition of place has largely come from within the sub-discipline of health geography where place is understood as a point of convergence between the physical and the social: as both an unbounded social space and as geographically anchored. Thus, places are defined as 'cultural and symbolic phenomena constructed through relationships between people and their settings' (Andrews and Moon, 2005: 56). By implication, people *constitute* the context and are not detached from it. Defining place as multifaceted raises the possibility of places having multiple identities. Thus, perceptions and meanings of place may differ according to people's social position. This more complex construction also presents a view of place as fluid, historically constituted and linked in various ways beyond the local geography through 'a distinct mixture of wider and more local social relations' (Massey, 1991: 29). The term 'landscape' has been used to describe these 'complex layerings of history, social structure and built environment that converge in particular places' (Kearns and Moon, 2002: 611). Overall, viewing place in these terms has the potential to lead to a more adequate understanding of how health emerges out of particular places during specific times.

The significance of place for public health

There continues to be considerable interest in understanding the relationship between places, people, and health, particularly at the local neighbourhood level and especially in relation to deprivation. New developments in technology, including the development of more powerful statistical tools, have stimulated quantitative research into place and its effects on health. The development of geographical information systems (GIS) technology (which allows the capture, analysis and display of geographically referenced – geocoded – data for use in computer mapping) has made it possible to link geographical patterns of health and disease with spatially referenced physical and social phenomena in a way that can provide aetiological clues about how places shape health and health inequality (Krieger, 2003). Quantitative studies have generated considerable debate in terms of the extent to which the association between place and health can be explained in compositional or contextual terms. Some argue that the poorer health of those living in areas of deprivation can be wholly explained by the density of disadvantaged people in those areas rather than any independent contextual effect (Sloggett and Joshi, 1994). These studies, especially those based on statistical regression techniques that isolate factors from each other, are limited in the extent to which they can study the inter-relationships between people, as well as between people and various dimensions of the places in which they live, particularly over time. Notwithstanding the many methodological limitations of these types of studies, there is a broad consensus that 'place' has a significant effect on health over and above individual-level factors (Chandola and Marmot, 2004).

Detailed qualitative research has shed light on the processes through which health might be shaped by place. This body of work reveals how people's sense of themselves is rooted in place (Frumkin, 2003). Even when living in deprived neighbourhoods people develop strong attachments, characterized by feelings of security with what is familiar (Batty *et al.*, 2011). Interestingly, neighbourhood problems tend not to be viewed as inherently attached to places, as policymakers are apt to suggest. Places thus provide a degree of stability in the everyday lives of people, likely to be particularly important to those who live with other (economic, for example) uncertainties. Proposals to change neighbourhoods in some way or being required to move neighbourhood (to seek employment, for example) represent potential disruptions that challenge these deeply held identities and attachments to surroundings.

Place-based resources, including informal support, are particularly valued by people (Batty *et al.*, 2011). Social affiliation is especially important for physical and mental health and well-being. How local environments enable social dynamics – through the positioning of amenities, the walkability of areas, street lighting, the general attractiveness of areas, and so on – is therefore significant. Social dynamics are also influenced by crime and the fear of crime, both of which might mediate the relationship between neighbourhood characteristics and mental health (Lorenc *et al.*, 2012). Fear is a key feature in people's accounts of how their health is affected by where they live (Parry *et al.*, 2007). It illustrates how neighbourhoods are not only constituted through their physical and social characteristics but that these are interdependent.

People's access to social, material and service-related resources has been central to explaining inequalities in health (Bernard *et al.*, 2007). Although places vary in the quality and quantity of resources, how people access them is not necessarily dependent on geographical proximity. In relation to access to healthy food, for example, interactions between people and their local food environment can be complex insofar as they are historically, culturally and economically constituted (Cummins *et al.*, 2007).

In England, successive governments since the 1960s have sought to revitalize declining areas. The UK's Labour government (1997–2010) specifically focused on place through its National Strategy for Neighbourhood Renewal, launched in 2001, in which it articulated its ambition that within 10 to 20 years 'no-one should be seriously disadvantaged by where they live' (Social Exclusion Unit, 2001: 8). Area-based initiatives – such as the New Deal for Communities and HAZs – were used to direct efforts and resources at deprived areas, primarily to improve the quality of services and facilities. Policymakers viewed these areas as detached from mainstream society in many ways. Thus far, conclusions from the **evaluation** of area-based initiatives are, at best, mixed (Bauld *et al.*, 2005; Beatty *et al.*, 2010). Drawing boundaries around areas defines them as 'problems' in need of intervention without necessarily understanding the physical and social complexity of places (Chatterton and Bradley, 2000). Moreover, it reinforces the view that solutions reside within the local area rather than with the broader economic system. As more complex conceptualizations of place suggest, local areas are not autonomous but are connected to wider networks of people, including local and central government, in a variety of ways. The limited success of area-based initiatives in relation to health, regeneration, sport development, **education** and so on has largely been attributed to the tendency of policymakers to simplify the complex causes of the problems they are seeking to address. In particular, strategies tend to emphasize the delivery of projects and services rather than seeking broader political solutions.

More recently in England, a broader role for local government in 'place shaping' has, been articulated. Lyons (2007) set out a far-reaching strategic role for local government that went beyond providing local services and funding small projects, to include the judicious investment in public infrastructure as well as the creative use of its planning powers to promote local people's health and well-being. The integration of public health teams into local government from 2013 in England has the potential to increase pressure on the local leadership to act as a 'place shaper'. The point to note here is that despite the constraint of central government policy, local government has some discretion over local policy and strategy. Moreover, focusing on economic regeneration on its own is unlikely to lead to broader health and social benefits (Shucksmith *et al.*, 2010). As indicated above, there is no shortage of empirical evidence to indicate what some of the better investments for health might be at a local level. The design of urban areas to include attractive public amenities that include green spaces, road design that is sensitive to the 'walkability' of neighbourhoods and includes the use of speed limits in residential areas, adequate street lighting, as well as affordable, high-quality housing have been shown to have a number of direct and indirect effects on health and well-being (Dorling, 2010; Frumkin, 2003). It remains to be seen how local governments use their powers under these new arrangements, especially during a period of sustained financial austerity.

Conclusion

Although there is a tendency to speak about the geographical expansion of social relations, place, particularly the local neighbourhood in which people live out their everyday lives, matters to people. Place also matters to health, although the mechanisms remain to be elucidated. In this regard, public health might benefit from a more direct engagement with empirical and theoretical work within health geography where the general starting point is that 'places form people as much as places are formed from people' (Tunstall *et al.*, 2004: 8).

POLICY

Context

Global institutions, governments and organizations produce policies that range from the relatively simple to the more complex. In doing so, they seek to influence the actions of those within their purview. Drawing on an earlier definition by Winslow in 1920, Acheson (1988: 4) defined public health as 'the science and art of preventing disease, prolonging life and promoting health through the organized efforts of society'. This oft-quoted and widely adopted definition conveys the view that public health is a field of practice that is action-oriented towards specific ends. Significantly, it also implies that the **determinants** of **health** are, at least theoretically, modifiable; that is to say, disease *can* be prevented, health *can* be promoted and life *can* be prolonged. Policy constitutes one way in which societies organize themselves towards particular goals. Because the determinants of health are policy-sensitive, understanding how policies are formulated and implemented is a central concern of contemporary public health.

Defining policy

Titmuss (1974: 23) provides a succinct definition of policy relating it to 'the principles that govern action directed towards given ends'. This definition implies that policies are concerned with change, aspiring to move from what is perceived as an unsatisfactory situation to that which is more satisfactory (Murphy, 1998: 104). Some policies might involve maintaining the status quo or making only small modifications to existing policies. Titmuss's definition links 'action' and 'ends' to 'principles' and in so doing infers that policies are – either implicitly or explicitly – underpinned by values and beliefs about how the policy issue has been understood as well as what is perceived to be the appropriate way to address it. Ham (2004) also draws attention to values in policies by arguing that while the goals of policy might generally be agreed, the means by which they are to be achieved are more likely to attract controversy. In the alcohol field for example, there is broad agreement that alcohol consumption in some groups is sufficiently high to damage health as well as generate social problems. The introduction of a policy to regulate the minimum price per unit of alcohol as a mechanism for reducing consumption has, however, been highly controversial. This example illustrates the distinction – often not clear-cut – between normative (value-based) and instrumental policy-making. Normative approaches in the public health policy field reflect a view that policymakers should intervene in regulating alcohol prices, for example. Instrumental approaches are based on the most effective way to reach desired ends and, in the public health field, draw on ideas relating to the use of **evidence** in policy-making (Smith and Katikreddi, 2013).

'Public policy' refers specifically to policies produced by governments (Buse *et al.*, 2005). Health policy, for example, refers to the policies produced by the Department of Health (in the UK). This covers policies relating to the health care system as well as public health. Health policy, however, frequently tends to focus on health *care* (and, in the UK, the NHS in particular) rather than public health. Having a separate public health department – such as the Folkehelse Directorate (public health department) within the Ministry of Health and Care Services, as in Norway – may have some advantages in prioritizing and protecting public health policy. From a public health perspective, however, policies developed by many, if not all, government departments have implications for public health. Foreign, defence, environment, transport, energy and economic policies, for example, have considerable power to act on the wider determinants of health, alongside social policies that more specifically relate to social security, health, **education**, housing and personal social services. This broader view of health policy is reflected in the concept of 'healthy public policy', first articulated as a key strategy for promoting health in the *Ottawa Charter for Health Promotion* (WHO, 1986) and subsequently developed by Milio (1988). Draper (1988: 217) argues that the goal of healthy public policy is to make government activity across the board contribute as much as possible to health development, while recognizing the trade-offs that are an inevitable and necessary part of the policy process. In a similar vein, Ståhl *et al.* (2006) coined the phrase, 'health in all policies'. Kickbusch (2013), however, prefers the terminology 'governance for health and wellbeing' to convey the same idea of concerted and co-ordinated policy development.

The significance of policy for public health

There has been a tendency to view the policy process as linear or rational, starting with the definition of the issue, identifying possible courses of action, objectively weighing up and choosing from alternatives, implementing actions and evaluating their consequences. This view is in keeping with the scientific and medical perspectives commonly expressed in the field of public health in general, and evidence-based policy in particular. To some extent, attachment to the model provides something of a safety blanket for those in public health who seek to avoid engaging with politics. Walt (1994) argues, however, that the rational model distorts the reality of policy as a more complex, contingent and dynamic *process*. In particular, the process is a political one; it involves those with power and authority making decisions about what does and what does not get onto the policy agenda and how policies take shape (Buse *et al.*, 2005). Policy is, therefore, more than legislation or regulation, although these may be outcomes of the policy process.

Policy formulation and policy implementation are the terms used to refer to key stages in the policy process. Policies tend to begin life as issues through a process of politicization, 'whereby an issue ceases to be a purely private concern, is debated in the public sphere, then becomes a matter for politicians to address' (Roberts 2009: 201). Violence, for example, has relatively recently been identified as a major public health issue. In the UK for example, domestic violence became a responsibility of health services in 2004 through the Domestic Violence Crime and Victims Act 2004. Yet women's groups had been dealing with the consequences for women and children of living in violent relationships since the 1960s. The opening up of a 'policy window' – an agenda-setting opportunity – emerges, according to Kingdon (1984), out of particular circumstances relating to complex interactions between the characteristics of the issue, the features of political institutions and perceptions that policy solutions are possible. The 'policy narrative' (the conventional wisdom) about domestic violence shifted significantly. Changing policy narratives about specific issues is difficult, however; they tend to persist in spite of evidence to the contrary. Evidence of limited effectiveness has failed to shift the policy emphasis on individual responsibility for **lifestyle** behaviours and the use of **behaviour change** approaches. Commercial interest groups also influence policy narratives, for example, by arguing against regulation by making reference to the idea of the 'nanny state'. As Sparks (2011) points out, this kind of 'misdirection' obfuscates the evidence that regulation saves lives. Commercial companies such as Coca-Cola spend considerable sums of money on marketing, often targeting children. In the USA, children's intake of sugared beverages surpassed that of milk (Brownell and Frieden, 2009). Without some form of regulation these trends are likely to continue. Nonetheless, anti-regulatory policy narratives tend to persist because they simplify complex problems and therefore make them appear more amenable to policy intervention (Exworthy *et al.*, 2003). Reflecting the political imperatives associated with electoral cycles the timescales for achieving desired changes tend to be short-medium term. Policymakers working in these circumstances tend to use ideas, rather than evidence, in a selective way 'filtering' and 'recycling' ideas that fit with ideological orientations (Smith, 2012).

Sometimes a policy window opens up quite quickly after a major event. Such was the case with the smoking ban on the London Underground in 1987 following the King's Cross station fire (Lang and Raynor, 2012). Policymakers at that time had considerable leverage, in part because there was a growing consensus about the undesirability of smoking in some public places. This example illustrates a further facet of the policy-making process in that policy decisions tend to be framed in particular ways through the use of specific language to convey a policy solution as 'obvious'. In this way, policy decisions can be depoliticized. The approach to the financial crisis of the coalition government in the UK since 2010 has been one of presenting its policy of financial austerity as the only 'sensible' and 'right' way to proceed: ergo, all other alternatives are not sensible and are wrong.

In recent years there has been a trend towards the growing importance of a wider number of interest (or pressure) groups in the policy formulation process. Of particular note, is the lobbying of the government by the commercial sector, the tobacco, alcohol and food industries especially. Business interests such as these, tend to be the most powerful of all interest groups, vital as they are to the economy and employment (Buse *et al.*, 2005). In the UK, the commercial sector has become increasingly involved in the development of policy relating to public health through the Responsibility Deal. The ferocity with which the tobacco industry protects its commercial interests has become evident in relation to the proposed introduction of plain packaging of cigarettes. Following its introduction in Australia, England planned to follow suit but recently reversed the decision, an act that led to a rise in tobacco share prices (Collin and Hill, 2013). This policy U-turn has raised a number of questions about the process through which the shift took place and the closeness of commercial organizations, such as the tobacco industry, to government. The lack of a statutory register of lobbyists, which would contribute to greater transparency in relations between government officials and outside organizations, has also been criticized (Collin and Hill, 2013).

Policies change as they move to the local level because those involved in implementation have, by degrees, some discretion in how they interpret policy initiatives. There is, in other words, room for slippage between policy intention and implementation, commonly referred to as the implementation gap (Dopson and Waddington, 1996). The degree to which policies succeed is, therefore, related to the process of implementation. This allows policymakers to distance themselves from policies that do not achieve their goals by pointing towards the problems of implementation. In so doing they avoid responsibility for framing what might be poor or inadequately resourced policies. The current emphasis on local strategies to improve health and narrow **inequalities** may be fundamentally limited in what can be achieved if many of the determinants of health are strongly shaped by national policies.

Policy implementation involves micropolitical processes that take shape in organizations such as schools, workplaces, hospitals and so on. Complex policies – such as those in the UK relating to economic regeneration – present particular challenges associated with **partnership** working. However, even smaller-scale changes can be difficult to implement. In an organizational context, policy implementation is often referred to as the management of change in which leadership based on consensus-building is important. That said, changing the practice of professional groups always tends to be difficult. Doctors in the USA and England, for example, have been reluctant to adopt clinical evidence-based guidelines, in spite of receiving training (Dopson, 2005; Elliott *et al.*, 2002). Having some kind of local discretion is not necessarily a bad thing, however. It provides opportunities to shape policies in particular ways that are better aligned with local or organizational cultures and priorities.

Policies often have unintended outcomes. A key area of contention has been the extent to which policies widen inequalities rather than narrow them through a process of levelling up as intended (Whitehead and Dahlgren, 2006). Individual strategies such as the use of health checks to screen for cardiovascular **risk** factors tend to widen inequalities because they rely of the mobilization of individuals' resources, which generally favour those better endowed with material and psychological reserves (Capewell and Graham, 2010). The use of a 'health in all policies' approach was adopted by the South Australian state government in 2007 to ensure population-level health was promoted alongside economic growth. This type of model includes a prospective assessment of the impact of policies and therefore has the potential to understand the consequences of policies (Fletcher, 2013).

Conclusion

Policies reflect political aspirations and may therefore be prone to the setting of unrealistic goals and targets. The growing interest in well-being and happiness as an explicit goal of policy is a reflection of this tendency (Bacon *et al.*, 2010). Policies may also overestimate the significance of policy – or any *one* policy – to bring about change. However, policies can shape the conditions in which people live and thus have the potential to improve health and narrow health inequalities. A critical understanding of the policy process is therefore central to contemporary public health practice.

PREVENTION

Context

In 1980, the World Health Assembly declared the world free from smallpox, the first and only disease in history to have been eradicated through concerted collaborative action: extensive vaccination, intense surveillance and rapid containment of outbreaks (Fenner, 1982). Other infectious diseases, such as malaria and polio, have been eliminated from specific countries or geographic regions but global eradication remains elusive, even though the scientific means are well-established. These advances in disease control throw into sharp relief the broader global picture of new and re-emerging diseases, as well as upward trends in non-infectious diseases such as cancers, CVD and other **health**-related problems associated with particular **'lifestyles'** (alcohol dependence, drug-related behaviours, obesity and so on). These trends have placed increasing demands on health care systems such that interest in prevention has been revitalized. In this context, prevention might seem an attractive and uncontentious idea, promising to avert human suffering as well as contain costs. However, debates about the purpose of prevention and the strategies used tend to be interwoven with political, ethical, economic and scientific arguments implying that prevention has, in practice, become a problematic and contested concept.

Defining prevention

Preventive **medicine** has traditionally been the field within which prevention has been developed, drawing on knowledge of the natural history of diseases (the clinical progression of disease processes over time in an individual) and **risk** factor **epidemiology**. Porta (2008: 192) defines prevention as 'Actions aimed at eradicating, eliminating, or minimizing the impact of disease and disability, or if none of these is feasible, retarding the progress of disease and disability'. This definition reflects the different levels at which prevention can occur – conventionally defined as primary, secondary and tertiary. Primary prevention aims to reduce the incidence (new cases) of disease by decreasing the risk of exposure. This might be by boosting individuals' resistance through, for example, improving their nutritional status or immunization against infectious diseases. Alternatively, prevention might be achieved by removing environmental risks by providing clean water or banning cigarette smoking in public places. At this level, prevention overlaps with an area of public health commonly referred to as health protection, which focuses primarily on the control of infectious diseases and environmental hazards. The term 'primordial prevention' (Beaglehole *et al.*, 1993) has been used to refer to the creation of conditions that limit the emergence and establishment of hazards known to increase the risk of disease, rather than simply reduce personal risk. This term overlaps with the term 'upstream' (McKinlay, 1981) or distal **determinants**, which both emphasize creating the preconditions for health. The distinction between the terms is perhaps ambiguous, although all imply actions aimed at keeping people healthy by limiting exposure to risks and enhancing protective factors.

Secondary prevention seeks to limit disease progression by early detection and intervention. Population-based targeted **screening** programmes are an example of secondary prevention and have been particularly directed at a number of cancers. The aim with secondary prevention is to detect early pathological changes at the cellular level, offer appropriate treatment and improve prognosis. Health checks for CVD, for example, also constitute a form of screening to assess CVD risk among those who may be unaware of their profile but who might benefit from some combination of lifestyle advice and medical intervention. Tertiary prevention is most commonly associated with recovery and rehabilitation. It aims to slow down progression of established disease, prevent further damage and improve quality of life. Cardiac rehabilitation programmes, for example, assist recovery from cardiovascular events. As with all frameworks and models however, they are best viewed as heuristic devices for thinking about phenomena. Classifying a preventive action at a particular level may not be straightforward and depends on the context. Treatment for HIV/AIDS (secondary prevention) reduces the risk of transmission (primary prevention) for example.

In recent years, the notion of prevention has expanded to include health-related phenomena other than medical illnesses and diseases and has been linked to the idea of 'early intervention' in a range of policy fields. This has become particularly evident in the field of child development where prevention has a dual meaning: early identification of an emerging problem as well as early intervention in the life course to avert problems in later life. In England, the development of Sure Start local programmes in areas of high **deprivation** in the late 1990s sought to deliver a comprehensive range of services to families with children under five years old. The aim was to ensure that children entered school ready to learn. Sure Start has been referred to as an 'upstream' approach (Gidley, 2007) insofar as it focused on trying to create the optimal family and **community** environment for healthy physical, cognitive, social and emotional development among children. The ultimate aim was to 'break the intergenerational transmission of poverty, school failure and social exclusion' (National Evaluation of Sure Start Team, 2010). Although seen as innovative in policy terms, it largely left untouched the fundamental **determinants** of area deprivation and family hardship, although it was anticipated that individuals might themselves improve their social position through employment and social mobility. Upstream approaches, although advocated, tend to be less common than downstream (secondary/tertiary) approaches to prevention.

The significance of prevention for public health

Public health problems, by definition, occur at a population level. Two approaches to prevention are frequently debated: a population-level strategy, which would include apparently healthy people, and a strategy that targets those at high risk. Rose (1981, 1985) has discussed the advantages and disadvantages of the two approaches in relation to CVD but his ideas have been more widely applied to a number of health phenomena, including the prevention of suicide (Knox *et al.*, 2004), gambling (Grun and McKeighue, 2000) and dental caries (Batchelor and Sheiham, 2002). Rose argued that population strategies should be the cornerstone of prevention on the basis that 'A large number of people exposed to a low risk is likely to produce more cases than a small number of people exposed to a high risk' (Rose, 1981: 1849). Recent estimates indicate that in Canada, 61 per cent of cases of diabetes mellitus will come from people at low or moderate risk (Manuel *et al.*, 2010). Population strategies aim to control the determinants of health and disease and shift the whole distribution of a risk variable in a more desirable direction, lowering the population mean through some measure in which all participate. Rose coined the term the 'prevention paradox' to describe the large benefits for the population compared to the small benefits for each individual. The logic of his argument applies to the case for immunization, as well as to nutritional supplementation of foodstuffs (Vitamin B in flour, for example) for protective factors. The aim is to alter norms of behaviour in relation to common determinants of health and disease (Rose, 1985).

The North Karelia CVD prevention project is a well-documented example of an intervention that was conceptualized and implemented as a community (population) problem related to the lifestyle of the *region* rather than to the lifestyles of a high risk group of individuals (Wagner, 1982). In the 1970s, the Finnish people in this region had some of the highest mortality rates from heart disease in the world. An integrated, multi-level approach was used to target general lifestyles through **education**, screening and changes to the environment. This led to marked reductions in lifestyle risks as well as reductions in rates of CVD during the five-year project (Puska, 2008). A similar strategy for HIV/AIDS control has been used in Brazil, which is widely credited with having averted a large number of AIDS cases, deaths and AIDs-related hospital admissions, with particular benefits for children (Ramos *et al.*, 2011). Since 1996, free universal access to antiretroviral therapy has been guaranteed (in law) to all those with AIDS. Although controversial and discouraged by many development agencies, including the World Bank, the strategy is believed to have reduced the stigma of AIDs, increasing people's willingness to be tested and increasing opportunities for risk behaviours to be addressed (Okie, 2006). Brazil's use of generic (rather than the more expensive patented) drugs made this initiative economically feasible. Alongside treatment, a diverse number of targeted strategies involving needle and syringe exchange programmes and condom distribution were used with vulnerable groups such as sex workers (prostitution is legal and regulated in Brazil), men who have sex with men, and injecting drug users, including those in prisons. Widespread public engagement with the programme was generated by the emerging AIDs movement, which emphasized the right to health and health care (enshrined in law in 1988) (Nunn *et al.*, 2009). These two examples illustrate how a multifaceted, sustained and well-resourced population-level programme, implemented in propitious domestic circumstances, can be an effective investment for disease control and health improvement.

The alternative high risk strategy has, nevertheless, become commonplace in many countries. Although such strategies have limited impact at a population level, the benefits to individuals are large. In England, CVD prevention in recent years has tended to emphasize pharmacological approaches to smoking cessation (nicotine replacement therapy), high blood pressure (antihypertensive drugs) and elevated cholesterol (statins) (Blackman, 2007), with the development of a 'polypill' (a fixed dose pill designed to reduce several CVD risk factors) being debated for use in primary, rather than second-ary prevention (Wald and Wald, 2010). Such developments have been described as the pharmaceuticalization of public health (Bell and Figert, 2012). This type of approach raises significant issues about drug costs, the potential for over-medication (partic-ularly for older people), as well as the **ethics** of preventing disease through the use of drugs, given their likely side-effects. Pharmaceuticalization also deflects attention and resources away from the fundamental causes of the unequal distribution of health and disease in the population; nor does it seek to change these. Although it is generally accepted that a combination of strategies is likely to be most effective, these debates are likely to intensify given the power of the pharmaceutical market and the likely appeal of personalized medicine.

Harm reduction policies and strategies are a particular form of prevention developed to minimize the harms associated with a behaviour, rather than seeking to change the behaviour itself. The central aim is to provide the *means* to minimize harm. Com-pulsory seat belt usage is an example of a population-based harm reduction policy, the aim of which was to reduce road trauma. In England, legislation passed in 1983 resulted in increased front passenger seat belt wearing from 40 to 95 per cent. Although offering individual protection to people in an accident, some have questioned the extent to which the legislation has reduced deaths to the level projected, either in England or elsewhere (Richens *et al.*, 2000). Part of the explanation put forward to account for this is 'risk compensation', whereby wearing a seat belt contributes to drivers feeling safer, increasing their likelihood of driving faster or more carelessly than they might other-wise do (Adams, 1994). This unintended consequence of preventive actions has been discussed widely in the field of sport and active recreation. Wearing helmets while skiing or cycling, for example, may alter people's perceptions of their vulnerability and shift their behaviour in a more risk-taking direction (Adams and Hillman, 2001). This issue has also been discussed in relation to the use of sunscreen to protect against melanoma (longer exposure times) and wearing condoms to protect against HIV transmission (more frequent sex and riskier practices) (Cassell *et al.*, 2006).

Targeted harm reduction programmes directed at specific groups have also been used. Needle and syringe exchange schemes, for example, aim to reduce the trans-mission of blood-borne infections (such as hepatitis C) associated with sharing drug-injecting equipment by providing access to sterile equipment. This type of harm reduction strategy has attracted considerable controversy, particularly in the prison setting. In 2010, just ten countries worldwide had introduced such programmes in prisons, in spite of the widely acknowledged prevalence of blood-borne diseases (Cook *et al.*, 2010). Similarly, the introduction of condoms into prisons to reduce transmission of HIV and other sexually transmitted infections remains uncommon globally in spite of research indicating that such a policy increases the use of protection during anal intercourse reducing the risk of infection transmission (Butler *et al.*, 2013). Although harm reduction is an official policy of the UN and is reasonably scientifically well-founded, its absence in prison environments is indicative of the ideological character of arguments relating to prevention. In these instances facts and values are often hidden and conflated (Tesh, 1988).

Harm reduction has been especially controversial in schools, sensitive as they are to charges of condoning or encouraging certain forms of behaviour through the provision of, for example, sex and relationship education and access to free condoms. However, other **settings** such as pharmacies and nightclubs have introduced a variety of harm reduction strategies that have directly sought to minimize the harms associated with young people's experimental, and often transient, risk-taking behaviours. In England since 2001, free emergency contraception has been available, including to those under sixteen judged competent to understand information. Pharmacies providing emergency contraception also offer sexual health advice, access to chlamydia screening and onward referral to relevant services. In a similar vein, nightclubs have been viewed as settings that can be made safer by, for example, providing free water to minimize the risk of dehydration for those using ecstasy, as well as seeking to make the environment safer by encouraging the use of shatterproof glass, and making condoms available and affordable (Bellis *et al.*, 2002).

The rationale for prevention is often couched in terms of reducing the demand for health care, as well as moderating wider social costs. Some have questioned this assumption, however, as prevention itself represents a cost. The increasing emphasis on the need for **evidence** of cost-effectiveness to inform preventive strategies can obscure the problematic nature of such **evaluation** methodologies when applied to the public health field. Even when robust evidence of cost-effectiveness is available, the political will to implement measures is often lacking. Although different social groups are more or less price-sensitive, there is strong evidence that price serves as an effective constraint on alcohol consumption (Ludbrook, 2009). However, debates about the introduction in England of a minimum price per unit of alcohol illustrate the complexity of prevention in practice, as arguments about the smoking ban in public places did earlier. These population-level measures challenge commercial interests as well as those of governments in relation to the labour market and excise revenue. In this context, research tends to be discredited by those with vested interests in maintaining the status quo, marginalizing scientific and humanitarian arguments in the process. With the exception of British Columbia in Canada, few states or countries have yet to implement a minimum pricing strategy for alcohol (Stockwell *et al.*, 2011). Some Scandinavian countries, such as Norway, run a state monopoly that controls price. Although there is currently some political commitment in the UK to introduce minimum pricing (Secretary of State for the Home Department, 2012) and the Scottish Parliament has passed relevant legislation to pave the way, representatives of the wine and spirits industry have mounted a legal challenge (Woodhouse and Ward, 2013). Conflicting ideologies, motives and priorities characterize these discussions, as illustrated by recent debates about gun control in the USA.

Population-level strategies also tend to provoke debate regarding where responsibility should lie for health. Obesity is widely recognized as a major driver of health care costs in the USA and elsewhere but calculations about the potential savings that could be made if prevention was prioritized tend to assume that attempts to change behaviour will be successful (Wilson, 2009). Nevertheless, population strategies, including legislation, can play a major role in supporting individual-level strategies by constraining the many and varied negative influences that shape behaviours, making it easier for people to act in more desirable ways.

Conclusion

Prevention can have a number of unintended consequences, including the creation of unforeseen new problems. In the case of legislation and other measures aimed at controlling smoking, tobacco companies are said to have marketed cigarettes more aggressively, especially in low-income countries. Tightening the control of tobacco has also meant that smoking has become more polarized within high-income countries, as cessation rates have fallen fastest in higher income groups, thus widening health **inequalities**. If successful, prevention can contribute to increases in life expectancy, which in turn can lead to increases in chronic conditions which pose their own problems. However, if preventive efforts were directed at the fundamental **determinants** of health there may be less need for specific preventive efforts. Put simply, social change towards greater equity might be the best preventative 'medicine' (Mackenbach, 2009).

PRIMARY HEALTH CARE

Context

Primary health care (PHC) is typically the first point of contact with the health care system for people. Although debates about PHC tend to orientate towards the 1978 *Alma-Ata Declaration* (WHO/UNICEF) the idea of PHC is not new. The Dawson Report, published in the UK in 1920, proposed the idea of primary health centres (Frenk, 2009) and Dawson himself was influenced by the idea of polyclinics first developed in the USSR after the Bolshevik Revolution (Berridge, 2008). Largely for financial reasons, Dawson's idea of a network of health centres was never implemented. The concept re-emerged, nevertheless, in the form of the Pioneer Health Centre, established in 1926 in Peckham as an 'experiment' to test out new ways of promoting family **health** and preventing disease by bringing together a range of services and activities, including sport and recreation (Baehr, 1944). This paved the way for other health centres to develop in London during the 1930s.

The health centre concept resurfaced in the UK in the 1960s. Around the same time, a reconsideration of the potential value of PHC in low-income countries was prompted by a realization of the limited value of using technology and specialist doctors to solve basic health problems. Cueto (2004) traces the term PHC to medical missionaries working in developing countries who emphasized the training of village workers to provide low cost, simple and effective health measures to communities. China's version of PHC took the form of 'barefoot doctors' – a crucial aspect of its rural health care system – which have been in decline since the late 1970s (Zhu *et al.*, 1989). The seemingly intractable health issues in low-income countries and the influence of ideas from elsewhere provided the context within which the *Alma-Ata Declaration* was developed. At that time, it was estimated that 2000 million people had no access to adequate health care amidst large-scale **inequalities** between and within countries. The Declaration provided the ideological basis for a revitalization of PHC. In so doing, it made the crucial link between PHC and public health, viewing the former as the means through which health for all might be achieved. This ambitious goal has not been achieved. Nonetheless, in 2008, *The Lancet* published a series of articles on PHC, arguing for the contemporary relevance of the *Alma-Ata Declaration* and a renaissance and re-visioning of PHC.

Defining primary health care

The *Alma-Ata Declaration* gives what might be viewed as an expanded definition of PHC:

> [E]ssential health care based on practical, scientifically sound and socially acceptable methods and technology made universally accessible to individuals and families in the **community** through their full participation and at a cost that the community and country can afford to maintain at every stage of their development in the spirit of self-reliance and self-determination.
>
> (WHO, 1978: 1 (emphasis added))

This definition, as well as the Declaration more broadly, reflects particular values – equity through universal access, community participation and ownership – as well as the importance the WHO attached to the need to reorient health care towards disease control, **prevention**, and **health promotion**. Such a shift necessitated collaboration with other sectors in order that adequate supplies of food, safe water and basic sanitation could be secured and maternal and child health care could be improved through better family planning and immunization coverage against the main infectious diseases. However, the varying ways in which this vision was interpreted illustrates many of the problems associated with turning ideas into actions.

The explicitly ideological character of the Declaration presented a challenge to the power and control of the medical profession as well as funding agencies, which saw their view of **economic development** leading to better health turned on its head. Rather than seeing its idealism as aspirational, the Declaration was criticized for being unrealistic. What followed in many low-income countries was 'selective primary health care' (selective PHC), funding agencies requiring a more medical, narrower form of PHC, leaving power and control in their hands rather than that of communities. Consequently, programmes were developed that focused on maternal and child health, specifically in relation to growth, oral rehydration therapy, breastfeeding and immunization (Cueto, 2004). These vertical, top-down programmes were seen by many as marginalizing PHC and creating dependency (Werner, 1995). Others have viewed them as necessary and complementary approaches particularly during an era of rapidly emerging HIV/AIDS and the outbreak of civil war in many countries (Chan, 2009). In some countries, there has been a shift to using selective PHC to strengthen broader health systems in order to enable them to deliver a more comprehensive range of services. The plethora of vertical programmes has, nevertheless, resulted in fragmentation, duplication and gaps in provision (Coovadia and Bland, 2008).

SAPs introduced by the IMF and the World Bank in the 1980s hastened the demise of PHC and consolidated selective PHC by setting in train health sector reform through the extension of the market alongside a concomitant reduction in state services (Hall and Taylor, 2003). The introduction of cost recovery (charging for oral rehydration salts and medicines, for example), user fees (for services) and caps on the number of nurses and doctors together reduced overall funding of systems and worsened access to health care for the poor (Lawn et al., 2008). Together these measures also affected household finances, limiting what could be spent on food (Werner, 1995). It is noteworthy that many countries have abandoned user fees (Johnson et al., 2012). Calls for the revitalization of PHC on the thirtieth anniversary of the *Alma-Ata Declaration* reflect this broader macroeconomic **policy** context, an outcome of which has been widening inequalities in health and a deterioration of health systems in some countries. As far as PHC is concerned, the ideology of the market and its attendant deregulation has come to be part of the problem rather than part of the solution for addressing health inequalities and inequities (Sanders et al., 2011).

The debate about the interpretation of PHC hinges, in part, on a particular issue that has resonance for all health care systems across the world. The term 'primary health care' and the term 'primary care' have tended to be used interchangeably (Muldoon *et al.*, 2006). Both suggest a 'first point of contact'. However, primary care has much in common with what in high-income countries is called general practice or family **medicine**, in which clinicians, typically doctors, provide person-centred care to address new needs and ongoing health problems (Starfield, 2011). In the UK, there has been criticism of the medical focus of much primary care over many years alongside calls for doctors to broaden the scope of their everyday interactions with patients, orientating their practice towards public health at an individual and population level (Hart, 1981; Stott and Davis, 1979). Similar to the *Alma-Ata Declaration* vision for PHC, Hart advocated primary care that was broad, comprehensive, and oriented towards the wider social **determinants** of health. Thus, the critical distinction between primary care and PHC is that the latter has an explicit reference point beyond the health care system (Rasanathan et al., 2011). Starfield (2011: 653) argues that the distinction is important because it turns on 'achieving greater equity in health through societal actions'.

The significance of primary health care for public health

Three broad themes can be identified in recent debates about the continuing role and purpose of PHC. These relate to the impact of PHC on health and health inequalities, who should deliver services, and, the orientation of PHC towards public health. Notwithstanding the limitations of cross-sectional studies, research in a number of high-income countries suggests that strong PHC systems are associated with a variety of improved health outcomes (Macinko et al., 2003). Moreover, good primary care experiences have been associated with buffering some of the adverse effects of income inequality (Shi et al., 2002) and more equitable distribution of health in a population (Rawaf et al., 2008). Starfield et al. (2005) found that states in the USA with a higher ratio of primary care doctors to population had lower rates of smoking and obesity. There is also broad agreement about the attributes of primary care that are likely to be important in leading to improved and more equitable population health: namely, free, universal access to a comprehensive range of services, person-centred (rather than disease-focused) and co-ordinated care (Starfield, 2011). A number of low- and middle-income countries with expanded primary care systems have also demonstrated several health gains, particularly in relation to maternal and child health: Thailand, Brazil, Cuba, Oman (Rawaf *et al.*, 2008), Gambia and Tanzania (Hall and Taylor, 2003). Gains over several years cannot be taken for granted, however, as fluctuating economic circumstances continue to threaten the extent and quality of provision, such as in Brazil (Kepp, 2008). China is endeavouring to turn back the clock and rebuild its primary care system having experimented with market-based reforms (Lui *et al.*, 2011), which it views as having failed to adequately control HIV/AIDS and CVD (Ma *et al.*, 2008).

The involvement of non-medically qualified practitioners in the planning and delivery of PHC was a central tenet of the *Alma-Ata Declaration*. A number of well-documented outreach models have been used in low- and middle-income countries: village health workers, barefoot doctors and birth assistants for example (Werner, 1984). Here, trained members of the community deliver prevention, care and treatment at low cost and using a low level of technology. Community health workers have been used in the USA and UK, particularly in areas where there are vulnerable, marginalized urban populations, helping people register to vote and escape from violence, as well as acting as advocates for their communities. Experimentation with creating new **settings** (such as healthy living centres) and roles (such as community volunteers and health trainers) in areas of **deprivation** in England has sought to engage 'the hard to reach', among whom **health needs** are judged to be greatest. Although explicitly funded to test out new ideas, limited **evaluation** means that their effectiveness remains uncertain. This might explain, at least in part, why community-based public health models such as these have remained something of a parallel development rather than influencing the shape of primary care more fundamentally.

The extent to which primary care can be oriented towards public health remains keenly debated in many high-income countries. In the UK, policy rhetoric continues to emphasize that not only are GPs and other primary care professionals ideally positioned to create opportunities in every patient encounter to discuss health-related issues that go beyond the initial presenting matter, they are also credible sources of advice. Beyond the policy field too, primary care has been identified as central to realizing health improvement and health inequalities targets (CSDH, 2008; Marmot, 2010; Royal College of Physicians, 2010; Wanless, 2004). It seems, nevertheless, that primary care in general, and GPs in particular, continue to individualize, medicalize and pharmaceuticalize patients' problems. Furthermore, the introduction of practice-based financial incentives in the UK has skewed activities towards those that attract payment while neglecting others (Peckham and Hann, 2008) – a matter worthy of note given current proposals in England to pay doctors to ask patients about their drinking habits (Secretary of State for the Home Department, 2012). **Evidence** from a number of countries suggests that primary care doctors may be reluctant to broaden their role to include health promotion activities because they lack the knowledge, skills and time to carry them out; they also question their value and appropriateness (McKinlay *et al.*, 2005; Schoen *et al.*, 2004). This echoes observations made in the late 1970s about doctors' reluctance to become more proactive and anticipatory in their patients' care

(Hart, 1981; Stott and Davis, 1979). Shifting public health work to other members of the PHC team may well leave unchanged the fundamental biomedical culture of PHC (Needle *et al.*, 2011). The location of social welfare services such as Citizens Advice Bureaux in PHC settings may provide a more effective model for how to expand public health work in primary care (Caiels and Thurston, 2005).

A variety of schemes have been introduced into primary care in many countries offering GPs alternatives or an adjunct to pharmaceutical interventions. Exercise on prescription schemes that use a 'prescription' for referral onto a programme of exercise have been particularly well-documented (Thurston and Green, 2004). The idea of providing a prescription has been extended to fruit and vegetable consumption (Kearney *et al.*, 2005) and to the arts to address mental health issues, including postnatal depression (Bungay and Clift, 2010; Perry *et al.*, 2008). These schemes link patients, via a prescription and referral process to community-based resources. The role of the GP (or other health professional) in the process is to initiate discussions and offer brief advice. A recent systematic review and meta-analysis of physical activity promotion in primary care (referral, advice and counselling interventions) concluded that schemes were effective in increasing self-reported activity at 12 months (Orrow *et al.*, 2012). Participation in regular low-impact exercise is a protective factor in a range of illnesses and diseases as well as having therapeutic benefits in some neurological disorders associated with ageing, including Alzheimer's disease (Lucia and Ruiz, 2011).

Conclusion

Globally, there is some consensus that the vision for PHC articulated in the *Alma-Ata Declaration* continues to be relevant to all countries if population health is to improve and health inequalities reduced. This seems particularly pertinent during periods of financial austerity, when those most vulnerable and marginalized face worsening circumstances, placing, in turn, additional strain on primary care services (Blane and Watt, 2012). In this regard, Chan (2009: 1586) argues that 'we will not be able to reach health-related MDGs unless we return to the values, principles, and approaches of primary health care'. Notwithstanding the continuing significance of PHC to public health, it seems likely, however, that change will be incremental, not least because of the power of elites such as the medical profession, national governments and global economic institutions. Some remain optimistic, however, noting that there are signs that market universalism is being challenged by global social movements. Incrementalism from the bottom up might, nonetheless, be engendered through those working in PHC seizing available opportunities.

RISK

Context

The application of science and technology in the public health field has lessened people's exposure to many risks (for example, through the purification of water, safe disposal of sewerage and preservation of foods). However, as Beck (1992) suggests in his much cited book *Risk Society*, new forms of risk have emerged that are themselves products of science and technology. He argues that these risks are all-pervasive, unavoidable and generated through global interdependencies. The Fukushima nuclear power plant accident in 2011 in Japan is an example. Other risks include those posed by **climate change**, genetically modified crops, living in the vicinity of an industrial complex, as well as medicine itself. Alongside the recognition of risks associated with science and technology, the individualization of risk locates a number of threats to **health** in people's genes and behaviours. Arising out of people's heightened awareness of risk has been the development of a culture of risk assessment and risk management. Paternalistic as these developments might seem – and driven in part by a fear of litigation – they have become a central feature of contemporary society in which the protection and promotion of health and well-being are primary goals. As a consequence, risk – its communication and management – has become a core concern of public health work.

Defining risk

Risk is a way of talking about events that are not certain: that is, they are viewed as being more or less likely. In the academic literature, two distinct ways of conceptualizing risk can be discerned. In **epidemiology** (and other quantitative sciences) objective, statistical notions of risk are used, based on a definition of risk as 'the probability that an event will occur' (Porta, 2008: 217). It follows from this that risk can be quantified in various ways, such that the magnitude of risk in relation to different activities or events can be calculated. In epidemiology, one commonly used measure is 'relative risk' (risk ratio, or numerical odds), defined as the ratio of the risk of an event among the exposed, to the risk among the unexposed (Porta, 2008: 213). Relative risk quantifies how much more likely someone is to develop a disease or other condition if they have been exposed compared to someone who has not. Relative risk has been used extensively to quantify various risks relating to different kinds of occupational exposure as well as 'behavioural risk factors', such as smoking. The *British Regional Heart Study*, for example, investigated the risk of smoking for myocardial infarction in men aged 40–59 years by comparing those who had ever smoked with those who had never smoked. They calculated a relative risk of 2.00, interpreted as those men who had smoked being twice as likely to have a myocardial infarction compared to those who never smoked (Petrie and Sabin, 2000). The odds ratio is a good estimate of the relative risk in situations where the disease is rare and there is no direct measure of the incidence of disease and is interpreted in the same way (Wassertheil-Smoller, 2004). A case-control study calculated an odds ratio of developing lung cancer among those who smoked 15–24 cigarettes a day compared to non-smokers, of 9.6. Both measures give an indication of the strength of the association, a criterion that is important in judging **causality**. A third measure of risk – absolute risk – is used to indicate an individual's probability of an event. One of the most commonly used measures of absolute risk is the Framingham score, often calculated during a CVD health check. This score predicts the 10-year risk of having a CVD event.

There has been extensive criticism of the statistical measurement of risk however. Sociologists, for example, tend to view risk as more-or-less socially constructed and culturally framed (Douglas and Wildavsky, cited in Hansson, 2010): that is to say, as a matter of perception unrelated to 'facts' and shaped by social norms. Integration of objective and subjective approaches presuppose that 'factual' risk information is made sense of subjectively, depending on people's context, values and social and economic location. The potential advantage of this integrated model is that it accounts for how risks can mean different things to different people depending on their situation. The risk of rain, for example, might be viewed and evaluated differently by a tourist and a farmer (Hansson, 2010).

Significance of risk for public health

In public health **policy** and practice, the tendency has been to apply the objective, factual and rational view of risk to health behaviour and decision-making. According to this view, people's health beliefs are influenced by quantitative risk information (their Framingham risk score and related **lifestyle** advice, for example) and their behaviour is modified accordingly. Research in the health field, however, indicates that people tend not to act in the ways that the objective risk model predicts (Bond and Nolan, 2011). Perception of risk has been studied quite extensively in relation to the uptake of preventive interventions such as vaccination and **screening**, as well as appraisals of disease risk. Unsurprisingly, perhaps, people's understanding of statistical risk tends to be limited.

Understanding the uptake of vaccinations has received renewed attention in recent years, particularly in the wake of the controversy over the safety of the MMR (measles, mumps, rubella) vaccine. In the late 1990s/early 2000s, the media drew attention to published scientific research that linked the MMR vaccine with risk of autism and Crohn's disease. During a long period of investigation (the outcome of which was that the research was judged to be fraudulent) there was a decline in vaccination uptake in the UK (from 92 per cent in the mid 1990s to 82 per cent in 2003 and as low as 75 per cent in London) and other countries such as the USA (Fitzpatrick, 2004). The success of mass vaccination programmes is dependent, however, on high uptake in order to maintain herd immunity; estimates suggest that coverage should be 92–95 per cent to prevent measles outbreaks, for example (Wright and Polack, 2006). Outbreaks of measles in some parts of Wales (UK) in 2013, where coverage was less than optimal indicated that parental concern about the vaccine had endured, in spite of the concerted efforts of health authorities to reassure parents (Public Health Wales, 2013). Indeed, parental refusal of vaccines seems to be increasing in some places even though vaccine risk is low (Chatterjee and O'Keefe, 2010). Insights from qualitative research suggest that vaccine safety is but one element informing parents' immunization decisions. Alongside vaccine risk are parents' perceptions of disease risk, the susceptibility or robustness of their child and perceptions of who is more or less at risk in their **community** (Bond and Nolan, 2011). This research suggests that appraisal of risk is better viewed as a complex and multifaceted process, rather than a one-off rational event. It involves subjective interpretations of authoritative 'factual' information made sense of in a personal context. This model of risk appraisal might be fruitfully applied to other vaccination-related 'conundrums' such as the limited uptake of influenza vaccination – which has few risks and demonstrable benefits associated with its use – by health care staff in many countries (Hollmeyer *et al.*, 2009).

Viewing the reduced take-up in terms of 'misperception' of risk oversimplifies a more complex phenomenon. Such a perspective will also tend to lead to a reliance on educational campaigns to 'correct' misperceptions. As the foregoing discussion implies, such an approach is likely to be limited in its impact. Parental anxiety about the MMR vaccination has endured and may well influence views about childhood vaccination more generally. Viewing risk as fluid rather than static suggests that people's perception of risk may well shift as their circumstances alter – a second child, a new partner, becoming unemployed, and so on. A simple categorization of parents into those who immunize their children and those who do not is likely to underestimate the opportunities for influencing vaccination uptake. The corollary to this, however, is that the communication of risk becomes much more challenging.

Insights into how people make sense of risk in relation to the causes of disease also indicates that objective, rational models of risk are likely to be limited in explaining risk-behaviours. 'Lay epidemiology' has been used as a concept to explain the ways in which people incorporate official messages about health risks with cultural beliefs, such as those relating to luck and fate. Discussing coronary heart disease, Davison *et al.* (1991) argue that lay epidemiology constitutes a rational way of accommodating potentially bothersome information in conditions of uncertainty. This view of risk re-frames 'rationality' as bound up with the emotional, day-to-day context of people's lives in which they make myriad decisions relating to a variety of competing phenomena. Risk management is thus an aspect of people's everyday lives. It also provides a way of understanding why conventional approaches to **behaviour change** based on communicating factual risk information are unlikely to succeed (Lawler *et al.*, 2003).

Applying a risk appraisal perspective (in which costs and benefits are analysed) to sport and physical activity illustrates some of the complexities involved in promoting particular forms of behaviour. The health benefits of regular physical activity have been extensively documented, particularly in relation to cardiovascular risk reduction and weight management. For children and youth, the accumulation of 60 minutes of at least moderate intensity physical activity daily has been internationally recommended (Janssen and LeBlanc, 2010). Nevertheless, participation in sport is not without risks; pain and injury, sometimes fatal injury, can be the outcome of being physically active, particularly in some high-impact contact-sports such as rugby. Injury is much less likely in moderate, rhythmical activities (Waddington, 2000). These outcomes incur a range of personal, social and economic costs, leading some to conclude that sports injuries are themselves a public health issue (Finch and Cassell, 2006). A study carried out in Flanders estimated the injury rate in a number of sports and found it ranged from 8.96 per cent for handball to 0.62 per cent for swimming (Cumps *et al.*, 2008). Direct medical costs amounted to 0.08 per cent of the health care budget. A systematic review of knee injuries among youth found that prevalence rates ranged between 10 and 25 per cent, knee injury tending to generate high economic costs (Louw *et al.*, 2007). An aspect of the professionalization of sports such as rugby has been to take steps to increase protective clothing to reduce injury. However, some argue that risk compensation is the outcome of these measures; players respond by being more physical in tackles and so on (Adams and Hillman, 2001).

These issues are particularly well-illustrated in the case of active travel, where the benefits associated with cycling to school or work tend to be emphasized – increases in physical activity, decline in traffic congestion and reduction in exhaust emissions, for example. Nonetheless, there are also potential costs such as exposure of cyclists to atmospheric pollution and accidents. Quantitative estimates suggest that the health benefits of cycling (months of life gained) were considerably larger than the risks associated with exposure to air pollution and traffic risks (De Hartog *et al.*, 2010). However, people's perception of the risks of cycling, particularly in urban areas where traffic may not be well controlled, may override objective cost-benefits analyses. With regard to children, there has been a trend in some countries towards children spending less time in outdoor play and active travel compared to previous generations (Wooley *et al.*, 2009). The reasons for this are manifold, but parental perceptions of risk in relation to 'strangers', road traffic and other hazards in the neighbourhood are relevant to understanding this trend (Carver *et al.*, 2008). Ironically, parents driving their children to school actively contribute to the dangers from which they are seeking to protect their children (Tranter and Pawson, 2001).

Risk perception and appraisal among young people has received considerable attention in recent years. Youth, it seems, tends to be a period of experimentation and, sometimes, deliberate risk-taking, in which there is a search for excitement and fun (Mitchell *et al.*, 2001). This suggests that risk may not necessarily be a negative phenomenon for young people (Austen, 2009) but rather a source of attraction related to the uncertainties (rather than predictability) found in some kinds of pastimes. Engaging in activities that have varying degrees of risk allows young people to express themselves, develop their identities and challenge boundaries, particularly those of authority. Participation in high-risk activities is, nevertheless, patterned along class and gender lines, as well as across different countries, reflecting different cultural norms and expectations. As far as sport is concerned, working class youth tend to be over-represented in fighting sports such as boxing and martial arts. Middle-class youth, on the other hand, are more likely to be involved in adventure sports, including extreme sports such as off-piste skiing and white water kayaking (Green, 2010). Other risks associated with styles of alcohol consumption and drug use tend to be more generally pervasive among youth. Here, young people tend to be aware of the risks associated with different activities and 'manage' them in various ways. For example, young people who use ecstasy are likely to be acquainted with the documented risks and take steps to minimize them (by avoiding dehydration for example) (Peters *et al.*, 2008). There has been a tendency in public health, however, to explain young people's smoking and alcohol consumption in terms of their perceptions of invulnerability, due to a lack of familiarity with severe health-related events. Research reveals, nonetheless, that risks can be perceived as 'worth it' because of the social benefits they bring (Denscombe and Drucquer, 1999). **Evidence** from a variety of countries indicates that adolescents who report having a positive connection to a trusted adult – parent or teacher – display fewer risky behaviours, are more socially competent and have higher self-esteem (Bynner, 2001).

Conclusion

Much of the debate in public health policy and practice about risk, risk avoidance through preventive action and risk-taking is presented in terms of individual behaviours. Less attention has been paid to understanding how people perceive and respond to risks in the environment. Exposure to risk is contoured according to the established patterns of inequality; people in lower socio-economic groups are not only more likely to experience being unemployed, live in a deprived neighbourhood, have poorer housing, live closer to hazards such a main roads, but also have less control over the risks emanating from these conditions. There may be a tendency for policymakers to rationalize such risks, obviating the need for policy action. The precautionary principle – better safe than sorry– is rarely applied in these contexts although often put forward as a tool for assessing and managing these types of environmental risks. It seems likely that risk assessment, communication and management will continue to be core aspects of public health work. Interpretive risk-perception approaches challenge established epidemiological approaches to this work but at the same time offer some ways forward for integrating lay and expert views on risk.

SCREENING

Context

Population-based screening is a well-established approach to secondary **prevention**. Most high-income countries have national screening programmes for CVD, various cancers, as well as a range of genetic factors. Screening contributes significantly to **health** service activity and costs. In England in 2011–2012, for example, 4.75 million screening tests for newborn babies and 5 million screening tests in pregnant women were carried out, and over 100,000 men were screened for abdominal aortic aneurysm (UK National Screening Committee (UK NSC), 2012). Alongside these programmes, opportunistic screening – for such things as hazardous alcohol consumption in Accident and Emergency (A&E) departments and high blood pressure in primary care – has expanded. The development of private sector organizations offering a range of screening tests – such as Doppler ultrasound examination of the carotid arteries and abdomen to test for peripheral artery disease (McCartney, 2012) – has added to the volume of screening opportunities. However, the proliferation of screening initiatives and tests within and beyond national health services may not be in an individual's best interests, particularly given the profit motive that underpins the market in screening. While screening has the potential to be a cost-effective strategy for preventing disease, extending life and reducing disability, it nonetheless carries **risks** and has a number of limitations. The need to scrutinize the costs and benefits of screening, as well as the ethical issues it raises, has been heightened by developments related to the human genome project as well as technology more generally.

Defining screening

One of the earliest formal definitions by the 1951 US Commission on Chronic Illness referred to screening as 'the presumptive identification of unrecognized disease or defect by the application of tests, examinations or other procedures which can be applied rapidly' (Porta, 2008: 224). The USA was one of the first high-income countries to expand its screening programmes, reflecting the technological developments that were taking place in **medicine** during the 1950s. Since then a number of definitions have emerged, reflecting the expansion of screening to cover a wide variety of diseases, disorders and conditions. Definitions have also sought to differentiate screening from other clinical interventions from which people might benefit. Wald for example, defines screening as

> the systematic application of a test or enquiry to identify individuals at sufficient risk of a specific disorder to benefit from further investigation or direct preventive action, among people who have not sought medical attention because of symptoms of that disorder.
>
> (Wald 2008: 50)

Despite originally adopting Wald's definition, the UK NSC's most recent definition placed greater emphasis on the choices that follow from a screening test result:

> [A] process of identifying apparently healthy people who may be at increased risk of a disease or condition [who] can then be offered information, further tests and appropriate treatment to reduce their risk and/or any complications arising from the disease or condition.
>
> (UK NSC, 2012: 8).

The advantage of Wald's (2008) definition is, however, that it encapsulates the three core elements of screening about which there is some agreement and from which flow a number of issues. The first element is the screening test, the purpose of which is to identify those who have an elevated risk of the disease or condition and which is judged to warrant further investigation (using a diagnostic test). Thus, the screening test is not itself diagnostic of disease. Depending on the outcome of the diagnostic test, treatment may follow. The second element of note is that screening involves *inviting* people to participate; in other words, individuals themselves have not sought medical attention because of symptoms relating to the disease or condition. Third, the key purpose of population-based screening is benefit to the individual. Wald (2008) points out that this element differentiates screening from surveillance activities designed to monitor trends in cases such as those related to mass anonymous testing for HIV.

The significance of screening for public health

The expansion of national screening programmes has been one of the more significant developments in public health in recent years, the underpinning rationale for which is that early detection and treatment increase the likelihood of better outcomes. In the UK, the NSC advises ministers and the NHS in all four countries on the case for implementing new population-based screening programmes. In 1968, Wilson and Jungner published the first set of criteria for judging whether or not a screening programme should be established and these are still considered the 'gold standard' (Andermann *et al.*, 2008). Drawing on these criteria, the UK NSC published an expanded version that broadly relate to: understanding of the condition; the effectiveness and reliability of screening and diagnostic tests and subsequent treatment; the organization of the screening programme itself; and, **evidence** of effectiveness and cost-effectiveness of the screening programme in reducing mortality or morbidity. These criteria (and other similar frameworks) were developed to ensure that screening was not undertaken where it might cause more harm than good and might constitute an unwise use of resources.

This means that whilst a valid and reliable screening test is a necessary element of a screening pathway (the term used to refer to the whole screening process from initial invitation, through to treatment if required), unless the condition is serious (rather than trivial), treatable and will benefit from earlier detection, the test should not be used because of its potential to increase people's anxiety and waste resources (Strong *et al.*, 2005). In relation to treatment, facilities should be adequate and treatment should be safe, effective (insofar as early treatment is more beneficial than treatment begun after the development of obvious disease) and acceptable. Serious shortages of surgeons, pathologists and oncologists, as well as a shortage of inpatient beds and theatre time can all lead to diagnostic delay. The criteria provide, therefore, a transparent framework for weighing up the case for a screening programme.

A particular concern is the validity of a screening test, in that it should correctly categorize those screened into individuals with or without the disease. This is not a straightforward task, in part because the cut off points for 'normal' and 'abnormal' can be quite arbitrary, particularly if there is limited knowledge of the way in which the factor of interest varies in the population. The measures of validity relevant to screening are sensitivity – the extent to which the test identifies *all* those with the disease – and, specificity – the extent to which the test identifies *only* those with the disease. In ideal circumstances a test would have high sensitivity and high specificity, as well as high predictive value – the probability of the disease given the results of the test (Porta, 2008). However, a feature of all screening tests is that they yield a number of 'false positives' (those whom the test shows as positive but who do not have the disease) and 'false negatives' (those whom the test shows as negative but who do in fact have the disease). The reason for recommending screening at specific intervals on many programmes is that a certain proportion of conditions such as cancers will be missed by a single screen. Without appropriate pre-test consultation and post-test follow-up people's understanding of their test result might be limited and give rise to either false reassurance (in the case of a false negative) or unnecessary anxiety and treatment (in the case of a false positive).

In the case of many cancers, prognosis is strongly linked to stage (size as well as the extent to which the cancer has spread) at diagnosis. Comparative studies of cancer survival rates have consistently shown the UK lagging behind other comparable European countries (Sant *et al.*, 2009), as well as Canada and Australia (Foot and Harrison, 2011). Part of the explanation for differences in survival has been the later stage at which cancers were diagnosed. National screening programmes for breast, cervical and bowel cancer, however, aim to increase early detection and improve survival. In the case of cervical cancer, five-yearly screening has been estimated to prevent 63–73 per cent of cancers in women over 50 years (Patnick, 2013). Diagnostic delay is, however, a reflection of whether or not patients attend for screening having been invited, as well as how quickly they are diagnosed and treated by the health care system (Foot and Harrison, 2011). Diagnostic delay is, therefore, a function of individual, doctor and other service factors. Although England is judged to have developed high quality screening programmes, uptake varies considerably by region (Weller and Campbell, 2009).

In national screening programmes, uptake (the proportion of those who, having been invited, attend and record a screening result) is a major determinant of success (Weller and Campbell, 2009). It can, however, be below the target level and thus compromise success, particularly if those at greater risk and with potentially more to gain are the ones least likely to attend. In some cases, the nature of the screening test itself may deter people from responding positively to an invitation. According to the criteria discussed above, the test should be simple, safe, valid and reliable, as well as acceptable to people. Screening for breast cancer (using mammography), cervical cancer (involving a cytological 'smear') and colorectal cancer (using a faecal occult blood test), however, have been shown to be perceived as involving unpleasant experiences (Jepson *et al.*, 2007). Test acceptability may well be an important factor in uptake. However, uptake is also patterned in relation to age, ethnic background, **deprivation** and gender. In England, uptake on the national Bowel Cancer Screening Programme has been 55–60 per cent outside London, and 40 per cent in London (target 60 per cent) (Logan *et al.*, 2011). Uptake among men and minority ethnic groups has been particularly low (Nnoaham *et al.*, 2010). Level of **education**, as well as ethnicity, have also been associated with uptake in the USA (Atar *et al.*, 2006). In relation to screening for breast cancer, socio-economic status is an important factor in explaining uptake, as well as ethnic group, with white women from higher socio-economic groups being more likely to attend (Weller and Campbell, 2009). Uptake of screening seems, therefore, to reflect broader patterns of inequality; overall, use of preventive services such as screening is less likely among disadvantaged groups.

Strategies to increase uptake have tended to focus on organizational aspects of the screening programme, such as sending reminder letters. The role of the media in bringing cervical cancer to the forefront of women's minds has been illustrated by the high public profile given to the diagnosis (in 2008) and subsequent death (in 2009) of Jade Goody (a reality television star) – subsequently referred to as the 'Jade Goody effect' (Lancucki *et al.*, 2012). Although screening rates for cervical cancer had been declining prior to 2008, particularly among younger women, there was a surge in attendances associated with the time of the broadcast of Goody's diagnosis and subsequent death (Bowring and Walker, 2010). About half a million additional cervical screening attendances were recorded in England between mid-2008 and mid-2009, representing relatively little over-screening but rather an increase among those for whom a smear was overdue (Lancucki *et al.*, 2012). Furthermore, women with fewer educational qualifications, from lower socio-economic groups and younger women were shown to have been particularly influenced by the publicity surrounding Goody's diagnosis and death (Marlow *et al.*, 2012). Although this example illustrates the way in which the media might be used to increase screening uptake it seems that the 'Goody effect' was relatively transient, with the increase in attendances not being sustained much beyond her death (Bowring and Walker, 2010).

Molecular and non-molecular technological developments have made it possible to detect an increasing number of diseases at the pre-clinical or pre-pathological stage (Andermann *et al.*, 2008). This has given rise to the expansion of online direct-to-consumer medical screening tests being offered to the public, which do not meet the established (Wilson and Jungner) criteria (Lovett *et al.*, 2012). Such legal but largely unregulated developments have the potential to cause harm (McCartney, 2012). Andermann *et al.* (2008) argue that the rise in the number of tests has also put pressure on health services to expand genetic screening programmes in particular. In most high-income countries screening for genetic conditions such as Down's syndrome and phenylketonuria, has become an established part of routine antenatal and early postnatal care. New disease genes, however, are being identified regularly through advances in technology associated with the human genome project. Genetic screening often raises complex issues because an individual's test result has implications for family members. Foetal genetic screening also raises questions about reproductive choices including termination of pregnancy. Developments in genomics have stimulated a re-evaluation of Wilson and Jungner's criteria.

The increase in opportunistic screening – screening offered during routine health care encounters – raises a number of issues, particularly where they involve screening for behaviours, such as hazardous drinking and, more recently, physical inactivity (NICE, 2013). **Primary health care** is often viewed as the setting for identification (of the 'condition') and brief advice (the 'treatment'). However, hospital A&E departments (for hazardous drinking) and maternity **settings** (for domestic violence/intimate partner violence) have also been used as sites for opportunistic screening. The **ethics** of screening in these types of locations are particularly contentious given that attendance is for reasons other than screening. The principle of informed consent may well be compromised in such situations (Getz *et al.*, 2003). The use of 'routine enquiry' for domestic violence in A&E, sexual health services as well as maternity settings has expanded in a number of countries in recent years. Avoiding potential harms to women and children has been shown to require a considerable shift away from the medical approach of 'detection' towards encouraging 'disclosure', training and support of clinicians and extensive partnership working with **community**-based services, including the police (Bacchus *et al.*, 2010).

Conclusion

The current screening context is volatile. Pressure for an expansion of national screening programmes is driven, at least in part, by new technological developments that hold out the promise of expanding preventive approaches in public health. In England, there have been calls for a national screening programme to detect atrial fibrillation in those over 65 years old to prevent premature death from stroke on the basis that it fulfils all the criteria set out by the UK NSC (Christie, 2012a). The development of an effective screening test for the early detection of lung cancer is also underway (Christie, 2012b). Beyond health care, screening has also been debated. In the sports arena, for example, the introduction of a pre-participation screening tool for all young competitive athletes to detect cardiovascular disorders has been discussed following a number of high profile sudden deaths or near-deaths during competitive events. From a public health perspective, the focus on prevention through early detection is likely to have a number of beneficial outcomes. Nonetheless, there is a danger that a focus on medically-based screening approaches shifts the focus away from the social **determinants** of, for example, hazardous drinking, domestic violence, lung cancer, CVD and so on, all of which are contoured in various ways in relation to social disadvantage.

SETTINGS

Context

Settings have long been targeted for intervention in public health through, for example, school-based **health education** and workplace campaigns. In 1986, however, the WHO signalled a change in thinking about settings, stating in the *Ottawa Charter* that 'health is created and lived by people within the settings of their everyday life; where they learn, work, play and love' (WHO, 1986: iii). Not only did this shift attention away from the health care system and individual responsibility for **health**, it also focused on the potential for developing health and well-being through creating supportive everyday environments. The WHO advocates settings-based approaches as conduits for operationalizing key **health promotion** principles and core values relating to empowerment, equity, participation and health creation. In other words, settings-based approaches are advocated as a particular means to a specified end. Such approaches have proliferated in many countries over the past two decades, becoming one of the more visible strategies for promoting health at a local level. The *Healthy Cities* project (the first settings-based initiative launched by the WHO in 1987), for example, has expanded from 11 European cities to a global network of some 1400 cities and towns. The WHO continues to advocate settings-based approaches relating to a variety of organizational contexts, including schools, workplaces, prisons and hospitals, as well as geographical spaces such as marketplaces and islands. In theory, these constitute pragmatic approaches for implementing multifaceted strategies; in practice, however, they pose considerable challenges.

Defining settings

A key distinction is made in the literature between a setting as simply a **place** to reach people and target interventions – the conventional approach – and the more complex vision articulated by the WHO. The WHO has not, however, extensively theorized the concept beyond its definition of a setting as a

> place or context in which people engage in daily activities in which environmental, organizational and personal factors interact to affect health and wellbeing ... where people actively use and shape the environment and thus create or solve problems relating to health.
>
> (Nutbeam, 1998: 19)

Implicit in this definition – and articulated more clearly in a number of related documents (WHO, 1986, 1999, 2009) – is the significance of supportive environments and, relatedly, the wider **determinants** of health – the social, economic, political, cultural and organizational influences in particular – that not only shape settings but are also recreated through settings. Drawing on ideas from ecology and animal behaviour, settings are presented as socio-ecological entities that comprise dynamic and complex interdependencies between human beings, as well as between them and their wider biophysical environment.

Systems theory has become one of the more prominent influences on theoretical discussions about settings in recent years (Paton *et al.*, 2005). Systems theorists conceptualize a setting as a 'whole' entity, comprising interrelationships that together create patterns of change and continuity. Moreover, systems are viewed as 'open' or permeable, connected in a variety of ways to local, regional, national and global influences. Theoretical discussions based on systems theory can sometimes tend, however, to reify settings, that is, to treat them as 'contexts' or 'systems' that exist apart from people. Conceptualizing settings as social networks of interdependent people counters this tendency. It also brings into focus the significance of social processes – human actions and interactions – that have the potential to be transformative through creating propitious conditions to support health. The balances of power residing in networks constitute a significant influence over how a settings-based initiative is framed and implemented in practice. Theorizing settings in terms of the potential for power struggles and conflict and complexity rather than linearity might enhance understanding of processes of implementation and their often unintended or limited consequences. Green *et al.*'s (2000: 23) definition captures a number of these ideas, arguing that settings are 'arenas of sustained interaction, with pre-existing structures, policies, characteristics, institutional values, and both formal and informal social sanctions on behaviours'. This definition is not only more congruent with the political reality of settings but is also applicable to a diversity of settings, more or less regardless of their size, complexity, mission and so forth.

The significance of settings for public health

Settings-based approaches have continued to have a relatively high profile globally, particularly within Europe, despite limited **evidence** of effectiveness (Dooris, 2005). Schools, workplaces, nightclubs, cities and towns, for example, are 'meso' institutions (Kickbusch, 2003) that offer the potential for population-based approaches for creating health. Although constrained in various ways by the broader social, economic and political environment, institutions have, by degrees, discretion over the organization of their everyday affairs. Settings-based approaches seek to maximize the health potential in these routine arrangements by working, often indirectly, but always concertedly, towards health. Underpinning the approach is the notion of health as a resource for life – living, working, learning and so on.

The WHO has been instrumental in supporting take-up of a settings-based approach to public health through establishing a variety of global networks. The Schools for Health in Europe Network (formerly the European Network for Health Promoting Schools), for example, supports a network of national co-ordinators from 43 countries. The Network advocates school health promotion based on a whole school approach, encouraging the health and education sectors to work together, using a positive concept of health and well-being and underpinned by the UN Convention on the Rights of the Child (www.schoolsforhealth.eu). National programmes further support schools in various ways, such as with resources and a framework to help them translate abstract ideas into practical and realistic programmes of work. The development of such programmes, alongside opportunities for accreditation and broader national requirements for school inspection that evaluate how the school supports health and well-being, have increased the attractiveness of settings-based approaches in some countries such as England. The values underpinning settings-based approaches are also consistent with educational philosophy making it relatively more straightforward to gain widespread commitment in schools by linking health and well-being with children's learning and school improvement more generally. The significance of the school ethos as a learning environment as well as one that supports health development is likely to find some support in many schools, particularly primary schools.

Applying a settings-based approach to prisons, on the other hand, poses major challenges. The health gains are potentially immense, particularly because a settings-based approach provides a means of accessing those who are 'hard to reach'. Not only are prisoners some of the most vulnerable people in society, they also tend to have complex physical and mental health conditions reflecting their chaotic **lifestyles** prior to incarceration. The permeability of prisons to wider networks of family and friends, especially following their release from confinement, has particular implications for the control of infectious diseases such as TB and HIV (Ginn, 2013). Release from prison also poses a major challenge when former prisoners have little support, no GP, nowhere to live and with few prospects of gaining a job or income (Woodall *et al.*, 2012). Prison environments in general and prison health services in particular have received intense criticism in recent years. In many countries prisons remain 'sick places' (de Viggiani, 2007: 115). Overcrowding is endemic and a regime of rules and rituals disempowers and undermines prisoners' mental health (Fraser *et al.*, 2009).

In 1995, the WHO Regional Office for Europe established its Health in Prisons Project (HIPP) in recognition of these enduring issues. The HIPP advocates a whole-prison approach, driven by health in all policies and informed by a rights-based perspective. The aim is to improve the assessment and treatment of undiagnosed conditions, support healthy lifestyles and mental health development, as well as focus on rehabilitation and release through developing alliances with relevant **community**-based organizations. Participation, empowerment and equity sit uncomfortably alongside a regime characterized by control, hierarchy and subservience and where the primary purpose is viewed as punishment rather than rehabilitation. As de Viggiani (2007: 115) concludes, 'health inequalities are enmeshed within the workings of the prison system itself'. Yet there are some exceptions to these general tendencies. Scandinavian countries are noted for their 'exceptionalism' in terms of their criminal justice systems, having low rates of imprisonment and relatively humane and 'civilized' conditions in prisons. In Norway, for example, prison health services have been fully integrated with local **primary health care** services since 1987. Financed and managed by health authorities, they maintain their independence (Bjørngaard *et al.*, 2009). These characteristics may well provide some of the preconditions within which a settings-based approach could be embedded.

Settings-based approaches bring into play the potential for conflict over values and may well limit the degree to which the approach is fully embraced. Giving children a voice through a school council is one thing; establishing a prisoner consultative forum is another. In schools, however, processes of consultation as well as wider policies and strategies to manage bullying effectively have been shown to influence relationships between staff and children in a positive direction and contribute to creating an ethos that supports school engagement and well-being (Thurston, 2006). If extended to prisons, similar benefits might well accrue. If a settings-based approach is viewed as a process of organizational development, a number of advantages for the organization may well emerge. A long-term commitment to embedding health and well-being into policies and facilitating greater participation and empowerment of those who tend to be more passive and marginalized might lead to better performing organizations. In other words, health is viewed as an asset closely related to the effective functioning of organizations (Dooris and Hunter, 2007). However, as Green *et al.* point out in relation to workplaces, resistance to implementing settings-based approaches may well reflect the competing internal agendas and interpretations of key 'gatekeepers' who hold the balance of power in specific settings and do not wish to see health promotion framed too broadly because it may call into question the status quo on which their power and material success rests.

(Green *et al.*, 2000: 24)

Leadership from senior managers is essential if the entire setting is to be developed. Some workplaces have shown enlightened self-interest in embracing settings-based approaches. Volkswagen (a leading car manufacturer) for example, has been described as a 'model of good practice' (Chu *et al.*, 2000: 158) by including health promotion and health protection as two of its corporate objectives. Workplaces vary considerably, however, and are constrained by the broader political and economic environment. Nonetheless, a settings-based approach provides opportunities for thinking through how investing in all employees may reap dividends in terms of absenteeism, accidents, employee turnover and so on.

The effectiveness of settings-based approaches has been extensively debated. As complex interventions, evaluating such approaches poses considerable methodological challenges. Deciding on appropriate indicators of success and timescales is also far from straightforward. National and local **evaluation** of the healthy schools programme in England concluded that a number of changes were made to organizational processes: introduction of schools councils, development of behaviour management policies, active playground management and so on. Whether or not these changes gave rise to improvements in health and well-being is less clear. Even if these did not improve, this does not necessarily render the approach unimportant or insignificant; it may point towards the limits of settings-based approaches and the stronger influence of other determinants. In the case of children, families are important. How a settings-based approach is implemented is also relevant to understanding effectiveness. Ideas are interpreted and re-interpreted by people in particular contexts, creating a complex interweaving of actions over which no one person has complete control. This characteristic of settings-based approaches can be overlooked in debates about effectiveness. Of most significance, perhaps, as an indicator of success is the extent to which the setting has, by degrees, embraced and operationalized the values of health promotion in its actions. In other words, are participation, empowerment, and equity of primary concern?

Conclusion

In reality, many settings pay scant regard to health, considering it to be unrelated to their core business. A settings-based approach therefore represents a public health strategy that has yet to fulfil its potential (Kickbusch, 2007). There are, however, indications that the idea continues to have currency, with an increasing number of settings being discussed – sports clubs and ecosystems, for example – not only as entry points for health promotion activity but as opportunities to re-consider how to better organize affairs with different interests, values, processes and outcomes in mind. In some cases this has involved the incorporation of additional agendas such as those relating to sustainable development where there is considerable convergence of interests and values. This indicates that there is still some interest in taking 'WHO philosophies and frameworks … off the shelves and onto the streets' (Ashton *et al.*, 1986: 319).

SOCIAL CAPITAL

Context

Social capital – in broad terms, who you know and are connected to – became particularly prominent in a number of **policy** fields, including public health, in the mid 1990s. A lack of social capital – or social cohesion – in deprived neighbourhoods was viewed as leading to social exclusion, which became at that time the preferred term for those who had been pushed to the margins of mainstream society (Roberts, 2009). Social exclusion specifically referred to people's limited participation in social life, politics, employment and so on, and was viewed as leading to a range of **health** and social problems. Policy solutions formulated to address social exclusion centred on strengthening disadvantaged communities through encouraging various forms of participation, in other words, by building social capital. In the UK, the emergence of this discourse reflected the shift towards framing health and social problems in (social) relational terms (Coalter, 2007a).

Considerable interest has been shown in social capital since the 1990s. The World Bank, for example, has been an advocate of the importance of social capital in advancing its **community** action work (http://go.worldbank.org/C0QTRW4QF0) and the OECD has co-ordinated developments relating to the measurement of social capital. There has, nevertheless, been extensive criticism of the concept, particularly on the grounds that it has been 'stretched, modified, and extrapolated to cover so many types of relationships at so many levels … that the term has lost all heuristic value' (Macinko and Starfield, 2001: 394). Nonetheless, it is an idea that has continued to have intuitive appeal and is likely to remain a part of the public health policy lexicon, in one guise or another for some time.

Defining social capital

Social capital is a concept that focuses on social relations. Several definitions can be found, with those offered by Bourdieu (1991), Coleman (2000), Putnam (1993), and Portes (1998) being commonly cited across a range of academic disciplines. These definitions have some commonality in that they all draw on ideas from sociology and economics. In economics, 'capital' refers to wealth in the form of money or other assets. Capital is thus something that can be invested and has the potential to lead to profit or gain. Sociologists, on the other hand, have long recognized that people form groups (networks) based on common beliefs, norms and identities, through which they share information and provide various forms of mutual support. Here 'capital' refers to assets – resources – that accumulate through people's mutually-oriented social relations. It thus differs from the concept of human capital (*individual* resources that can be developed through such processes as **education**) insofar as it accrues through interaction with others (Macinko and Starfield, 2001). Social capital also infers much more than the volume of social contact: what matters is the types of social capital residing in networks and how valuable they prove to be (Roberts, 2009). In other words, the significance lies in the extent to which they enable, rather than constrain access to benefits and opportunities. Acquiring social capital is also not without its costs. Time and energy are required to develop and maintain networks wherein the stock of social capital resides (Hawe and Shiell, 2000).

Definitions also differ in some important respects. Bourdieu and Wacquant (1992: 167) define social capital as the 'sum of resources, actual or virtual, that accrue to a group by virtue of possessing a durable network of more or less institutionalized relationships of mutual acquaintance and recognition'. Thus, social capital is a group-level resource that can be drawn on by individuals for instrumental purposes. Bourdieu argues that dominant groups (or elites) control access to networks, excluding members of other groups from potentially beneficial resources, maintaining their own relative advantages, and, in the process, perpetuating social **inequalities** (Stephens, 2008). For others, such as Portes (1998: 12), social capital resides with individuals (rather than groups), that is to say it is 'the capacity of individuals to command scare resources by virtue of their membership in networks or broader social structures'. Portes' definition gives greater conceptual clarity to social capital because it specifies quite tightly the core elements: resources, membership and networks. He also provides a framework that elaborates his definition by differentiating social processes (trusting relationships and feelings of reciprocity, for example) from the creation of social capital (the ability of an individual to secure benefits through membership of a group) and the consequences – positive and negative – that flow therefrom (Macinko and Starfield, 2001). Other definitions conflate these different dimensions of social capital (see, for example, Putnam, 1993).

Putnam's conceptualization has been especially influential in the public health and social policy fields. He defines social capital as 'features of social life such as networks, norms and social trust that facilitate co-ordination and co-operation for mutual benefit' (Putnam, 1993: 85). This definition emphasizes trust reciprocity and the expectations and obligations that arise therefrom, enabling people to call in favours, circulate valued information, facilitate access to opportunities, and so on (Hawe and Shiell, 2000). The popularity of Putnam's definition among policymakers may relate to his framing of the concept as a community-level resource that can engender co-operation and be used for collective action, and, by extension, increase civic engagement. As such, social capital is presented as a 'public good' that binds communities together in a socially inclusive manner. This communitarian perspective emphasizes the community as the basis for self-help and self-reliance, an idea that has been politically attractive in recent years (Coalter, 2007a). The OECD definition of social capital as 'networks together with shared norms, values and understandings that facilitate co-operation within and among groups' (Healy and Côté, 2001: 41) draws heavily on Putnam's definition. In the UK, the ONS adopted this definition as a basis for developing measures of social capital (Foxton and Jones, 2011). The preference for communitarian perspectives on social capital has meant that network-based approaches emphasizing access to power and resources (reflected in the definitions of Bourdieu and Portes) have been neglected (Moore *et al.*, 2006). However, network approaches have been applied in the health inequalities field as they directly link the structure and composition of social relations to broader societal patterns. They provide an account, therefore, of why networks are patterned in relation to class, gender and ethnicity in a way that gives advantages to some and not others (Stephens, 2008).

The significance of social capital for public health

Although social capital continues to be viewed as a somewhat ambiguous and contested concept it has undergone significant theoretical development. Putnam

(1995), for example, proposed two forms of social capital: localized or bonding social capital and bridging social capital. Bonding social capital describes the close ties that accumulate through informal and everyday interactions between people in local communities, including among family members. Putnam emphasizes the development of trust based on familiarity and closeness, which he sees as maintaining a strong in-group loyalty while reinforcing specific identities (Coalter, 2007a). Although policymakers have been concerned with the presumed weakness of social capital in disadvantaged neighbourhoods, levels of bonding social capital can be high. The provision of social support among friends and families – a particular kind of beneficial resource in these informal networks – can be especially important in disadvantaged neighbourhoods. In conceptualizing bonding social capital, however, Putnam acknowledged the potentially negative side of strong social ties insofar as they might both unite and segregate at one and the same time. Strong bonds within networks may also give rise to certain kinds of obligations and demands for conformity that preserve a group's subordinate status (Macinko and Starfield, 2001). Bridging social capital on the other hand refers to weaker ties with those beyond the familiar everyday pattern of interaction – with colleagues and friends of friends, for example – although still on the same horizontal level in terms of social position. Such connections might open up new information and opportunities for advancement than might be present in closer, more tightly bounded networks. Szreter and Woolcock (2004) proposed a third form – linking social capital – used to refer to vertical connections between different social strata, including those beyond the immediate community. If, as Portes (1998) argues, resources in some social networks are limited because people interact with others like themselves who are similarly under-endowed with assets (other unemployed people, for example), access to these wider networks has the potential to leverage a much broader range of resources (Forrest and Kearns, 2001).

Because of the importance that has been attached to levels of social capital in neighbourhoods and among groups, developing ways of measuring social capital has become a preoccupation of government statistics departments in many countries, as well as global institutions such as the OECD and World Bank. In the UK, for example, the ONS has developed a standardized set of questions that relate to the identified core dimensions of social capital in Putnam's definition (Babb, 2005). Questions on civic participation (perception of ability to influence events, for example), social networks and support (frequency of seeing or speaking to relatives, friends and neighbours), social participation (volunteering activity, for instance), reciprocity and trust (confidence in key institutions, including government, for example), and views on the local area (such as, enjoyment of living in the area) have been developed and incorporated into a number of national surveys (such as the General Household Survey from 2004/5) (Foxton and Jones, 2011). Because of a desire to compare measurement of social capital across nations, the OECD has co-ordinated efforts to harmonize social capital indicators. In some countries such as the UK, a desire to measure the social impacts of policy has meant that social capital has remained of interest to policymakers and academics alike. Although quantitative (survey-based) approaches to the measurement of social capital have proliferated, they continue to be viewed sceptically in some quarters. Several commentators have raised questions about the validity and reliability of measures that treat social capital as a single explanatory variable (Li, 2010; Macinko and Starfield, 2001; Szreter and Woolcock, 2004). More fundamentally perhaps, the validity of measuring social capital has been questioned on the basis that, conceptually, it relates primarily to the *qualitative* dimensions of social relations (Coalter, 2007a). Survey approaches are necessarily limited because they take a snapshot of a dynamic and unfolding phenomenon. In other words, social capital as a construct describes social relations that are always in flux.

Nevertheless, survey-based approaches to exploring the relationship between social capital and various health outcomes have become commonplace in recent years. The results from such studies have been inconsistent, however, probably reflecting the use of different ways of measuring social capital, among the many other methodological differences alluded to above. However, a recent longitudinal analysis of the British Household Panel Survey concluded that higher levels of social capital enhanced people's healthiness, happiness and perceived life satisfaction independently of other relevant factors (Li, 2007). Few studies have operationalized social capital in terms of bonding and bridging forms. The results from a community-based study of self-rated health in Japan, however, found that 'women benefited more from bridging social capital than men, whereas men may benefit more from bonding social capital than women' (Iwase *et al.*, 2012: 559). Although cultural differences between Japan and other similarly developed countries may limit the relevance of these findings elsewhere, the study is a reminder that the social capital-health relationship is likely to be multi-faceted and complex. The findings from Iwase *et al.*'s study, however, may explain, at least in part, why men's health is more likely to benefit from marriage compared to women. The benefits of social support for people's health and welfare may increase 'relational strain' for those who provide such support (Lynch *et al.*, 2000).

The role of social capital in explaining social **inequalities in health**, particularly in relation to income inequalities, has attracted considerable discussion and debate in recent years. Wilkinson (1996), for example, proposed that once societies reached a certain level of **economic development** health status was determined by social inequality rather than material disadvantage. A number of studies have explored empirically the relationship between income inequality and health using social capital as a key variable (see for example, Kawachi *et al.*, 1997; Marmot, 2005). These have produced mixed results, however (Dahl and Malmberg-Heimonen, 2010). Yet, interest in theorizing how social capital might mediate the relationship between income inequality and health remains. Drawing on ideas central to Putnam's work, psychosocial explanations (underpinned by various physiological mechanisms relating to immune and neuroendocrine responses to particular social environments) have been proposed. These speculate that income inequality gives rise to declining levels of actual and perceived social connectedness and trust, generating feelings of anxiety, isolation and stress, which in turn have a number of consequences for health and health behaviours (Wilkinson and Pickett, 2010). Perceptions of relative social position and status have also been included in psychosocial explanations. This body of research has, however, drawn extensive criticism on methodological, theoretical and political grounds (Dahl and Malmberg-Heimonen, 2010).

Although Putnam's work has been pre-eminent in the public health field, there has been a growing interest in the work of Bourdieu (Stephens, 2008). Bourdieu's emphasis on the differences in resources across social groups has highlighted the potential role of bridging and, in particular, linking social capital (Szreter and Woolcock, 2004). Qualitative research carried out in the UK, the USA and New Zealand suggests that external links beyond the immediate neighbourhood are potentially more beneficial to well-being than social connections within the neighbourhood (Stephens, 2008). The development of trusting and respectful relationships with influential people connected to formal institutions (education, healthcare and so on) is particularly important for those living in disadvantaged communities for welfare support as well as the opportunities and resources they might bring. As Szreter and Woolcock explained:

> [I]f relationships of trust and respect deteriorate between the poor and the range of more privileged people in their lives who are involved in delivering the essential public services of education, health and social security, then the capacity of the poor to acquire, utilize and benefit from health enhancing material goods will be seriously compromised.
>
> (Szreter and Woolcock, 2004: 662)

Bourdieu's work is also of interest because it provides a way of integrating material (economic), social and cultural capital into explanations relating to health and inequality. Cultural capital is broadly defined as the stock of knowledge, skills, beliefs, habits and tastes developed through a person's social milieu (Roberts, 2009). This implies that the form of cultural capital is interdependent with the types of social networks people develop and vice versa. Thus, social capital and cultural capital formation create, maintain and reproduce social inequalities. Getting a good job, for example, is easier if you have the 'right' social and cultural capital, and getting a good job is the primary way of generating economic capital. This suggests that the pattern of income inequality that has become a feature of many high-income countries gives rise to a particular pattern, form and content of social relations that give advantage to some and not others. Economic capital and social capital are important insofar as they facilitate access to cultural capital (Roberts *et al.*, 2009). Bourdieu argued that economic, cultural and social capital together forged social class positions (Graham, 2007). It seems that social capital is not declining but becoming class specific (Coalter, 2007b).

Conclusion

Szreter and Woolcock (2004) argue that within the public health field there is some consensus that social capital 'matters' but there is disagreement about how it might mediate better health. However, policymakers' attempts to create social capital are likely to be unsuccessful 'as social capital is based on activities, relationships and norms freely engaged in by individuals' (Coalter, 2007b: 553); in other words, it is an aspect of everyday social life. More fundamentally, it is debatable whether or not social capital adds anything new that is not already adequately represented by the concept of social class (Roberts, 2009).

SOCIAL MARKETING

Context

The idea of social marketing can be traced back to a paper published in 1952 by Wiebe, who analysed four social campaigns and concluded that 'brotherhood', as an example of a society's aspirations, could be sold just like soap – that is to say, through the astute application of marketing approaches (Walsh *et al.*, 1993). This idea was developed further by Kotler and Zaltman (1971) in a systematic examination of the applicability of marketing concepts to the promotion of social objectives, such as safe driving and family planning. They defined social marketing as 'the design, implementation and control of programs calculated to influence the acceptability of social ideas and involving considerations of product planning, pricing, communication, distribution, and marketing research' (1971: 5).They concluded that a number of specific social causes – pollution control and drug use for example – could benefit from 'market thinking' and planning.

The concept of social marketing has diffused extensively in the intervening years. Some of the earliest examples of the application of social marketing approaches to public health occurred in low-income countries in the 1960s and 1970s. Here, much of the significant research and development work on social marketing was related to immunization and family planning. Social marketing approaches continue to be used by non-governmental and other not-for-profit organizations in promoting contraception use and immunization uptake in these countries. In 1988, the WHO published a handbook on social marketing, the aim of which was 'to stimulate and assist' staff in applying social marketing to the promotion of **health** and health for all (Birkinshaw, 1998: i). These developments suggest a degree of acceptance that the primary goal of social marketing is not simply to promote *ideas* (as reflected in Kolter and Zaltman's definition) but rather to bring about **behaviour change** (Andreasen, 2002).

In England, social marketing emerged as an approach to improving population health alongside a continuing emphasis on behaviour change. The public health White Paper *Choosing Health: Making Healthy Choices Easier* (DH, 2004) identified the potential of social marketing as a tool to improve the effectiveness of health-related interventions. French (2009: 265) argued that this represented something of a shift at a government level towards a more 'personalized choice-based approach to the promotion of health'. The subsequent establishment of the National Social Marketing Centre (NSMC) in 2006 was followed by a series of publications that cumulatively expressed the desire for all public health work to be informed by an understanding of what motivated people and to embed social marketing principles into all health improvement work. One consequence of this was that health organizations in England invested an increasing proportion of their resources into social marketing work. The most recent public health White Paper in England (Secretary of State for Health, 2010) signals an intent to publish a social marketing strategy to support the government's efforts to change behaviours.

Defining social marketing

Since Kotler and Zaltman's (1971) description of social marketing, definitions have tended to include specific reference to behaviour change. In England, the concept of social marketing has mainly been developed and promoted by the NSMC. In 2006, it defined social marketing as 'the systematic application of marketing alongside other concepts and techniques to achieve specific behavioural goals, for a social or public good' (French and Blair-Stevens, 2006). The social or public goods referred to here are health-related goals – such as practising safe sex or giving up smoking. Building on

Andreasen's (2002) six characteristics of social marketing approaches, the NSMC provides eight benchmark criteria, the purpose of which is to establish demarcation lines between what is, and what is not, social marketing. According to these eight criteria, social marketing: has a strong orientation to 'customers' to ensure that interventions are shaped in relation to their current needs and desires; has a clear focus on behavioural goals; is informed by behaviour theory; is based on 'insight' into what moves and motivates people; uses the idea of 'exchange' to maximize the potential 'offer' and minimize the 'costs' of changing a specific behaviour; uses the idea of internal and external competition to understand the factors that influence people's ability to change their behaviour; targets specific audience groups using segmentation; considers a 'mix' of intervention methods (French, 2009). Thus, social marketing is seen as much more than communicating a message. As Blair-Stevens (2010: 66) argues 'At its heart, it's about developing a deeper contextual understanding and insight into people's lives, and then using this to craft interventions and approaches that are valued by those being addressed, which can achieve measurable impacts in what people actually do – their behaviour.' To date, the majority of social marketing interventions have been directed at individuals – the so-called 'end user'. However, Bloom and Novelli (1981) point out that social marketing could be used by profit-making organizations such as alcohol manufacturers to encourage responsible drinking.

The more recent definition of social marketing published by the NSMC marks a departure point in that any direct reference to 'marketing' has been removed: 'an approach used to develop activities aimed at changing or maintaining people's behaviour for the benefit of individuals and society as a whole' (Hopwood and Merritt, 2011: 40). This may reflect something of a desire to distance the concept from the idea of marketing.

The significance of social marketing for public health

Advocates of social marketing emphasize the use of a systematic approach to planning and reviewing an intervention. The five stage process – scope, develop, implement, evaluate, review – is referred to as the Total Process Planning model (French and Blair-Stevens, 2006). Considerable emphasis is put on the scoping stage in order to understand the audience and guide the development of the initiative. Scoping starts with the collection of geographic (where people live, normally based on their postcode) and demographic (age, sex, marital status and so on) information – hence the term geo-demographics. This is then supplemented with data – from interviews, focus groups and surveys – on how people think, feel and act in relation to the issue in question, the aim of which is to generate insight into their **lifestyles,** attitudes and other personality factors – so-called psychographic variables (Walsh *et al.*, 1993). Next, the process of formal audience segmentation begins, a process that has been used extensively in the commercial sector to understand 'the rich mixture of the population who may have different wants and needs, acknowledging that what appeals to one individual will not necessarily appeal to another' (Carlin *et al.*, 2008: 3). The aim of segmentation is to organize the audience into clusters of apparently like-minded people who *behave* in similar ways, share similar *beliefs,* and have similar expressed *needs* (Abbas *et al.*, 2009). French (2009) has argued that segmentation is a more sophisticated process of grouping people than the traditional approach used in public health of targeting groups based on much more limited information, such as living in areas of **deprivation** (identified through IMD scores of Super Output areas). In recent years, it has become possible to access large datasets from commercial companies. MOSAIC UK, for example, is a commercial dataset owned by Experian Ltd, described as a leading global provider of consumer classifications. Experian claims that MOSAIC UK provides consumer classification categories that are based on

> over 850 million pieces of information across 450 different data points (which) are condensed using the latest analytical techniques to identify 15 summary groups and 66 detailed types that are easy to interpret and understand … (giving) an accurate reflection of the UK consumer of today, and tomorrow.
>
> (Experian, 2014: 3)

An example of the use of audience segmentation to address problematic alcohol consumption is described by Carlin *et al.* (2008). Nine profiles (for example, *Urban Intelligence, Symbols of Success, Rural Isolation*) were developed using geo-demographic information from the Experian system combined with other consumer and regional public health data, including lifestyle surveys. Fairly detailed profile descriptions were developed that revealed lifestyles and habits in relation to alcohol use. The largest of the Mosaic groups in the region was *Ties of Community*. Those assigned to the *Ties of Community* category lived in well-established, but old-fashioned communities, and tended to marry young. The drinking pattern for the group is one of drinking outside the home, particularly for men. Audience segmentation has also been used by Sport England, the government agency responsible for sport strategy. It has developed the online Sport Market Segmentation Tool (http://segments.sportengland.org). Using data from Sport England's *Active People Survey*, the Department of Culture, Media and Sport's *Taking Part Survey* and the Mosaic Tool from Experian, 19 sporting segments have been constructed, which include Leanne the supportive single; Ben the competitive male urbanite; and Elaine the empty nest career lady (Coalter, 2013).

Such segments are used to tailor interventions to bring about behaviour change. The intervention design and development stage is informed by two key ideas. First, approaches tend to be based on an explicit theory of behaviour change. Recent social marketing initiatives have made use of Locke and Latham's goal-setting theory and the Health Action Process Approach to address obesity (Thomas, 2009), but other models such as the TTM (Prochaska and Diclemente, 1983) have also been used in relation to reducing hazardous drinking (Thurston *et al.*, 2010). Second, intervention methods are underpinned by the concept of exchange theory. This refers to how the benefits from changing a behaviour are presented relative to the costs, with the aim of tipping the balance in favour of benefits. This might involve the use of incentives to encourage the desired behaviour as well as the removal of barriers to change. The concept of 'competition' is also used to inform intervention strategies, in that an analysis is carried out to identify all the factors that compete with the desired behaviour. These ideas have much in common with those underpinning behavioural economics (nudging).

In England in recent years, there has been a relatively rapid increase in social marketing activity directed at a number of public health issues. Social marketing approaches directed at reducing alcohol consumption, particularly among specific groups, continue to be advocated (Secretary of State for the Home Department, 2012). There are signs, however, that social marketing approaches are being applied to an increasing range of health issues, by a diverse number of organizations. Evans and McCormack (2008) describe how social marketing has been used in the USA in 'tobacco countermarketing', the aim of which has been to counter the marketing messages of tobacco companies. The American Legacy Foundation 'truth®' researched the beliefs and attitudes of young people in order to identify factors that might encourage them to reject smoking as a socially desirable behaviour. The Foundation specifically branded anti-smoking messages in order to promote a smoke-free lifestyle. Evans and McCormack also discuss how social marketing can be used to develop effective communication between doctors and patients when **evidence** is ambiguous and messages are complicated as with **screening** for prostate cancer.

Despite the appeal and pervasiveness of social marketing, concerns remain about its effectiveness in bringing about behaviour change – the so-called 'bottom line' for social marketers (Andreasen, 2002). Notwithstanding the problems of **evaluation**, some studies have reported that interventions in relation to healthy eating, increasing physical exercise, smoking cessation, reducing substance misuse and decreasing littering have been effective, at least in the short term (Gordon *et al.*, 2006; Robertson, 2008; Hopwood and Merritt, 2011). Others, nevertheless, report equivocal findings (see, for example, Winters, 2009). Although evaluation is an important aspect of the social marketing process, limitations on funding as well as the methodological problems of carrying out evaluation, particularly over the longer term, tend to preclude systematic, independent and detailed evaluation. Furthermore, as Winters (2009) states, the enthusiasm for social marketing may have led to unduly optimistic expectations regarding what it might achieve. In the commercial world, shifting behaviours a few percentage points might be counted as success. However, given the size of many public health problems, larger scale movements of change are required.

In its relatively short history, social marketing has attracted substantial interest alongside considerable controversy. For some critics, the very idea of applying marketing ideas and methods to health improvement is fundamentally at odds with the core values of public health (Walsh, *et al.*, 1993). Marketing health can also be viewed as commodification insofar as health is packaged as a 'product' to be sold in various ways. Marketing is viewed as guided by commercial values where the 'hard sell' can involve accentuating the positive aspects of changing behaviour and minimizing the costs, thus manipulating and even coercing people towards behaviour change. However, as Kotler and Zaltman (1971: 8) argue, the issue is not

> whether a particular approach suits one's taste, but whether it works. If a 'hard' marketing style raises more money for cancer research than a 'soft' style it must be respected by those who think cancer research is more important than personal aesthetics.

These debates reflect particular ethical and value positions, in the sense of judgements about how health should or should not be promoted and protected. Many of the early writers on social marketing emphasized the need for responsibility and accountability to people (Walsh *et al.*, 1993). These issues remain contentious. Furthermore, social marketing emphasizes individual responsibility and views behaviours as aspects of an individual **lifestyle** chosen freely rather than as constrained and enabled by the social, political and economic conditions. All in all, because marketing drives consumption, it is viewed by some as part of the problem rather than part of the solution (Walsh *et al.*, 1993). Others have argued that social marketing can help revitalize and refocus **health promotion**, because they share a similar theory and practice base (Griffiths *et al.*, 2009). It is difficult to be persuaded by this argument, however, given the explicit values of health promotion wherein empowerment occupies a central position. Others have raised the problem of selecting certain groups for intervention, something at odds with the work of many agencies whose mission is based on ideas of egalitarianism, anti-discrimination and equity (Bloom and Novelli, 1981).

In addition to these overarching concerns a number of specific issues have been raised in relation to social marketing methods. One criticism relates to the use of geo-demographics in characterising segments of the population. Roberts (2009: 109) argues that 'geodemographic identities seem unlikely to be as stable or to become as deeply rooted as those associated with ethnicity, gender and social class'. Coalter makes a similar point in relation to the market segments used by Sport England (2013: 4) to characterize population sub-groups, the result of which is that issues of structure and culture are ignored 'and we are presented with ... a wholly individualized exploration of meaning and motivation'. The discourse of audience segmentation seems to have displaced the discourse of social stratification and **inequalities** in health. The logic of audience segmentation is that 'personalized' and 'individually tailored' health improvement projects can be delivered to specific population segments. Sociologists might describe this as a postmodern 'solution' in an increasingly pluralistic society. Nonetheless, the fact remains that academic research on **inequalities** in health continues to reveal the importance of class, gender and ethnicity in explaining the patterns of health and illness. Audience segmentation obscures wider patterns of inequality. In this regard, it is worth noting that in England, social marketing in public health came to prominence during the Labour government (1997–2010), a government that expressed a desire to address health inequalities but without mentioning the word 'class'. Social marketing provides a suitable tool for such a strategy. Although social marketing has been presented as a technical and rational approach that makes it attractive to governments (Blair-Stevens, 2010), like all interventions, it is underpinned by an implicit ideology. The ideology of social marketing is that of individualism and lifestylism, both of which emphasize personal responsibility. Andreasen (2002) questions, however, whether individual-level behaviour change is always the right (ethical) approach.

Conclusion

Social marketing approaches have endured with some success in the developing world, particularly in relation to the promotion of family planning and contraception. Perhaps this is an example of an issue where there is a clear overarching *national* need – such that less attention is given to audience segmentation. There is also a clear 'product' – condoms and oral pills that can be offered at a discounted price. Changing behaviour may also be more straightforward because motivation is likely to be high, particularly among women. Elsewhere, however, questions remain about its effectiveness and relevance. It may well be the case that social marketing offers a potentially useful approach for addressing some issues in some situations, rather than being promoted as a panacea to a whole range of complex health problems and behaviours.

SOCIALIZATION

Context

Socialization is a well-established (albeit contested) term within the social sciences but one that has received less attention within public health until relatively recently. Yet the process by which human beings become, more or less, competent members of society is relevant to understanding all human actions, including those that relate directly and indirectly to **health**. Socialization involves the acquisition of knowledge, skills, views, values, attitudes and general predispositions. In contrast to the idea of innate behaviours and personality traits, socialization infers that 'the learning process that human children undergo in their interactions with others largely consists of expanding and refining inborn abilities' (de Swann, 2001: 56). This implies that the development of particular dispositions is not inevitable. Rather, they might be better understood as reflecting a lifelong process of social development. This opens up a variety of possibilities for improving health and preventing disease, particularly in relation to families and schools, both of which have come under increasing scrutiny over the past decade or so as **settings** for **health promotion**.

Defining socialization

Early definitions of socialization tended to emphasize pattern, predictability and uniformity, and imply that it provides a mechanism for limiting people's actions to a narrow, acceptable range appropriate to the group within which they are located. Critics point out, however, that this view of socialization is deterministic, crowding out notions of change, unpredictability and creativity, based, as it is, on an over-socialized conceptualization of human beings (Wrong, 1961). More recent definitions and interpretations emphasize the dynamic interweaving of complex socialization *processes*, with different people and groups (such as friends) being more or less influential in different settings at various points in time. Thus, the developmental trajectories that emerge cannot be directly controlled or predicted. However, central to all definitions of socialization is the idea that it is *people* who shape and form *other people*, such that 'society actually becomes part of the individual, who internalizes the knowledge and beliefs, and builds a personality, enabling him or her to become a full member of society' (Roberts, 2009: 270). This is perhaps most readily understood in relation to parents – especially mothers, but increasingly fathers too – who are expected to take responsibility for the initial (primary) socialization of a child. Secondary socialization refers to processes beyond the family – at school, with friends, at work, through social media, for example – indicating that socialization tends to be viewed as a lifelong process, with later stages expanding the foundations formed early on (Roberts, 2009). Families and schools, comprised as they are of networks of people, are key settings for socialization, and parents, teachers and friends key agents of socialization.

Learning – a fundamental mechanism in socialization – takes place through inter-actions with others, more or less casually and more or less informally, so that things are learnt, unlearnt, and rejected (de Swann, 2001). Formal, intentional processes of socialization involve various forms of constraint and pressure (persuasion through to punishment) intended to influence behaviour. Parents' child-rearing practices can include the use of various forms of pressure to help children learn to control and direct their own actions in relation to social norms such that they internalize expected ways of behaving (particularly in relation to the control of drives and emotions), which over time become tantamount to 'second nature'. Alongside these intentional efforts are informal, unintentional processes whereby everyday interactions within the family transmit a variety of subliminal messages through which children learn how things are done, what is valued, how events are coped with, what the consequences of certain actions are, and so on. In the case of schools, the terms 'hidden' and 'informal' curriculum have been used to describe these aspects of how children learn norms of behaviour beyond the family. The blend of formal and informal processes of learning varies according to the setting. As children move into the teenage years, parental significance diminishes while that of friends increases, shifting the emphasis towards more negotiated processes of learning – something viewed as integral to the development of young people's emerging identities. Formal and informal socialization processes are also important in professional work settings. Junior doctors, for example, learn how to be doctors by spending time on hospital wards, not only to assimilate technical knowledge and skills but also 'tacit knowledge and "craft" skills, norms and values and "professional" modes of conduct' (Gabe *et al.*, 2004: 169).

Socialization implies that 'personality' is developed and socially constructed. Habitus is the term used by sociologists, such as Bourdieu, to describe the 'durable perceptions, understandings and predispositions to action' (Roberts, 2009: 20). In keeping with the idea of socialization as a lifelong process, habitus can change but invariably builds on existing predispositions. Thus, developmental trajectories are best understood in terms of that which has gone before. This is significant for public health because the character of early lives appears to delimit future possibilities. However, in spite of the intentions of significant others such as parents and teachers to socialize children with specific goals in mind, the habituses they develop reflect the interweaving of many (sometimes conflicting) influences leading to a variety of unplanned and unintended outcomes. Thus, habitus attributes to people greater degrees of flexibility than more deterministic notions of personality. Because learning takes place through interactions with others it will qualitatively differ from one milieu to the next, reflecting the social networks of which people are a part. This means that differences in social-ization are socially inherited (de Swann, 2001). Bourdieu argues that different social classes develop different and distinctive habituses with predispositions for certain tastes and preferences according to the cultural capital transmitted by their parents. According to this view, choices are socially generated through a class-specific habitus (Abel and Frohlich, 2012). Furthermore, class differences tend to be perpetuated because of the relative ease with which social bonds are formed between those with similar habituses. People tend to choose partners with similar habituses and of similar social class and level of **education** (Nilsen *et al.*, 2012), furthering the reproduction of class differences.

The significance of socialization for public health

In general terms, socialization has particular significance for public health because it sheds light on the development of health-related predispositions, behaviours and norms. At the same time, it draws attention to the significance of the social milieu into which people are born, develop and mature. In this respect, it expands the settings-based ideas prominent in the health promotion literature by providing an explanation for how settings, as social networks, create the conditions and possibilities for health development. Socialization has also been used to explain two more specific and interrelated issues of relevance to public health. First, socialization processes during the formative years of children's lives appear important in terms of developing a range of capacities and vulnerabilities that have implications for future health and well-being. Second, socialization has been proposed as part of the explanation for social **inequalities** in health (Singh-Manoux and Marmot, 2005).

Socialization offers a mechanism for understanding how parents (more or less systematically and strategically) imbue their children with cultural capital – a developing repertoire of knowledge, skills, tastes and values that become part of their habitus. Thus, the formation of educational and professional aspirations (potential choices), contoured by the gendered socialization practices of parents, are a feature of cultural capital. Such aspirations are particularly significant for girls, as starting a family tends to be delayed with higher educational achievement. The support given to children in relation to their education – reading to children, visiting school, talking about their teachers and so forth (Schoon and Bynner, 2003) – implicitly transmits a variety of messages about the value of education. Increasingly it seems, middle-class parents engage in 'concerted cultivation of children' (Chambers, 2012: 85), enrolling them in a diverse array of organized, enriching activities. Working class and poorer parents on the other hand, are more likely to view their child's development as a 'natural' process in which their role is to nurture, love and support (Lareau, 2002). This illustrates how early socialization can give rise to forms of cultural capital that lead to different class- and gender-based developmental trajectories. Forms of cultural capital can also help explain the engagement of children and youth in health-related practices that collectively come to represent a form of **lifestyle**. Childhood and youth are the life-stages during which the foundations for long-term uses of leisure, for example, are laid (Green, 2010). The best predictor of individuals' sports participation at any given time is whether or not they have played in the past (Roberts and Brodie, 1992). This example indicates that parents have a key role in the development of sporting capital (Kay and Spaaij, 2012) through the transmission of particular types of cultural practices; post-childhood experiences are less significant in this regard (Birchwood *et al.*, 2008).

Parents are the most important influences on young children's attitudes to alcohol, many children becoming familiar with parental drinking – and the associated home rules, norms and practices – from a young age (Valentine *et al.*, 2010). Children learn, it seems, not through direct discussion with parents but informally: through experiences associated with parental supervision and monitoring, as well as through observing the unfolding of everyday home life. Eadie *et al.* (2010) concluded that children's observation of parents' and other adult relatives' drinking meant that even young children (7–12 years) developed a relatively sophisticated understanding of alcohol and its effects, including knowledge of their parents' drinking preferences. Parents, especially mothers, tend to emphasize learning to drink at home in a safe environment (Valentine *et al.*, 2010), emphasizing moderation through their own behaviour (Eadie *et al.*, 2010). Furthermore, supervised drinking at home, as well as observing relatives drinking moderately, seems to limit the likelihood of teenagers drinking to excess later (Velleman, 2009). However, parents' socializing practices vary by class, alcohol consumption taking place more overtly in working class families, including drunkenness at home and in the local **community** (Eadie *et al.*, 2010). Parents' stance on alcohol tends to be more nuanced and ambiguous than in relation to smoking and illicit drug use. As children become more sensitive to the influence of their friends, however, parental authority diminishes (Sondhi and Turner, 2011; Velleman, 2009). Nevertheless, it seems that drinking behaviour is mediated by social context. Young adults are more likely to drink to excess with friends, actively pursuing drunkenness as an aspect of having fun, forming and reinforcing friendships, while showing more restraint in the company of family members (Seaman and Ikegwuonu, 2010).

The interdependent relationship between parents and children suggests that children can influence their parents' parenting practices. Children's disapproval of their parent's alcohol consumption, for example, can act as a socializing influence on their parents' behaviour (Eadie *et al.*, 2010). In the USA, children have also been shown to pressurize parents to spend on their behalf, particularly as they become sensitive to the relative spending power of their friends' parents (Chambers, 2012). Consumption increasingly permeates children's relationships, playing a central part in identity formation, particularly during youth. Sociologists recognize the possibility of self-socialization, people selecting situations that will facilitate their development into 'the persons they wish to become' (Roberts 2009: 170). McCreanor *et al.* (2005) discuss young people's identity formation and alcohol marketing. They argue that young people increasingly use branded alcohol as a way of signifying their identity and place in the world, a matter exploited by the alcohol industry. Exposure to frequent youth-oriented and pro-drinking promotional messages contours youth identities towards the consumption of alcohol as an aspect of a particular lifestyle that gives meaning and significance to young people's lives. This reveals the relevance of agents of socialization beyond parents and teachers at critical periods in the **lifecourse**, as well as the complexity and ambiguity associated with notions of conscious choice.

Parenting practices can also give rise to various kinds of vulnerabilities in children. For example, children who have experienced early parental neglect are more likely to experience emotional difficulties in later life, including a limited capacity to form close ties with others (Bynner, 2001). Longitudinal studies covering the period from birth to adulthood have shown the cumulative consequences of disadvantaged life histories and the 'vicious and virtuous circles' that children living in different social circumstances experience (Schoon and Bynner, 2003: 22). How parents socialize their children, however, reflects not only their own socialization but also the socio-economic circumstances in which they endeavour to parent their children. Linking socialization processes to these wider conditions shifts the analysis away from simply blaming parents for their perceived inadequacies. Parents' interactions with their children can be put under strain if, for example, they experience unemployment as humiliating and degrading (Christoffersen, 2000). Parenting under stress has also been documented in areas of **deprivation** (Spijkers *et al.*, 2011) where living in poverty and experiencing mental illness can go hand in hand (Gilbert *et al.*, 2008). However, supportive social policies such as those in Nordic countries can ameliorate some of the consequences of these circumstances by helping parents cope with adversity (Chambers, 2012; Graham, 2002).

Conclusion

Children's vulnerability to an array of persistent adverse social and economic circumstances is well-established. Socialization provides a conceptual framework for understanding how such circumstances shape personal attributes and give rise to durable developmental consequences with implications for adult health and well-being. Perhaps what is less well understood is how children develop resilience and the capacity to rise above their backgrounds, succeeding against the odds (Schoon and Bynner, 2003). The concept of socialization would suggest that this is in some way linked to parenting practices and processes of socialization more broadly. According to this view, socialization links social inequalities in health via the social **determinants** of child development (Kendall and Li, 2005). From a **policy** perspective this points to the importance of primary **prevention** and early intervention, for example, through Sure Start local programmes, implemented in England from 1997, which focused on families with children aged 0–4 years. However, significant changes can occur in later life, if the social context changes. Adult delinquent behaviour, for example, can change through marriage to a non-delinquent spouse (Bynner, 2001). This suggests that socialization processes unfold throughout the lifecourse, opening up possibilities for change in later adulthood.

THE WELFARE STATE

Context

A broad consensus has emerged in recent years that **health** in general, and health **inequalities** in particular, are strongly influenced by how society is organized (Grøholt *et al.*, 2007). At a national level, a key aspect of social organization is the form of a country's welfare state. During the twentieth century, the welfare states of most high-income countries expanded, especially during the post-war period. Before that time, the state had little involvement in regulating the economy or providing welfare (Fraser, 2009). The welfare state mediates access to publicly-funded services (through direct and indirect taxation) such as housing, and support in the form of benefits during times of hardship. In so doing, the welfare state acts on the wider **determinants** of health and influences the degree of inequality that people experience (Graham, 2007). Inequalities are, therefore, 'policy sensitive' rather than inevitable, since the social policies governments pursue influence 'people's educational opportunities, their employment and earnings and their income and wealth' (Graham, 2007: 160). Political debate since the 1970s, however, has centred on the question of the 'affordability' of public social spending programmes (that is to say, spending on the welfare state) rather than 'social progress'. These debates have gathered considerable momentum since the 2007/8 global financial crisis. In the UK, the coalition government has embarked on an unprecedented, fundamental and rapid restructuring of the welfare state in response to the economic downturn. While the expressed aim is to reduce its public debt, the outcome will be to contract the state, with a concomitant shift in the balance of social rights (Taylor-Gooby, 2012). **Evidence** from countries that have undergone similar restructuring – such as Canada and New Zealand – suggests that this is likely to have considerable negative implications for the poor and vulnerable. It is against this background that discussions about the role of the welfare state in improving public health and reducing health inequalities take place.

Definition

Although definitions vary, there is some agreement that the welfare state 'involves state responsibility for securing some basic modicum of welfare for its citizens' (Esping-Andersen, 1990: 18–19), a central aspect of which is to act as a buffer against the consequences of labour market processes which generate inequalities (Graham, 2007). In the UK, the Beveridge Report (1942) set out the principles (subsequently implemented) for the development of a welfare state in Britain, which included the creation of the NHS. However, core services go beyond heath care to include **education** and housing, for example. The welfare state also includes systems to conserve people's incomes during unemployment, sickness (through various kinds of benefits) and old age (through a state pension). The idea of services in 'cash and kind' is reflected in Miller's (2003: 95) definition of the welfare state as comprising 'the set of institutions and policies that distribute both money and essential goods and services to citizens on a non-market basis'. This definition illustrates the central principle of 'decommodification': citizens are freed from dependence on the labour market to sustain their standard of living (Esping-Anderson, 1990). It also alludes implicitly to the 'redistribution' of resources across an individual's lifespan, a key aim of welfare states. Redistribution across social groups, however, is contentious in many welfare state systems (Graham, 2007).

Within the OECD, social spending has increased, on average, from 19 to 22 per cent of GDP (the standard measure of the value of final goods and services produced by a country during a period) between 2007/08 and 2012 in real terms (that is to say, adjusted for increases in prices) (OECD, 2012). The main increase took place between 2007 and 2009. The increase reflects both a greater need for social support (in relation to unemployment, for example) and stagnating GDP. Nonetheless, the proportion of GDP varies by country. In 2009, France (32.1 per cent) and Denmark (30.2 per cent) spent most on their welfare states. The UK (24.1 per cent) and Norway (23.3 per cent) were around the OECD average, while Korea (9.4 per cent) and Mexico (8.2 per cent) spent least. Overall, however, historical trends indicate that welfare states in many countries have more than doubled in size since the 1960s. The reasons for this relate to an expansion of social programmes, more generous benefits and demographic pressure from an ageing population in relation to pensions and health and social care (OECD, 2012). Exactly how these different elements combine in different welfare systems, however, is dependent on broader political processes.

The varying proportions of welfare state spending over time reflect the influence of different (political) ideologies – general sets of ideas and beliefs that are used to justify policies and actions – relating to the role of the state in welfare provision. In this regard, typologies of welfare state regimes have been developed, one of the most commonly cited of which is that of Esping-Anderson (1990). Although this has been criticized, his three-fold typology of liberal, conservative, and social democratic welfare state regimes can be used as a starting point for making sense of a complex field (see for example Bambra, 2007). According to Esping-Anderson, liberal (neo-liberal) welfare states (for example, those of the UK, USA, Canada, Australia) are characterized by minimal state provision, means-tested benefits (eligibility assessed on the basis of income) with strict entitlement criteria, deregulation of the market and privatization of state enterprise. Conservative (Bismarckian) welfare states (Finland, Germany, France) are characterized by a minimal welfare state, an emphasis on the family and regulation of the market. Social democratic welfare states (Denmark, Norway, Sweden) have the stated goal of providing uniform social protection and a democratic right to adequate living conditions for the whole population, including an aspiration towards full employment. This latter type of welfare state is based on an expanded view of citizenship to incorporate the idea of 'social rights' (as well as political and civil rights) which give all citizens universal access to relatively generous services and benefits. The state is strongly interventionist and redistributive, creating a compressed wage structure that combines with taxes and public transfers to further equalize incomes (Grøholt *et al.*, 2007).

Typologies, such as that of Esping-Anderson, obscure variations within each 'ideal type', as well as understate the dynamic character of welfare states over time. A significant point to note is the global trend towards governments adopting neo-liberal policies, encouraged and supported by international institutions such as the World Bank, the WTO and the IMF. Neo-liberals believe in free markets, favouring global free trade, low taxes, a restricted role for the state in welfare and work to protect individual liberties against the state (Roberts, 2009). This ideology has underpinned the restructuring of welfare states in New Zealand, Canada and more recently the UK (Taylor-Gooby, 2012). According to this analysis, welfare state capitalism is constructed to enable a capitalist system to benefit the capitalist class, rather than the poor (Bambra, 2009). Economic policy thus drives social policy.

The significance of welfare states for public health

A key interest for those in public health has been the extent to which welfare state regimes differentially affect population health and health inequalities. Mackenbach (2012) notes the persistence of health inequalities in a number of countries during the period of welfare state expansion. Furthermore, health inequalities are not necessarily smaller in countries with the most generous social programmes. Norway is a case in point. Although Norwegians experience good health, inequalities have not been eradicated despite initial assumptions to the contrary (Grøholt *et al.*, 2007). However, some studies have found that countries with a social democratic welfare state regime tend to do better on a number of indicators, such as infant mortality and low birth weight (Chung and Muntaner, 2007) and self-reported health (Eikemo *et al.*, 2008). A recent review concluded that social democratic regimes had better population health compared to others, implying that universalism rather than means-testing is beneficial (Brennenstuhl *et al.*, 2012). It concluded, nonetheless, that there was little evidence that such regimes had smaller inequalities, proposing that universal policies benefit all groups. Part of the inconsistency between studies may relate, at least in part, to the differential impact of specific policies on specific groups. Popham *et al.* (2013) concluded from their comparative study of 37 countries that the Nordic countries had the smallest inequalities in mortality for men but not women.

Graham (2007) points out, nevertheless, that welfare systems were not specifically designed to reduce health or social inequalities. Rather than focus on the welfare state regime – a complex, shifting, multi-layered construct – attention to specific policy measures and related outputs might provide a more valid approach (Brennenstuhl *et al.*, 2012). Studies have found that some forms of welfare state can reduce gender inequalities in income through specific policy instruments. In the UK, cash benefits have played a major role in equalizing incomes and living standards (Graham, 2007). In this respect, the welfare state can play a role in preventing and reducing poverty, particularly in relation to children. Childhood is a period of amplified susceptibility to poverty, particularly when families are persistently poor (Holmes and Kiernan, 2013). Both UK government enquiries into inequalities in health – the Black Report and the Acheson Inquiry – made recommendations relating to the reduction of child poverty. Some welfare states, such as those of Finland, Norway and Sweden are much more effective in lifting children out of poverty compared to the USA and UK (Bradshaw, 2002; Mackenbach, 2011b). Sweden in particular has been successful at keeping child poverty low even during its significant economic downturn in the 1990s. Studies have indicated that it matters less what country you live in if your parents have a higher level of education. However, it matters more for children in the UK or USA if their parents have a low level of education compared to children living in Finland (Wilkinson and Pickett, 2010). This illustrates the significance of national policies rather than global economic forces (Graham, 2007). Universal systems rather than means-testing are particularly pro-poor and thus important in preventing poverty (Horton and Gregory, 2010). They also reduce stigma and improve take-up of awards (Baumberg *et al.*, 2012).

The extent to which the welfare state ameliorates disadvantage is also relevant to understanding the impact of targeted **behaviour change** interventions to improve health. A number of studies have shown that this type of intervention widens inequalities because those in higher socio-economic groups benefit most. Smoking cessation interventions, for example, have been more effective in higher socio-economic groups (Ferguson *et al.*, 2005) and Sure Start local programmes have been found to benefit less disadvantaged parents (Belsky *et al.*, 2006). Graham (2007: 163) argues that 'policies that reduce inequalities in life chances and living standards may therefore be a precondition for progress in reducing inequalities in proximal risk factors'. This may be particularly important given the shifting pattern of health behaviours such as smoking and low physical activity, both of which are skewed towards those in lower socio-economic groups. This might account for the limited progress on reducing health inequalities even where welfare provision has improved (Pega *et al.*, 2012).

Health care tends to receive one of the largest budgets in state welfare provision. In the UK, health spending accounted for 9.8 per cent of GDP in 2009, slightly above the OECD average of 9.6 per cent. Here, the public sector continues to pay 84 per cent of all health spending (OECD, 2011a). Nonetheless, concerns about a movement towards a US-style insurance-based health system (17.6 per cent of GDP in 2010, 48.2 per cent of which is publicly financed) have heightened since 2010, especially since the passing of the Health and Social Care Act (2012). This Act has the potential to extend the role of the private sector in the delivery of health care (shrinking the public sector in the process) through the use of competitive tendering processes to commission required services. The acceleration of a mixed economy of health care has been driven by neo-liberal ideology interwoven with ideas about consumer choice, value for money and increasing performance, including driving down waiting times. The application of neo-liberal ideology to the NHS is seen as undermining the egalitarian principles on which is has been founded, especially important for those who are poor and vulnerable.

A major criticism of advanced health care systems relates to their costs. In England, a relatively small proportion is spent on public health and **prevention** – approximately 4 per cent (£3.7 billion, 2006/7) of the total health budget (£93.5 billion, 2006/7) – which is above the OECD average of 2.8 per cent (Butterfield *et al.*, 2009). This budget covers maternal and child health and family planning; school health services; prevention of infectious diseases; occupational health care; and, environmental surveillance (but excludes preventive pharmaceuticals). Easing the pressures on health care systems (and costs) requires a greater emphasis on prevention and better chronic disease management. Yet, conventionally 'health policy' is, in effect, health *care* policy, in which public health is viewed as a lower priority (Hunter *et al.*, 2010). The escalation of obesity rates in many countries since 1980 has put additional pressure on curative health systems that could be addressed through a range of public health measures (OECD, 2011b). In England, the current restructuring of the health service and the relocation of public health and **health promotion** to local government may lead to its further marginalization, particularly given the financial pressures and the relatively short-term financial objectives being pursued.

Public health itself constitutes an important part of the welfare state outside the health care system, particularly in relation to local government. In England, the Local Government Act (2000) gave local authorities specific powers to promote social, economic and environmental well-being (Hunter, 2010). Regardless of national policy, local government has discretionary powers in a number of areas that can influence health and well-being, such as air quality management, schools meals, speed limits, and using its planning function to design walking and cycling routes (Dorling, 2010). Loft (2010) also draws attention to the role of local authorities in enforcing environmental health and trading standards, which include reducing alcohol and tobacco-related harm and maintaining acceptable standards of private rented housing, food standards and safety. Hunter (2010: 11), however, argues that 'For various reasons and with some exceptions local authorities as a whole have not seen their health enhancing role as uppermost in their thinking or central to their core business.' Consequently, opportunities to promote health and well-being at a local level may well be overlooked.

Conclusion

Navarro (2011) argues that politics tends to be avoided in public health. Yet it is clear that the size, shape and form of a welfare state are determined by a nation-state's prevailing political ideology. Moreover, the post-war consensus relating to the necessity for governments to manage market economies actively and provide welfare has all but disintegrated (Graham, 2007). Some countries (notably the Nordic countries) have, however, so far maintained a large degree of consensus, actively seeking to reduce poverty and narrow incomes through concerted policy measures. It is a moot point – what Bambra (2011) refers to as a 'puzzle' and Mackenbach (2011a) a 'paradox' – whether or not their impact on social inequalities translate into smaller health inequalities. The considerable methodological and conceptual challenges may preclude a resolution of this question. Nonetheless, recent challenges to neo-liberal ideology (particularly in relation to the negative consequences of deregulation of the market and reduction in the size of the state in welfare provision) have not diminished enthusiasm for its application to all aspects of public policy in England and elsewhere (Krugman, 2013). Against this background, however, is the decline in support for the welfare state among the general public in the UK (Duffy *et al.*, 2013).

REFERENCES

Abbas, J., Carlin, H., Cunningham, A., Dedman, D. and McVey, D. (2009) *Geodemographic Segmentation. Technical Briefing 5*, York: Association of Public Health Observatories.

Abel, T. (2008) 'Cultural capital and social inequality in health', *Journal of Epidemiology & Community Health*, 62: e13. doi:101136/jech.2007.066159

Abel, T. and Frohlich, K. (2012) 'Capitals and capabilities: linking structure and agency to reduce health inequalities', *Social Science & Medicine*, 74: 236–44.

Abel, T., Cockerham, C. and Neimann, S. (2000) 'A critical approach to lifestyle and health', in J. Watson and S. Platt (eds) *Researching Health Promotion* (pp. 54–77), London: Routledge.

AbouZahr, C., Adjei, S. and Kanchanachitra, C. (2007) 'From data to policy: good practices and cautionary tales', *The Lancet*, 369: 1039–46.

Acheson, D. (1988) *Public Health in England: The Report of the Committee of Inquiry into the Future Development to the Public Health Function*, (Cm 28), London: HMSO.

Acheson, D. (1998) *Independent Inquiry into Inequalities in Health Report*, London: The Stationery Office.

Adam, E. and Kumari, M. (2009) 'Assessing salivary cortisol in large-scale epidemiological research', *Psychoneuroendocrinology*, 34: 1423–6.

Adams, J. (1994) 'Seatbelt legislation: the evidence revisited', *Safety Science*, 18: 135–52.

Adams, J. and Hillman, M. (2001) 'The risk compensation theory and bicycle helmets', *Injury Prevention*, 7: 89–91.

Ahnquist, J., Wamala, S. and Lindstrom, M. (2012) 'Social determinants of health – a question of social or economic capital? Interaction effects of socioeconomic factors on health outcomes', *Social Science & Medicine*, 74: 930–9.

Ajzen, I. (1985) 'From intentions to actions: a theory of planned behaviour', in J. Kuhl and J. Beckman (eds) *Action-Control: From Cognition to Behaviour* (pp. 11–39), Heidelberg: Springer.

Aldridge, H., Kenway, P., Macinnes, T. and Parekh, A. (2012) *Monitoring Poverty and Social Exclusion 2012*, York: Joseph Rowntree Foundation.

Allen, P., Black, N., Clarke, A., Fulup, N. and Anderson, S. (2001) *Studying the Organization of Health Services: Research Methods*, London: Routledge.

Allin, S., Grignon, M. and Le Grand, J. (2010) 'Subjective unmet need and utilization of health care services in Canada: what are the equity implications?', *Social Science & Medicine*, 70: 465–72.

Andermann, A., Blancquaert, I., Beauchamp, S. and Déry, V. (2008) 'Revisiting Wilson and Jungner in the genomic age: a review of screening criteria over the past 40 years', *Bulletin of the World Health Organization*, 86(4): 317–19.

Anderson, L., Shinn, C., Fullilove, M., Scrimshaw, S., Fielding, J., Normand, J. and Carande-Kulis, V. (2003) 'The effectiveness of early childhood development programs. A systematic review', *American Journal of Preventive Medicine*, 24(3S): 32–46.

Anderson, P., Chisholm, D. and Fuhr, D. (2009) 'Effectiveness and cost–effectiveness of policies and programmes to reduce the harm caused by alcohol', *Lancet*, 373: 2234–46.

Anderson, R. and Funnell, M. (2005) 'Patient empowerment: reflections on the challenge of fostering the adoption of a new paradigm', *Patient Education and Counseling*, 57: 153–7.

Andersson, R. and Musterd, S. (2005) 'Area-based policies: a critical appraisal', *Tidschrift voor Economische en Sociale Geografie*, 96(4): 377–89.

Andreasen, A. (2002) 'Marketing social marketing in the social change marketplace', *Journal of Public Policy and Marketing*, 21(1): 2–13.

Andrews, G. and Moon, G. (2005) 'Space, place, and the evidence base: Part 1 – an introduction to health geography', *Worldviews on Evidence-Based Nursing*, 2(2): 55–62.

Andrews, T. (1999) 'Pulled between contradictory expectations: The Norwegian mother/child service and the 'new' public health', *Critical Public Health*, 9(4): 269–85.

Andrews, T. (2006) 'Conflicting public health discourses – tensions and dilemmas in practice: the case of the Norwegian mother and child health service', *Critical Public Health*, 16(3): 191–204.

Antonovsky, A. (1996) 'The salutogenic model as a theory to guide health promotion', *Health Promotion International*, 11: 11–18.

Armitage C. and Connor, M. (2000) 'Social cognition models and health behaviour: a structured review', *Psychology & Health*, 15(2): 173–189.

Asbridge, M. (2004) 'Public place restrictions on smoking in Canada: assessing the role of the state, media, science and public health advocacy', *Social Science & Medicine*, 58: 13–24.

Ashton, J. (2007) 'Grasping defeat: health promotion is a doing word, not a proper noun', *Journal of the Royal Society for the Promotion of Health*, 127(5): 207–8.

Ashton, J. (2010) 'Inequalities, assets and local government – opportunities for democratic renewal posed by the global economic crisis', in F. Campbell (ed.) *The Social Determinants of Health and the Role of Local Government* (pp. 62–64), London: IDeA.

Ashton, J. and Seymour, H. (1988) *The New Public Health*, Milton Keynes: Open University Press.

Ashton, J., Grey, P. and Barnard, K. (1986) 'Healthy cities: WHO's new public health initiative', *Health Promotion International*, 1(3): 319–24.

Atar, A., Elzey, J., Insaf, T., Grau, A., Stain, S. and Ahmed, N. (2006) 'Colorectal cancer prevention: adherence patterns and correlates of tests done for screening purposes with the United States populations', *Cancer Detection and Prevention*, 30: 134–43.

Atkinson, R. and Kintrea, K. (2001) 'Disentangling area effects: evidence from deprived and non–deprived neighbourhoods', *Urban Studies*, 38: 2277–98.

Atkinson, S. (2011) 'Moves to measure wellbeing must support a social model of health', *BMJ*, 343: d7323.

Attree, P., French, B., Milton, B., Povall, S., Whitehead, M. and Popay, J. (2011) 'The experience of community engagement for individuals: a rapid review of evidence', *Health and Social Care in the Community*, 19(3): 250–60.

Audit Commission (1998) *A Fruitful Partnership. Effective Partnership Working*, Abingdon, Oxon: Audit Commission Publications.

Austen, L. (2009) 'The social construction of risk by young people', *Health, Risk & Society*, 11(5): 451–70.

Azjen, I. and Fishbein, M. (1980) *Understanding Attitudes and Predicting Social Behavior*, Englewood Cliffs, NJ: Prentice Hall.

Babb, P. (2005) *Measurement of Social Capital in the UK*, London: Office for National Statistics.

Bacchus, L., Bewley, S., Vitolas, C., Aston, G., Jordan, P. and Murray, S. (2010) 'Evaluation of a domestic violence intervention in the maternity and sexual health services of a UK hospital', *Reproductive Health Matters*, 18(36): 147–57.

Bacon, N., Brophy, M., Mguni, N., Mulgan, G. and Shandro, A. (2010) *The State of Happiness. Can Public Policy Shape People's Wellbeing and Resilience?* London: The Young Foundation.

Baehr, G. (1944) 'The Peckham Experiment', *The Millbank Memorial Fund Quarterly*, 22(2): 352–7.

Bailey, N. and Livingston, M. (2007) *Population Turnover and Area Deprivation*, Basingstoke: The Policy Press.

Baker, D. (2006) 'The meaning and the measure of health literacy', *Journal of General Internal Medicine*, 21: 878–83.

Ball, S. (2010) 'New class inequalities in education: why education policy may be looking in the wrong place! Education policy, civil society and social class', *International Journal of Sociology and Social Policy*, 30(3): 155–66.

Bambra, C. (2007) 'Going beyond the three worlds of welfare capitalism: regime theory and public health research', *Journal of Epidemiology &Community Health*, 61: 1098–102.

Bambra, C. (2009) 'Welfare state regimes and the political economy of health', *Humanity & Society*, 33: 99–117.

Bambra, C. (2011) 'Health inequalities and welfare state regimes: theoretical insights on a public health "puzzle"', *Journal of Epidemiology & Community Health*, 65: 740–5.

Bambra, C. (2012) 'Reducing health inequalities: new data suggest that the English strategy was partially successful', *Journal of Epidemiology & Community Health*, 66(7): 662.

Bandura, A. (1998) 'Health promotion from the perspective of social cognitive theory', *Psychology & Health*, 13(4): 623–49.

Barbour, R. (2011) 'The biographical turn and the 'sociologization' of medicine', *Medical Sociology Online*, 6(1): 15–25.

Barker, D. (1998) *Mothers, Babies and Health in Later Life*, Edinburgh, UK: Churchill Livingstone.

Barnes, M., Matka, E. and Sullivan, H. (2003) 'Evidence, understanding and complexity', *Evaluation*, 9(3): 265–84.

Barr, B., Taylor–Robinson, D. and Whitehead, M. (2012) 'Impact on health inequalities of rising prosperity in England 1998–2007 and implications for performance incentives: longitudinal ecological study', *BMJ*, 335: e7831.

Bartley, M. (2012a) 'Explaining health inequality: evidence from the UK', *Social Science & Medicine*, 74: 658–60.

Bartley, M. (ed.) (2012b) *Life Gets under your Skin*, London: UCL Research Department of Epidemiology and Public Health.

Bartley, M., Blane, D. and Montgomery, S. (1997) 'Health and the life course: why safety nets matter', *BMJ*, 314: 1194–6.

Barton, H. and Grant, M. (2006) 'A health map for the local human habitat', *The Journal for the Royal Society for the Promotion of Health*, 125(6): 252–3.

Bassett, M. (2003) 'Editor's Choice. Public Health Advocacy', *American Journal of Public Health*, 93(8): 1204.

Batchelor, P. and Sheiham, A. (2002) 'The limitations of a "high–risk" approach for the prevention of dental caries', *Community Dental Oral Epidemiology*, 30: 302–12.

Batty, E., Cole, I. and Green, S. (2011) *Low Income Neighbourhoods in Britain. The Gap between Policy Ideas and Residents' Realities*, York: Joseph Rowntree Foundation.

Bauld, L., Judge, K., Barnes, M., Benzeval, M., Mackenzie, M. and Sullivan, H. (2005) 'Promoting social change: the experience of Health Action Zones in England', *Journal of Social Policy*, 34(3): 427–45.

Baum, F. (2011) 'From norm to Eric: avoiding lifestyle drift in Australian health policy', *Australian & New Zealand Journal of Public Health*, 35(5): 404–6.

Baum, F., Laris, P., Fisher, M., Newman, L. and MacDougall, C. (2013) '"Never mind the logic, give me the numbers": former Australian health ministers perspectives on the social determinants of health' *Social Science & Medicine*, 87: 138–146.

Baumberg, B., Bell, K. and Gaffney, D. (2012) *Benefits Stigma in Britain*, Elizabeth Finn Care/University of Kent.

Bayer, R. (2008) 'Stigma and the ethics of public health: not can we but should we' *Social Science & Medicine*, 67: 463–72.

Beaglehole, R., Bonita, R. and Kjellström, T. (1993) *Basic Epidemiology*, Geneva: World Health Organization.

Beattie, A. (1991) 'Knowledge and control in health promotion: a test case for social policy and social theory', in M. Bury, M. Calnan and J. Gabe (eds) *The Sociology of the Health Service* (pp. 162–202), London: Routledge.

Beatty, C., Foden, M., Lawless, P. and Wilson, I. (2010) 'Area based regeneration partnerships and the role of central government: the New Deal for Communities programme in England', *Policy & Politics*, 38(2): 235–51.

Beauchamp, D. (1976) 'Public health as social justice', *Inquiry*, 13: 1–14.

Beauchamp, T. and Childress, J. (2009) *Principles of Biomedical Ethics*, Oxford: Oxford University Press.

Beck, U. (1992) *Risk Society: Towards a New Modernity*, London: Sage.

Becker, M. (1974) *The Health Belief Model and Personal Health Behaviour*, New Jersey: Thorofare.

Bell, S. and Figert, A. (2012) 'Medicalization and pharmaceuticalization at the intersections: looking backward, sideways and forward', *Social Science & Medicine*, 75(5): 755–83.

Bellis, M., Hughes, K. and Lowey, H. (2002) 'Healthy nightclubs and recreational substance use: from harm minimisation to a healthy settings approach', *Addictive Behaviour*, 27: 1025–35.

Belsky, J., Melhuish, E., Barnes, J., Romaniuk, H. and the NESS Research Team. (2006) 'Effects of Sure Start local programmes on children and families: early findings from a quasi–experimental, cross–sectional study', *BMJ*, 332: 1476–78.

Bennett, I., Chen, J., Soroui, J. and White, S. (2009) 'The contribution of health literacy to disparities in self–rated health status and preventive health behaviours in older adults', *Annals of Family Medicine*, 7(3): 204–11.

Ben-Shlomo, Y. and Kuh, D. (2002) 'A life course approach to chronic disease epidemiology: conceptual models, empirical challenges and interdisciplinary perspectives', *International Journal of Epidemiology*, 31: 293.

Benzeval, M. and Judge, K. (2001) 'Income and health: the time dimension', *Social Science & Medicine*, 52: 1371–90.

Benzeval, M., Judge, K. and Whitehead, M. (eds) (1995) *Tackling Inequalities in Health: An Agenda for Action*, London: King's Fund.

Bernard, P., Charafeddine, R., Frohlich, K., Daniel, M., Kestens, Y. and Potvin, L. (2007) 'Health and inequalities and place: a theoretical conception of neighbourhood', *Social Science & Medicine*, 65: 1839–52.

Bernburg, J. (2010) 'Relative deprivation theory does not imply a contextual effect of country-level inequality on poor health: a commentary on Jen, Jones and Johnston (68:4, 2009)', *Social Science & Medicine*, 70: 493–5.

Berridge, V. (2008) 'Polyclinics: haven't we been there before?', *BMJ*, 336: 1161–2.

Berridge, V. (2010) 'The art of medicine. Thinking in time: does health policy need history as evidence?' *The Lancet*, 375: 798–9.

Berridge, V., Christie, D. and Tansey, E. (eds) (2006) Public health in the 1980s and 1990s: decline and rise? The transcript of a witness seminar held by the Wellcome Trust Centre for the History of Medicine at UCL, London, on 12 October 2004, Volume 26, London: Wellcome Trust Centre for the History of Medicine.

Berthoud, R. and Bryan, M. (2011) 'Income, deprivation and poverty: a longitudinal analysis, *Journal of Social Policy*, 40(1): 135–56.

Bettcher, D. and Lee, K. (2002) 'Globalisation and public health', *Journal of Epidemiology & Community Health*, 56: 8–17.

Bhopal, R. (2008) *Concepts of Epidemiology. Integrating the Ideas, Theories, Principles and Methods of Epidemiology*, Oxford: Oxford University Press.

Bigdeli, M. and Ir, P. (2010) *A Role for User Charges? Thoughts from Health Financing Reforms in Cambodia. Background Paper 42*, Geneva: World Health Organization.

Birchwood, D., Roberts, K. and Pollack, G. (2008) 'Explaining differences in sport participation rates among young adults: evidence from the South Caucasus', *European Physical Education Review*, 14(3): 283–98.

Birkinshaw, M. (1998) *Social Marketing for Health*, Geneva: World Health Organization.

Bjørngaard, J., Rustad, A. and Kjelsberg, E. (2009) 'The prisoner as patient: a health services satisfaction survey', *BMC Health Services Research*, 9: 176. doi:10.1186/1472-6963-9-176

Bjørnskov, C. (2010) 'Do elites benefit from democracy and foreign aid in developing countries?', *Journal of Development Economics*, 92: 115–24.

Black, D., Morris, J., Smith, C., Townsend, P. and Whitehead, M. (1988) *Inequalities in Health: The Black Report: The Health Divide*, Penguin: London.

Black, N. (2001) 'Evidence-based policy: proceed with care', *BMJ*, 323: 275–9.

Blackburn, J. (2000) 'Understanding Paolo Freire: reflections on the origins, concepts, and possible pitfalls of his educational approach', *Community Development Journal*, 35(1): 3–15.

Blackman, T. (2007) 'Statins, saving lives and shibboleths', *BMJ*, 334: 902.

Blackman, T., Elliott, E., Greene, A., Harrington, B., Hunter, D., Marks, L., Mckee, L., Smith, K. and Williams, G. (2009) 'Tackling health inequalities in post–devolution Britain: do targets matter?' *Public Administration*, 87(4): 762–78.

Blair–Stevens, C. (2010) 'Integrating social marketing into what we do', in F. Campbell (ed.) *The Social Determinants of Health and the Role of Local Government* (pp. 65–67), London: IDeA.

Blamey, A. and Mckenzie, M. (2007) 'Theories of change and realistic evaluation. Peas in a pod or apples and oranges?', *Evaluation*, 13(4): 439–55.

Blanden, J., Gregg, P. and Machin, S. (2005) *Intergenerational Mobility in Europe and North America. A Report Supported by the Sutton Trust*, London: Centre for Economic Performance, University College London.

Blane, D. (1985) 'An assessment of the Black Report's "explanations of health inequalities"', *Sociology of Health & Illness*, 7(3): 423–42.

Blane, D. and Watt, G. (2012) *GP Experience of the Impact of Austerity on Patients and General Practices in Very Deprived Areas: A report for GPs at the Deep End*. Available online at www.gla.ac.uk/departments/generalpracticeprimarycare/deepend/ (accessed 26 May 2012).

Blane, D., White, I. and Morris, J. (1996) 'Education, social circumstances and mortality', in D. Blane, E. Brunner and R. Wilkinson (eds) *Health and Social Organisation. Towards a Health Policy for the Twenty–first Century* (pp. 171–184), London: Routledge.

Blaxter, M. (1990) *Health and Lifestyles*, London: Routledge.

Blaxter, M. (1997) 'Whose fault is it anyway? People's own conceptions of the reasons for health inequalities', *Social Science & Medicine*, 44(6): 747–56.

Blaxter, M. (2010) *Key Concepts in Health*, Cambridge: Polity Press.

Bloom, D. and Canning, D. (2007) 'Commentary: the Preston curve 30 years on: still sparking fires', *International Journal of Epidemiology*, 36: 498–9.

Bloom, P. and Novelli, W. (1981) 'Problems and challenges in social marketing', *The Journal of Marketing*, 45(2): 79–88.

Blouin, C., Chopra, M. and van der Hoeven, R. (2009) 'Trade and social determinants of health', *The Lancet*, 373: 502–7.

Böckerman, P., Johansson, E., Saarni, S. I. and Saarni, S. E. (2013) 'The negative association of obesity with subjective well–being: is it all about health?', *Journal of Happiness Studies*, doi:10.1007/s10902-013-9453-8.

Boerma, J. and Stansfield, S. (2007) 'Health statistics now: are we making the right investments?', *The Lancet*, 369: 779–86.

Bond, L. and Nolan, T. (2011) 'Making sense of perceptions of risk of diseases and vaccinations: a qualitative study combining models of health beliefs, decision–making and risk perception', *BMC Public Health*, 11: 943.

Bongaarts, J. (2009) 'Human population growth and the demographic transition', *Philosophical Transactions of The Royal Society B*, 364: 2985–90.

Bosley, S. (2009) 'Compulsory vaccination urged after measles outbreak', *The Guardian* 3 June, 2009.

Bostock, S. and Steptoe, A. (2012) 'Association between low functional health literacy and mortality in older adults: longitudinal cohort study', *BMJ*, 344: e1602. doi:10.1136/bmj. e1602

Bourdieu, P. (1984) *Distinction: a Social Critique of the Judgement of Taste*, London: Routledge and Kegan Paul.

Bourdieu, P. (1991) 'The forms of capital', in J. Richardson (ed.) *Handbook of Theory and Research for the Sociology of Education* (pp. 241–58), New York: Greenwood.

Bourdieu, P. and Wacquant, L. (1992) *Invitation to Reflexive Sociology*, Chicago: University of Chicago Press.

Bowden-Jones, H. and Smith, N. (2012) 'The medical management of problem gamblers', *BMJ*, 344: e1559. doi:10.1136/bmj.e1559

Bowring, J. and Walker, P. (2010) 'The "Jade Goody effect": what now for cervical cancer protection?', *Journal of Family Planning and Reproductive Health Care*, 36: 51–4.

Boyce, T. and Hunter, D. (2009) *Improving Partnership Working to Reduce Health Inequalities*, London: The King's Fund.

Bradshaw, J. (1972) 'A taxonomy of social need', *New Society*, 19: 459–568

Bradshaw, J. (1994) 'The conceptualization and measurement of need: a social policy perspective', in J. Popay and G. Williams (eds) *Researching the People's Health* (pp. 45–58), London: Routledge.

Bradshaw, J. (2002) 'Child poverty and child outcomes', *Children & Society*, 16: 131–40.

Branfield, F. and Beresford, P. (2006) *Making User Involvement Work. Supporting Service User Networking and Knowledge*, York: Joseph Rowntree Foundation.

Branson, C., Duffy, B., Perry, C. and Wellings, D. (2012) *Acceptable Behaviour? Public Opinion on Behaviour Change Policy*, London: Ipsos Mori Social Research Institute. Available online at www.ipsos–mori.com/researchpublicaitons/publiations/1454/Acceptable–Behaviour. aspx (accessed 2 April 2012).

Braveman, P. (2006) 'Health disparities and health equity: concepts and measurement', *Annual Review of Public Health*, 27: 167–94.

Braveman, P. and Gruskin, S. (2003) 'Defining equity in health' *Journal of Epidemiology & Community Health*, 57: 254–8.

Braveman, P. and Tarimo, E. (2002) 'Social inequalities in health within countries: not only an issue for affluent nations', *Social Science & Medicine*, 54: 1621–35.

Brennenstuhl, S., Quesnel–Vallée, and McDonough, P. (2012) 'Welfare regimes, population health and health inequalities: a research synthesis', *Journal of Epidemiology & Community Health*, 66: 397–409.

Breslow, L. (1999) 'From disease prevention to health promotion', *Journal of the American Medical Association*, 281(11): 1030–3.

Breton, E., Richard, L. and Gagnon, F. (2007) 'The role of health education in the policy change process: lessons from tobacco control', *Critical Public Health*, 17(4): 351–64.

Brimicombe, A. and Café, R. (2012) 'Beware, win or lose: domestic violence and the World Cup', *Significance*, 9(5): 32–5.

Bronfenbrenner, U. (1986) 'Ecology of the family as a context for human development: research perspectives', *Developmental Psychology*, 22(6): 723–742.

Brown, C., Lloyd, S. and Murray, S. (2006) 'Using consecutive rapid participatory appraisal studies to assess, facilitate and evaluate health and social change in community settings', *BMC Public Health*, 6(68). doi:10.1186/1471-2458-6-68

Brown, G. (1984) 'Depression: a sociological view', in N. Black, D. Boswell, A. Gray, S. Murphy, and J. Popay (eds) *Health and Disease. A Reader*, Milton Keynes: Open University Press.

Brown, P. and Zavestoski, S. (2004) 'Social movements in health: an introduction', *Sociology of Health & Illness*, 26(6): 679–94.

Brown, T., Cueto, M. and Fee, E. (2006) 'The World Health Organization and the transition from "International" to "Global" public health', *American Journal of Public Health*, 96(1): 62–72.

Brownell, K. and Frieden, T. (2009) 'Ounces of prevention: the public policy case for taxes on sugared beverages', *New England Journal of Medicine*, 360: 1805–8.

Brunner, E. (1997) 'Socioeconomic determinants of health: stress and the biology of inequality', *BMJ*, 314: 1472–6.

Bryden, A., Petticrew, M., Mays, N., Eastmure, E. and Knai, C. (2013) 'Voluntary agreements between government and business. A scoping review of the literature with specific reference to the Public Health Responsibility Deal', *Health Policy*, 110: 186–97.

Buck, F. and Frosini, F. (2012) *Clustering of Unhealthy Behaviours Over Time: Implications for Policy*, London: The King's Fund.

Bungay, H. and Clift, S. (2010) 'Arts on prescription: a review of practice in the UK', *Perspectives in Public Health*, 130(6): 277–81.

Bunker, J. (2001) 'The role of medical care in contributing to health improvements within societies', *International Journal of Epidemiology*, 30: 1260–3.

Burkett, I. (2011) 'Appreciating assets: a new report from the International Association for Community Development', *Community Development Journal*, 46(4): 573–8.

Bury, M. (2005). *Health and Illness*, Cambridge: Polity Press.

Buse, K., Mays, N. and Walt, G. (2005) *Making Health Policy*, Maidenhead: Open University Press/McGraw Hill.

Butler, C., Simpson, S., Hood, K., Cohen, D., Pickles, T., Spanou, C., McCambridge, J., Moore, L., Randell, E., Alam, M. F., Kinnersley, P., Edwards, A., Smith, C., Rollnick, S. (2013) 'Training practitioners to deliver opportunistic multiple behaviour change counselling in primary care: a cluster randomised trial', *BMJ*, 346, f1191. doi:10.1136/bmj.f1191

Butler, T., Richters, J., Yap, L. and Donovan, B. (2013) 'Condoms for prisoners: no evidence that they increase sex in prison, but they increase safe sex', *Sexually Transmitted Infections*, doi:10.1136/sextrans-2012-050856

Butterfield, R., Henderson, J. and Scott, R. (2009) *Public Health and Prevention Expenditure in England*, London: Department of Health.

Bynner, J. (2001) 'Childhood risks and protective factors in social exclusion', *Children & Society*, 15: 285–301.

Caiels, J. and Thurston, M. (2005) *Evaluation of the Warrington District CAB GP Outreach Project*, Chester: University of Chester, Centre for Public Health Research.

Caldwell, J. (1986) 'Routes to low mortality in poor countries', *Population and Development Review*, 12(2): 171–220.

Calnan, M. (1987) *Health and Illness: the Lay Perspective*, New York: Tavistock.

Calnan, M. and Williams, S. (1991) 'Style of life and the salience of health: an exploratory study of health related practices in households from differing socio–economic circumstances', *Sociology of Health and Illness*, 13(4): 506–29.

Cameron, E., Mathers, J. and Parry, J. (2008) '"Health and well–being": questioning the use of health concepts in public health policy and practice', *Critical Public Health*, 18(2): 225–32.

Campaner, R. (2011) 'Mechanistic causality and counterfactual-manipulative causality: recent insights from philosophy of science', *Journal of Epidemiology & Community Health*, 65, 1070–4.

Capewell, S. and Graham, H. (2010) 'Will cardiovascular disease prevention widen health inequalities?', *PLoS Medicine*, 7(6): e1000320.

Carlin, H., Morleo, M., Cook., P. and Tocque, K. (2008) *Using Geodemographics to Segment the Market for Hazardous and Harmful Drinkers in Cheshire and Merseyside*, Liverpool: Northwest Public Health Observatory.

Carlisle, S. (2000) 'Health promotion, advocacy and health inequalities: a conceptual framework', *Health Promotion International*, 15(4): 369–76.

Carlisle, S. (2010) 'Tackling health inequalities and social exclusion through partnership and community engagement? A reality check for policy and practice aspirations from a Social Inclusion Partnership in Scotland', *Critical Public Health*, 20(1): 117–27.

Carmona, R. (2006) 'Health literacy: a national priority', *Journal of General Internal Medicine*, 21: 803.

Carr–West, J. (2010) *Community Empowerment: What is it and Where is it Going?*, London: IDeA.

Carstairs, V. (1995) 'Deprivation indices: their interpretation and use in relation to health', *Journal of Epidemiology & Community Health*, 49(Suppl 2): S3–S8.

Carter–Pokras, O. and Baquet, C. (2002) 'What is a "health disparity"?', *Public Health Reports*, 117: 426–34.

Carver, A., Timperio, A. and Crawford, D. (2008) 'Playing it safe: the influence of neighbourhood safety on children's physical activity: a review', *Health & Place*, 14, 217–27.

Cassell, M., Halperin, D., Shelton, J. and Stanton, D. (2006) 'Risk compensation: the Achilles' heel of innovation in HIV prevention', *BMJ*, 332: 605–7.

Cavanagh, S. and Chadwick, K. (2005) *Health Needs Assessment: a Practical Guide*, London: Health Development Agency.

Chambers, D. (2012) *A Sociology of Family Life. Change and Diversity in Intimate Relations*, Cambridge: Polity Press.

Chan, M. (2009) 'Primary care as a route to health security', *The Lancet*, 373: 1586–7.

Chandola, T. and Marmot, M. (2004) 'Social epidemiology', in W. Ahrens, and I. Pigeot (eds) *Handbook of Social Epidemiology* (pp. 893–916), Berlin: Springer.

Chandola, T., Brunner, E. and Marmot, M. (2006) 'Chronic stress at work and the metabolic syndrome: prospective study', *BMJ*. doi:10.1136/bmj.38693.435301.80

Chandy, L. and Gertz, G. (2011) *Poverty in Numbers: the Changing State of Global Poverty from 2005 to 2015*, Washington DC: The Brookings Institution.

Chapman, S. (2001) 'Advocacy in public health: roles and challenges', *International Journal of Epidemiology*, 30: 1226–32.

Chapman, S. (2004) 'Advocacy for public health: a primer', *Journal of Epidemiology & Community Health*, 58: 361–5.

Chatterjee, A. and O'Keefe, C. (2010) 'Current controversies in the USA regarding vaccine safety', *Expert Review of Vaccines*, 9(5): 497–502.

Chatterton, P. and Bradley, D. (2000) 'Bringing Britain together? The limitations of area-based regeneration policies in addressing deprivation', *Local Economy*, 15(2): 98–111.

Cheraghi-Sohi, S. and Calnan, M. (2013) 'Discretion or discretions? Delineating professional discretion: the case of English medical practice', *Social Science and Medicine*, 96: 52–9.

Cheshire, J. (2012) 'Lives on the line: mapping life expectancy along the London Tube network', *Environment & Planning A*, 44: 1525–8.

Childress, J., Faden, R., Gaare, R., Gostin, L., Kahn, J., Bonnie, R., Kass, N., Mastroianni, N., Moreno J. and Nieburg, P. (2002) 'Public health ethics: mapping the terrain', *Journal of Law, Medicine & Ethics*, 30: 170–8.

Chinn, D. (2011) 'Critical health literacy: a review and critical analysis', *Social Science & Medicine*, 73: 60–7.

Christie, B. (2012a) 'People over 65 should be screened for atrial fibrillation, say stroke specialists', *BMJ*, 344: e1644.

Christie, B. (2012b) 'Screening trial of blood test for lung cancer is set to start in Scotland' *BMJ*, 344: e2312.

Christoffel, K. (2000) 'Public health advocacy: process and product', *American Journal of Public Health*, 90(5): 722–6.

Christoffersen, M. (2000) 'Growing up with unemployment. A study of parental unemployment and children's risk of abuse and neglect based on national longitudinal 1973 cohorts in Denmark', *Childhood*, 7(4): 421–38.

Chu, C., Breucker, G., Harris, N., Stitzel, A., Gan, X. and Dwyer, S. (2000) 'Health-promoting workplaces: international settings development', *Health Promotion International*, 15(2): 155–67.

Chung, H. and Muntaner, C. (2007) 'Welfare state matters: a typological multilevel analysis of wealthy countries', *Health Policy*, 80: 328–39.

Coalter, F. (2007a) *A Wider Social Role for Sport: Who's Keeping the Score?*, London: Routledge.

Coalter, F. (2007b) 'Sports clubs, social capital and social regeneration: 'ill–defined' interventions with hard to follow outcomes', *Sport in Society*, 10(4): 537–59.

Coalter, F. (2013) 'Game plan and The Spirit Level: the class ceiling and the limits of sports policy?', *International Journal of Sport Policy and Politics*, 5(1): 3–19.

Cochrane, A. (1972) *Effectiveness and Efficiency. Random Reflections on Health Services*, London: Nuffield Provincial Hospitals Trust.

Cochrane, A. (1984) 'Effectiveness and efficiency', in N. Black, D. Boswell, A. Gray, S. Murphy, and J. Popay (eds) *Health and Disease. A Reader* (pp.115–21), Milton Keynes: Open University Press.

Cockerham, W. (2000) 'Health lifestyles in Russia', *Social Science & Medicine*, 51: 1313–24.

Cockerham, W. (2005) 'Health lifestyle theory and the convergence of agency and structure', *Journal of Health and Social Behaviour*, 46: 51–67.

Cohen, B. and McKay, M. (2010) 'The role of public health agencies in addressing child and family poverty: public health nurses' perspectives', *The Open Nursing Journal*, 4: 60–71.

Coleman, J. (1990). *Foundations of Social Theory*, Cambridge, MA: Harvard University Press.

Collin, J. and Hill, S. (2013) 'Corporate involvement in public health policy is being obscured', *BMJ*, 346: f3429. doi:1136/bmjf3429

Collin, J. and Lee, K. (2007) 'Globalization and public health policy', in A. Scriven and S. Garman (eds) *Public Health: Social Context and Action* (pp. 105–15), Maidenhead: Open University Press/McGraw Hill.

Collins, C., Alagiri, P., Summers, T. and Morin, S. (2002) 'Abstinence only vs. comprehensive sex education. What are the arguments? What is the evidence?', *Policy Monograph Series March 2002*, University of California, AIDS Research Institute.

Colvin, C. (2011) 'Think locally, act globally: developing a critical public health in the global South', *Critical Public Health*, 21(3): 253–6.

Commission on the Social Determinants of Health (2008) *Closing the Gap in a Generation: Health Equity through Action on the Social Determinants of Health*, Geneva: World Health Organization.

Connell, J. and Kubisch, A. (1998) 'Applying a theory of change approach to the evaluation of comprehensive community initiatives: progress, prospects and problems', in K. Fulbright-Anderson, A. Kubisch, L. Schorr and C. Weiss (eds) *New Approaches to Evaluating Community Initiatives: Volume 2, Concepts, Methods and Contexts* (pp. 15–44), Washington DC: Aspen Institute.

Constantine, N. (2012) 'Regression analysis and causal inference: cause for concern?', *Perspectives on Sexual and Reproductive Health*, 44(2): 134–7.

Cook, C., Bridge, J. and Stimson, G. (2010) 'The diffusion of harm reduction in Europe and beyond', in T. Rhodes and D. Hedrich, (eds) *European Monitoring Centre for Drugs and Drug Addiction. Harm Reduction: Evidence, Impacts and Challenges. Monograph Series No 10* (pp. 37–56), Luxembourg: Publications Office of the European Union.

Coovadia, H. and Bland, R. (2008) 'From Alma-Ata to Agincourt: primary health care in Aids', *The Lancet*, 372: 866–8.

Coulter, A. (1987) 'Lifestyles and social care: implications for primary care', *Journal of the Royal College of General Practitioners*, 37: 533–6.

Coulter, A. and Ellins, J. (2007) 'Effectiveness of strategies for informing, educating and involving patients', *BMJ*, 335: 24–7.

Costello, A., Abbas, M., Allen, A. Ball, S., Bell. S., Bellamy, R., Friel, S., Grace, N., Johnson, A., Kett, M., Lee, M., Levy, C., Maslin, M., McCoy, D., McGuire, D., McGuire, B., Montgomery, H., Napier, D., Pagel, C., Patel, J., Antonio, J., de Oliveira, P., Redclift., N., Rees, H., Rogger, D., Scott, J., Stephenson, J., Twigg, J., Wolff, J. and Patterson, C. (2009) 'Managing the health effects of climate change', *The Lancet*, 373: 1693–733.

Cox, B., Blaxter, M., Buckle, A. *et al.* (1987) *The Health and Lifestyle Survey*, London: Health Promotion Research Trust.

Craig, P., Dieppe, P., Macintyre, S., Michie, S., Nazareth, I., Petticrew, M. (2008) 'Developing and evaluating complex interventions: the new Medical Research Council guidance', *BMJ*, 337: 979–83.

Craig, P., Cooper, C., Gunnell, D., Haw, S., Lawson, K., Macintyre, S., Ogilvie, D., Petticrew, M., Reeves, B., Sutton, M. and Thompson, S. (2011) *Using Natural Experiments to Evaluate Population Health Interventions: Guidance for Producers and Users of Evidence*, MRC. Available online at www.mrc.ac.uk/naturalexperimentsguidance (accessed 11 March 2013).

Crawford, R. (1977) 'You are dangerous to your heath: the ideology and politics of victim blaming', *International Journal of Health Services*, 7(4): 663–80.

Crawford, R. (1980) 'Healthism and the medicalization of everyday life', *International Journal of Health Services*, 10(3): 365–88.

Crawford, R. (2006) 'Health as a meaningful social practice', *Health: An Interdisciplinary Journal for the Social Study of Health, Illness and Medicine*, 10(4): 401–20.

Crawshaw, P., Bunton, R. and Gillen, K. (2003) 'Health Action Zones and the problem of community', *Health and Social Care in the Community*, 11(1): 36–44.

Crissman, H., Adanu, R. and Harlow, S. (2012) 'Women's sexual empowerment and contraceptive use in Ghana', *Studies in Family Planning*, 43(3): 201–12.

Cueto, M. (2004) 'The origins of primary health care and selective primary health care', *American Journal of Public Health*, 94(11): 1864–74.

Culyer, A. (1998) 'Need: is a consensus possible?', *Journal of Medical Ethics*, 24: 77–80.

Cummins, S., Curtis, S., Diez-Roux, A. and Macintyre, S. (2007) 'Understanding and representing "place" in health research: a relational approach', *Social Science & Medicine*, 65: 1825–38.

Cumps, E., Verhagen, E., Annemans, L. and Meeusen, R. (2008) 'Injury rate and socioeconomic costs resulting from sports injuries in Flanders: data derived from sports insurance statistics 2003', *British Journal of Sports Medicine*, 42: 467–77.

Cutler, D. and Lleras–Muney, A. (2006) 'Understanding differences in health behaviours by education', *Journal of Health Economics*, 29: 1–28.

Daghofer, D. (2011). *Communicating the Social Determinants of Health: Scoping Paper*. Wellspring Strategies Inc. Available online at http://med.sums.ac.ir/icarusplus/export/ sites/medical_school/departments/clinical_sciences/community-medicine/resourse-page/download/sdh_scoping_paper_-_final_with_ex_summ_-_25april2011.pdf (accessed 20 November 2011).

Dahl, E. and Malmberg-Heimonen, I. (2010) 'Social inequality and health: the role of social capital', *Sociology of Health & Illness*, 32(7): 1102–19.

Dahlgren, G. and Whitehead, M. (1991) *Policies and Strategies to Promote Social Equity in*

Health. Stockholm: Institute for Futures Studies.

Dahlgren, G., Nordgren, P. and Whitehead, M. (eds) (1996) *Health Impact Assessment of the EU Common Agricultural Policy*, Stockholm: Swedish National Institute of Public Health.

Davey Smith, G. and Ebrahim, S. (2001) 'Epidemiology: is it time to call it a day?', *International Journal of Epidemiology*, 30: 1–11.

Davey Smith, G., Shipley, M. and Rose, G. (1990) 'Magnitude and causes of socioeconomic differentials in mortality: further evidence from the Whitehall Study', *Journal of Epidemiology & Community Health*, 44(4): 265–70.

Davidson, R., Kitzinger, J. and Hunt, K. (2006) 'The wealthy get healthy and the poor get poorly? Lay perceptions of health inequalities', *Social Science & Medicine*, 62: 2171–82.

Davies, J. (2009) 'The limits of joined–up government: towards a political analysis', *Public Administration*, 87(1): 80–96.

Davis, A., Hirsch, D., Smith, N., Beckhelling, J. and Padley, M. (2012) *A Minimum Income Standard for the UK in 2012: Keeping Up in Hard Times*, York: Joseph Rowntree Foundation.

Davison, S., Davey Smith, G. and Frankel, S. (1991) 'Lay epidemiology and the prevention paradox: the implications of coronary candidacy for health education', *Sociology of Health & Illness*, 13(1): 1–19.

Dawson, A. and Verweij, M. (2007) *Ethics, Prevention and Public Health*, Oxford: Oxford University Press.

Deaton, A. (2002) 'Policy implications of the gradient of health and wealth', *Health Affairs*, 21(2): 13–30.

DeFilippis, J. (2001) 'The myth of social capital in community development', *Housing Policy Debate*, 12(4): 781–806.

Denscombe, M. and Drucquer, N. (1999) 'Critical incidents and invulnerability to risk: young people's experience of serious health-related incidents and their willingness to take health risks', *Health, Risk & Society*, 1(2): 195–213.

Department for Communities and Local Government (2011) *The English Indices of Deprivation 2010*, London: Department for Communities and Local Government.

Department for Work and Pensions (2012) *Child Poverty in the UK: The report on the 2010 Target*, London: The Stationery Office.

Department of Health (2004) *Choosing Health: Making Healthy Choices Easier*. Cm. 6374, London: Department of Health.

Department of Health (2011) *Health in a Global Context: An Outcomes Framework for Global Health 2011–2015*, London: UK Government.

Department of Health (2013) *Statutory Guidance on Joint Strategic Needs Assessments and Joint Health and Wellbeing Strategies*, London: Department of Health.

Department of Health and Social Security (1980) *Inequalities in Health: The Black Report*, London: HMSO.

Derkzen, P., Franklin, A. and Bock, B. (2008) 'Examining power struggles as a signifier of successful partnership working: a case study of partnership dynamics', *Journal of Rural Studies*, 24: 458–66.

Diamond, J. (2006) 'Au revoir to partnerships: where next?', *International Journal of Public Sector Management*, 19(3): 278–86.

Dickinson, H. and Glasby, J. (2010) 'Why partnership working doesn't work', *Public Management Review*, 12(6): 811–28.

Diderichsen, F., Andersen, I. and Manuel, C., Andersen, A.-M., Bach, E., Baadsgaard, M. Brønnum-Hansen, H., Jeune, B., Jørgensen, T. and Søgaard, J. (2012). Health inequality: determinants and policies', *Scandinavian Journal of Public Health*, 40 (Suppl 8): 12–105.

Ding, Q. and Hesketh, T. (2006) 'Family size, fertility preferences, and sex ratio in China in the era of the one child family policy: results from national family planning and reproductive health survey', *BMJ*, 333: 371–73.

Doll, R. and Hill, A. (1950) 'Smoking and carcinoma of the lung', *BMJ*, 2(4682): 769–82.

Doll, R. and Hill, A. (1954) 'The mortality of doctors in relation to their smoking habits', *BMJ*, 1(4877): 1451–5.

Doll, R. and Hill, A. (1964) 'Mortality in relation to smoking: ten years' observations of British doctors', *BMJ*, 1(5396): 1399–410.

Donaldson, C. and Mooney, G. (1991) 'Needs assessment, priority setting and contracts for health care: an economic view', *BMJ*, 303: 1529–30.

Dooris, M. (2005) 'Healthy settings: challenges to generating evidence of effectiveness', *Health Promotion International*, 21(1): 55–65.

Dooris, M. and Hunter, D. (2007) 'Organisations and settings for promoting public health', in C. Lloyd, S. Handsley, J. Douglas, S. Earle and S. Spurr (eds) *Policy and Practice in Promoting Public Health* (pp. 95–125), London: Sage Publications.

Dopson, S. (2005) 'The diffusion of medical innovations: can figurational sociology help?', *Organization Studies*, 26(8): 1125–44.

Dopson, S. (2006) 'Debate: why does knowledge stick? What we can learn from the case of evidence–based health care', *Public Money and Management*, 26(2): 85–6.

Dopson, S. and Waddington, I. (1996) 'Managing social change: a process–sociological approach to understanding organisational change within the National Health Service', *Sociology of Health & Illness*, 18: 525–50.

Dorfman, L., Wallack, L. and Woodruff, K. (2005) 'More than a message: framing public health advocacy to change corporate practices', *Health Education & Behavior*, 32(3): 320–36.

Dorling, D. (2010) 'Using the concept of "place" to understand and reduce health inequalities', in F. Campbell (ed.) *The social Determinants of Health and the Role of Local Government* (pp. 16–25), London: IDeA.

Dorling, D. (2012) 'Editorial – inequality and injustice: some news from Britain', *Urban Geography*, 33(5): 621–9.

Dorling, D., Rigby, J., Wheeler, B., Ballas, D., Thomas, B., Fahmy, E., Gordon, D. and Lupton, R. (2007) *Poverty, Wealth and Place in Britain 1968–2005*, Bristol: Policy Press.

Dowling, B., Powell, M. and Glendinning, C. (2004) 'Conceptualising successful partnerships', *Health and Social Care in the Community*, 12(4): 309–17.

Doyal, L. and Gough, I. (1991) *A Theory of Human Need*, Basingstoke: Macmillan.

Draper, R. (1988) 'Healthy public policy: a new political challenge', *Health Promotion International*, 2(3): 217–18.

Due, P., Krølner, R., Rasmussen, M., Andersen, A., Damsgaard, M., Graham, H. and Holstein, B. (2011) 'Pathways and mechanisms in adolescence contribute to adult health inequalities', *Scandinavian Journal of Public Health*, 39(Suppl 6): 62–78.

Duffy, B., Hall, S., Pope, S. and O'Leary, D. (2013) *Generation Strains. A Demos and Ipsos MORI Report on Changing Attitudes to the Welfare State*, London: Demos.

Dunne, A., Scriven, A. and Furlong, C. (2012) 'Funding linked to evidence: what future for health promotion?', *Perspectives in Public Health*, 132: 109–10.

Durkheim, E. (1897, 1970) *Suicide: a Study in Sociology*, London: Routledge.

Eadie, D., MacAskill, S., Brooks, O., Heim, D., Forsyth, A. and Punch, S. (2010) *Pre–teens Learning About Alcohol: Drinking and Family Contexts*, York: Joseph Rowntree Foundation.

Eikemo, T., Bambra, C., Judge, K. and Ringdal, K. (2008) 'Welfare state regimes and differences in self–perceived health in Europe: a multi–level analysis', *Social Science & Medicine*, 66, 2281–95.

Elias, N. (1991) *The Society of Individuals*, New York: Continuum.

Elliott, L., Nerney, M., Jones, T. and Friedmann, P. (2002) 'Barriers to screening for domestic violence', *Journal of General Internal Medicine*, 17: 112–16.

Elton, L. (2004) 'Goodhart's Law and performance indicators in higher education', *Evaluation & Research in Education*, 18: 120–8.

Eriksen, M., Mackay, J. and Ross, H. (2012) *The Tobacco Atlas*, 4th edn, Atlanta: American Cancer Society.

Eriksson, M. and Lindstrom, B. (2008) 'A salutogenic interpretation of the *Ottawa Charter*', *Health Promotion International*, 23(2): 190–9.

Esping-Andersen, G. (1990) *The Three Worlds of Welfare Capitalism*, London: Polity Press.

Experian Marketing Services (2014) Mosaic. The consumer classification solution for consistent cross-channel marketing, Experian Ltd. Available online at http://experian.co.uk/marketing-services/products/mosaic/mosaic-in-detail.html (accessed 23 May 2014).

Evans, D. (2003) '"Taking public health out of the ghetto": the policy and practice of multi-disciplinary public health in the United Kingdom', *Social Science & Medicine*, 57: 959–67.

Evans, D. and Knight, T. (eds) (2006) "There was no plan!" The origins and development of multidisciplinary public health in the UK. Report of the witness seminar held at the University of the West of England, Bristol on 7 November 2005, Bristol: University of the West of England. Available online at http: //hsc.uwe.ac.uk/hsc/index.asp?pageid=843 (accessed 28 March 2013).

Evans, W. and McCormack, L. (2008) 'Applying social marketing in health care: communicating evidence to change consumer behaviour', *Medical Decision Making*, 28: 781–92.

Ewles, L. (1996) 'The impact of the NHS reforms on specialist health promotion in the NHS', in A. Scriven and J. Orme (eds) *Health Promotion: Professional Perspectives* (pp. 66–74), Basingstoke: Macmillan Press Ltd.

Exworthy, M. (2011) 'The illness narratives of health managers: developing an analytical framework', *Evidence and Policy: A Journal of Research, Debate and Practice*, 793: 345–58.

Exworthy, M., Blane, D. and Marmot, M. (2003) 'Tackling health inequalities in the United Kingdom: the progress and pitfalls of policy', *Health Services Research*, 38(6): 1905–19.

Faden, R. and Shebaya, S. (2010) 'Public health ethics', in Edwards N. Zalta (ed.) *The Stanford Encyclopedia of Philosophy* (Summer 2010 Edition). Available online at http://plato.stanford.edu/archives/sum2010/entries/publichealth–ethics/ (accessed 18 March 2013).

Fehr, R., Hurley, F., Mekel, O. and Mackenbach, J. (2012) 'Quantitative health impact assessment: taking stock and moving forward', *Journal of Epidemiology & Community Health*, 66(12): 1088–91.

Fenner, F. (1982) 'A successful eradication campaign. Global eradication of smallpox', *Reviews of Infectious Diseases*, 40(5): 916–30.

Ferguson, J., Bauld, L., Chesterman, J. and Judge, K. (2005) 'The English smoking treatment services: one–year outcomes', *Addiction*, 100(Suppl.2): 59–69.

Finch, C. and Cassell, E. (2006) 'The public health impact of injury during sport and active recreation', *Journal of Science and Medicine in Sport*, 9: 490–7.

Fishbein, M. and Ajzen, I. (1975) *Belief, Attitude, Intention and Behaviour: an Introduction to Theory and Research*, Reading, MA: Addison-Wesley.

Fitzpatrick, M. (2004) 'MMR: risk, choice, chance', *British Medical Bulletin*, 69: 143–53.

Fletcher, A. (2013) 'Working towards "health in all policies" at a national level', *BMJ*, 346: f1096.

Font, J., Hernández-Quevedo, C. and McGuire, A. (2011) 'Persistence despite action? Measuring the patterns of health inequality in England (1997–2007)', *Health Policy*, 103: 149–59.

Foot, C. and Harrison, T. (2011) *How to Improve Cancer Survival: Explaining England's Relatively Poor Rates*, London: The King's Fund.

Foot, J. and Hopkins, T. (2010) *A Glass Half Full: How an Asset Approach can Improve Community Health and Wellbeing*, London: IDeA.

Foreman, A. (1996) 'Health needs assessment', in J. Percy–Smith (ed.) *Needs Assessment in Public Policy* (pp. 66–81), Buckingham: Open University Press.

Formby, E. and Wolstenholme, C. (2012) '"If there's going to be a subject that you don't have to do …" Findings from a mapping study of PSHE education in English secondary schools', *Pastoral Care in Education*, 30(1): 5–18.

Fornara, F., Carrus, G., Passafaro, P. and Bonnes, M. (2011) 'Distinguishing the sources of normative influence on pro-environmental behaviours: the role of local norms in household waste recycling', *Group Processes and Intergroup Relations*, 15(5), 623–35.

Forrest, R. and Kearns, A. (2001) 'Social cohesion, social capital and the neighbourhood', *Urban Studies*, 38(12): 2125–43.

Fosse, E. (2009) 'Norwegian public health policy: revitalization of the social democratic welfare state?', *International Journal of Health Services*, 39(7): 287–300.

Foxton, F. and Jones, R. (2011) *Social Capital Indicators Review*, London: Office for National Statistics.

Frankel, S. (2001) 'Commentary – Medical care and the wider influences upon population health: a false dichotomy', *International Journal of Epidemiology*, 30: 1267–8.

Fraser, A., Gatherer, A. and Hayton, P. (2009) 'Mental health in prisons: great difficulties but are there opportunities?', *Public Health*, 123: 410–14.

Fraser, D. (2009) *The Evolution of the British Welfare State: A History of Social Policy since the Industrial Revolution*, Basingstoke: Palgrave Macmillan.

Freebody, P. and Luke, A. (1990) '"Literacies" programs: debates and demands in cultural context', *Prospect*, 5: 7–16.

Freire, P. (1972) *Pedagogy of the Oppressed*, Harmondsworth: Penguin.

French, J. (2009) 'The nature, development and contribution of social marketing to public health practice since 2004 in England', *Perspectives in Public Health*, 129: 262–7.

French, J. and Adams, L. (1986) 'From analysis to synthesis: theories of health education', *Health Education Journal*, 45(2): 71–74.

French, J. and Blair–Stevens, C. (2006) *Social Marketing Pocket Guide*, London: National Consumer Council.

Frenk, J. (2009) 'Reinventing primary health care: the need for systems integration', *The Lancet*, 373: 170–3.

Freudenberg, N. (2005) 'Public health advocacy to change corporate practices: implications for health education practice and research', *Health Education & Behaviour*, 32(3): 298–319.

Fried, L., Bentley, M., Buekens, P., Burke, D., Frenk, J. and Klag, M. (2010) 'Global health is public health', *The Lancet*, 375: 535–7.

Friedli, L. (2013) '"What we've tried hasn't worked": The politics of assets based public health', *Critical Public Health*. 23(2): 131–145.

Friel, S., Dangour, A., Garnett, T., Lock, K., Chalabi, Z., Roberts, I., Butler, A., Butler, C., Waage, J., McMichael, A. and Haines, A. (2009) 'Public health benefits of strategies to reduce greenhouse-gas emissions: food and agriculture', *The Lancet*, 374: 2016–25.

Frumkin, H. (2003) 'Healthy places: exploring the evidence', *American Journal of Public Health*, 93(9): 1451–6.

Gabe, J., Bury, M. and Elson, M. (2004) *Key Concepts in Medical Sociology*, London: Sage Publications.

Getz, L., Sigurdsson, J. and Hetlevik, I. (2003) 'Is opportunistic disease prevention in the consultation ethically justifiable?' *BMJ*, 327: 498–500.

Giddens, A. (2008) *The Politics of Climate Change: National Responses to the Challenge of Global Warming*, London: Policy Network Paper.

Gidley, B. (2007) 'Sure Start: an upstream approach to reducing health inequalities', in A. Scriven and S. Garman (eds) *Public Health: Social Context and Action* (pp. 144–53), Maidenhead: Open University Press.

Gilbert, R., Widom, C., Browne, K., Fergusson, D., Webb, E. and Janson, S. (2008) 'Burden and consequences of child maltreatment in high-income countries', *The Lancet*. doi:10.1016/S0140-6736(08)61706-7

Gilman, S. (2012) 'The successes and challenges of life course epidemiology: a commentary on Gibb, Fergusson and Horwood', *Social Science & Medicine*, 75: 2124–8.

Ginn, S. (2013) 'Promoting health in prison', *BMJ*, 346: f2215. doi:10.1136/bmj.f2216

Glass, N. (2006) 'Sure Start: where did it come from; where is it going?', *Journal of Children's Services*, 1(1): 51–7.

Global Health Strategies Initiatives (2012) 'Shifting paradigm. How the BRICs are reshaping global health and development'. Available online at www.ghsinitiatives.org/downloads/ghsi_brics_report.pdf (accessed 9 December 2012).

Goldman, D. and Smith, J. (2011) 'The increasing value of education to health', *Social Science & Medicine*, 72: 1728–37.

Goldthorpe, J. (2010) 'Analysing social inequality: a critique of two recent contributions from economics and epidemiology', *European Sociological Review*, 26(6): 731–44.

Gomm, M., Lincoln, P., Pikora, T. and Giles-Corti, B. (2006) 'Planning and implementing a community-based public health advocacy campaign: a transport case study from Australia', *Health Promotion International*, 21(4): 284–92.

Goodwin, P. (2008) *Policy Incentives to Change Behaviour in Passenger Transport*, Centre for Transport & Society, University of the West of England, Bristol. OECD International Transport Forum, Leipzig, May 2008 Transport and Energy: The challenge of climate change. Available online at www.internationaltransportforum.org/topics/workshops/ws2goodwin.pdf (accessed 25 November 2011).

Gordon, D. (2010) 'Determinants of health equity in developing nations', *Social Alternatives*, 29(2): 28–32.

Gordon, R., McDermott, L., Stead, M. and Angus, K. (2006) 'The effectiveness of social marketing interventions: what's the evidence?', *Journal of Public Health*, 120: 1133–9.

Gostin, L. and Mok, E. (2009) 'Grand challenges in global health governance', *British Medical Bulletin*, 90: 90–118.

Gostin, L., Freidman, E., Ooms, G., Gebauer, T., Gupta, N., Sridhar, D., Chenguang, w., Røttingen, J.-A. and Sanders, D. (2011) 'The joint action and learning initiative: towards a global agreement on national and global responsibilities for health', *Plos Medicine*, 8(5): e1001031. doi:10.1371/journal.pmed.10001031

Gough, I. (2003) *Lists and Thresholds: Comparing our Theory of Human Need with Nussbaum's Capabilities Approach*, WeD Working Paper 01, The Wellbeing of Developing Countries Research Group, University of Bath. Available online at http://eprints.lse.ac.uk/36659 (accessed 6 July 2013).

Graham, H. (1989) 'Women and smoking in the United Kingdom: the implications for health promotion', *Health Promotion*, 3(4): 371–82.

Graham, H. (2002) 'Building an inter-disciplinary science of health inequalities: the example of lifecourse research', *Social Science & Medicine*, 55: 2005–16.

Graham, H. (2004) 'Social determinants and their unequal distribution: clarifying policy understandings', *Millbank Quarterly*, 82(1): 101–24.

Graham, H. (2007) *Unequal Lives: Health and Socioeconomic Inequalities*, Maidenhead: Open University Press/McGraw Hill.

Graham, H. and Kelly, M. (2004) *Health Inequalities: Concepts, Frameworks and Policy*, London: Health Development Agency.

Graham, H. and Power, C. (2004) 'Childhood disadvantage and health inequalities: a framework for policy based on lifecourse research', *Child: Care, Health & Development*, 30(6): 671–8.

Graham, H., Hawkins, S. and Law, C. (2010) 'Lifecourse influences on women's smoking before, during and after pregnancy', *Social Science & Medicine*, 70: 582–7.

Graham, H., Inskip, H., Francis, B. and Harman, J. (2006) 'Pathways of disadvantage and smoking careers: evidence and policy implications', *Journal of Epidemiology & Community Health*, 60(Suppl II): ii7–ii12.

Green, J. (2008) 'Health education: the case for rehabilitation', *Critical Public Health*, 18(4): 447–56.

Green, J. and South, J. (2006) *Evaluation*, Milton Keynes: Open University Press.

Green, J. and Tones, K. (2010) *Health Promotion: Planning and Strategies*, London: Sage Publications Ltd.

Green, K. (2010) *Key Themes in Youth Sport*, Oxon: Routledge.

Green, L., Poland, B. and Rootman, I. (eds) (2000) *Settings for Health Promotion: Linking Theory and Practice*, Thousand Oaks, CA: Sage.

Greene, M., Joshi, S. and Robles, O. (2012) *By Choice not by Chance: Family Planning, Human Rights and Development*, New York: United Nations Population Fund.

Greenhalgh, T. (2010) *How to Read a Paper. The Basics of Evidence-Based Medicine*, 4th edn, Chichester: John Wiley and Sons.

Greenhalgh, T. and Wessley, S. (2004) '"Health for me": a sociocultural analysis of healthism in the middle classes', *BMJ*, 69: 197–213.

Griffiths, J., Blair–Stevens, C. and Parish, R. (2009) 'The integration of health promotion and social marketing', *Perspectives in Public Health*, 129: 268–71.

Grifo, F., Halpern, M. and Hansel, P. (2012) *Heads They Win, Tails we Lose. How Corporations Corrupt Science at the Public's Expense*, Cambridge, MA: UCS. Available online at www.ucsusa.org/scientific_integrity (accessed 11 March 2012).

Grøholt, E., Dahl, E. and Elstad, J. (2007) 'Health inequalities and the welfare state', *Norsk Epidemiologi*, 17(1): 3–8.

Grol, R. and Wensing, M. (2004) 'What drives change? Barriers to and incentives for achieving evidence-based practice', *The Medical Journal of Australia*, 180: S57–S60.

Grun, L. and McKeigue, P. (2000) 'Prevalence of excessive gambling before and after introduction of a national lottery in the United Kingdom: another example of the single distribution theory', *Addiction*, 95(6): 959–66.

Hacking, J., Muller, S. and Buchan, I. (2011) 'Trends in mortality from 1965 to 2008 across the north–south divide: comparative observational study', *BMJ*, 342: d508. doi:10.1136/bmjd508

Haines, A. and Patz, J. (2004) 'Health effects of climate change', *Journal of the American Medical Association*, 291(4): 99–103.

Hale, D., Coleman, J. and Layard, R. (2011) *A Model for the Delivery of Evidence–Based PSHE (Personal Wellbeing) in Secondary Schools*, Discussion Paper No 1071, London: Centre for Economic Performance, London School of Economics/Economic & Social Research Council.

Hall, J. and Taylor, R. (2003) 'Health for all beyond 2000: the demise of the *Alma-Ata Declaration* and primary health care in developing countries', *Medical Journal of Australia*, 178: 17–20.

Hallin, D., Brandt, M. and Briggs, C. (2013) 'Biomedicalization and the public sphere: newspaper coverage of health and medicine, 1960–2000s', *Social Science and Medicine*, 96: 121–8.

Ham, C. (2004) *Health Policy in Britain. The Politics and Organisation of the National Health Service*, New York: Palgrave Macmillan.

Ham, M., Hedman, L., Manley, D. and Coulter, R. (2012) *Intergenerational Transmission of Neighbourhood Poverty in Sweden: an Innovative Analysis of Individual Neighbourhood Histories*, Discussion Paper No 6572, Bonn, Germany: IZA.

Hansen, E. and Easthope, G. (2007) *Lifestyle in Medicine*, Oxford: Routledge.

Hansson, S. (2010) 'Risk: objective or subjective, facts or values', *Journal of Risk Research*, 13(2): 231–8.

Hart, J. T. (1971) 'The inverse care law', *The Lancet*, 1: 405–12.

Hart, J. T. (1981) 'A new kind of doctor', *Journal of the Royal Society of Medicine*, 74: 871–83.

De Hartog, J., Boogaard, H., Nijland, H. and Hoek, G. (2010) 'Do the health benefits of cycling outweigh the risks?', *Environmental Health Perspectives*, 118(8): 1109–16.

Harvey, F. (2012) 'UK makes biggest emissions cuts in Europe', *The Guardian*, 24 October. Available online at www.guardian.co.uk/environment/2012/act/24/uk–eu–carbon–emission–cuts (accessed 24 October 2012).

Hawe, P. and Shiell, A. (2000) 'Social capital and health promotion: a review', *Social Science & Medicine*, 51: 871–85.

Hawton, K. (2002) 'United Kingdom legislation on pack size of analgesics. Background, rationale, and effects on suicide and deliberate self–harm', *Suicide and Life-Threatening Behaviour*, 32(3): 223–9.

Hayes, S., Mann, M., Morgan, F., Kelly, M. and Weightman, A. (2012) 'Collaboration between local health and local government agencies for health improvement', *The Cochrane Database of Systematic Reviews*, Issue 10. Art. No.: CD007825. doi:10.1002/14651858.CD007825.pub6

Head, A. (1979) 'Community development in post–industrial society', in D. Chekki (ed.) *Community Development* (pp. 101–15), New Delhi, India: Vikas Publishing House.

Health Promotion (1986) 'A discussion document on the concept and principles of health promotion', *Health Promotion*, 1(1): 73–6.

Healy, T. and Côté, S. (2001) *The Well-Being of Nations: The Role of Human and Social Capital*, Paris: Centre for Educational research & Innovation, Organisation for Economic Co-operation and Development. Available online at www.oecd.org/edu/innovation-education/1870573.pdf (accessed 22 May 2013).

Henderson, M., Wright, D., Raab, G., Abraham, C., Parkes, A., Scott, S. and Hart, G.(2006) 'Impact of a theoretically based sex education programme (SHARE) delivered by teachers on NHS registered conceptions and terminations: final results of cluster randomised trial', *BMJ*, 3334(7585). doi:10.1136/bmj.39014.503692.55

Hertzman, C., Siddiqi, A., Hertzman, E., Irwin, E., Vaghri, L., Houweling, Z., Tanja, A., Bell, R., Alfredo, T. and Marmot, M. (2010) 'Tackling inequality: get them while they're young', *BMJ*, 340: 346–8.

Herzlich, C. (1973) *Health and Illness: A Social Psychological Analysis*, London: Academic Press.

Heuveline, P. and Weinshenker, M. (2008) 'The international child poverty gap: does demography matter?', *Demography*, 46(1): 173–91.

Hill, A. (1965) 'The environment and disease: association or causation?', *Proceedings of the Royal Society of Medicine*, 58: 295–300.

Hinote, B., Cockerham, W. and Abbott, P. (2009) 'The spectre of post communism: women and alcohol in eight post-Soviet states', *Social Science & Medicine*, 68: 1254–62.

HLS-EU Consortium. (2012) *Comparative Report of Health Literacy in Eight Members States*. The European Health Literacy Survey HLS-EU Online Publication. www.health–literacy.eu

Hollmeyer, H., Hayden, F., Poland, G. and Buchholz, U. (2009) 'Influenza vaccination of health care workers in hospitals: a review of studies on attitudes and predictors', *Vaccine*, 27: 3935–44.

Holmes, J. and Kiernan, K. (2013) 'Persistent poverty and children's development in the early years of childhood', *Policy and Politics*, 41(1): 19–42.

Holt, T. (2008) 'Official statistics, public policy and public trust', *Journal of the Royal Statistical Society*, A, 171, Part 2: 323–46.

Hood, C. (2006) 'Gaming in targetworld: the targets approach to managing British public services', *Public Administration Review*, 66(4): 515–21.

Hopewell, S., McDonald, S., Clarke, M. and Egger, M. (2008) 'Grey literature in meta-analyses of randomized trials of health care interventions', *Cochrane Database of Systematic Reviews 2007*, Issue 2. Art. No.: MR000010. doi:10.1002/14651858.MR000010.pub3

Hopwood, T. and Merritt, R. (2011) *Big Pocket Guide to Using Social Marketing for Behaviour Change*. Available online at www.thensmc.com/sites/default/files/Big_Pocket_guide_2011.pdf (accessed 20 October 2012).

Horton, T. and Gregory, J. (2010) 'Whose middle is it anyway? Why universal welfare matters', *Public Policy Research*, December 2009–February 2010: 218–25.

House of Commons Public Administration Select Committee (2013) *Public Trust in Government Statistics. A Review of the Operation of the Statistics and Registration Service Act 2007*, London: The Stationery Office Limited.

House of Lords Science and Technology Select Committee (2011) *Behaviour Change*, London: The Stationery Office Limited.

Huber, M., Knottnerus, J., Green, L., van der Horst, H., Jadad, A., Kromhout, D., Leonard, B., Lorig, K., Loureiro, L., van der Meer, J., Schnabel, P., Smith, R., van Weel, C. Smid, H. (2011) 'How should we define health?', *BMJ*, 343: 234–7.

Hughner, R. and Kleine, S. (2004) 'Views of health in the lay sector: a compilation and review of how individuals think about health', *Health*, 8: 395–422.

Huijts, T., Eikemo, T. A. and Skalická, V. (2010) 'Income–related health inequalities in the Nordic countries: examining the role of education, occupational class and age', *Social Science & Medicine*, 71: 1964–72.

Humphreys, K. and Piot, P. (2012) 'Scientific evidence alone is not sufficient basis for health policy', *BMJ*, 344: e1316. doi:10.1136/bmj.e1316

Hunter, D. (2010) 'What makes people healthy and what makes them ill?', in F. Campbell (ed.) *The Social Determinants of Health and the Role of Local Government* (pp. 11–15), London: IDeA.

Hunter, D. and Perkins, N. (2012) 'Partnership working in public health: the implications for governance of a systems approach', *Journal of Health Services Research & Policy*, 17(Suppl 2): 45–52.

Hunter, D., Marks, L. and Smith, K. (2010) *The Public Health System in England*, Bristol: The Policy Press.

Husain, M. (2010) 'Contribution of health to economic development: a survey and overview', Economics, 4(2010–14). Available online at http://dx.doi.org/10.5018/economics-ejournal. ja.2010–14 (accessed 27 February 2012).

Illich, I. (1975) 'The medicalization of life', *Journal of Medical Ethics*, 1: 73–7.

Institute of Medicine. (2004) *Health Literacy: A Prescription to End Confusion*, Washington DC: National Academies Press.

Intergovernmental Panel on Climate Change (2007) *Fourth Assessment Report*, New York: Cambridge University Press.

Intergovernmental Panel on Climate Change (2012) *Managing the Risks of Extreme Weather Events and Disasters to Advance Climate Change Adaptation: Summary for Policy Makers*, Cambridge: Cambridge University Press.

Intergovernmental Panel on Climate Change (2013) Human Influence on Climate Clear, IPCC Report Says. Press release, 27 September. www.ipcc.ch/news_and_events/docs/ar5_wgi_en.pdf

Ipsos-Mori (2013) 'In an age of big data and focus on economic issues, trust in the use of statistics remains low'. Available online at www.ipsos-mori.com/researchpublications/ researcharcive/3175/in-an-age-of-big-data-and-focus-on-economic-issues-trust-in-the-use-of-statistics-remains-low.aspx (accessed 14 July 2013).

Iwase, T., Suzuki, E., Fujiwara, T., Takao, S., Doi, H. and Kawachi, I. (2012) 'Do bonding and bridging social capital have differential effects on self–rated health? A community based study in Japan', *Journal of Epidemiology & Community Health*, 66: 557–62.

Jama, D. and Dugdale, G. (2012) *Literacy: State of the Nation: A Picture of Literacy in the UK Today*, London: National Literacy Trust. Available online at www.literacytrust.org.uk/ assets/0001/2847/Literacy_State_of_the_Nation_-_2_Aug_2011.pdf (accessed 1 June 2013).

Janssen, I. and LeBlanc, A. (2010) 'Systematic review of the health benefits of physical activity and fitness in school-aged children and youth', *International Journal of Behavioural Nutrition and Physical Activity*, 7: 40.

Jepson, R., Hewison, J., Thompson, A. and Weller, D. (2007). 'Patient perspectives on information and choice in cancer screening: a qualitative study in the UK', *Social Science & Medicine*, 65: 890–9.

Johnson, A., Goss, A., Beckerman, J. and Castro, A. (2012) 'Hidden costs: the direct and indirect impact of user fees on access to malaria treatment and primary care in Mali', *Social Science & Medicine*, 75: 1786–92.

Jolly, R., Emmerij, L. and Weiss, T. (2009) 'The UN and human development', *Briefing Note Number 8*, 1–6. Available online at www.UNhistory.org (accessed 21 September 2013).

Joyce, J. (2004) 'Williamson on evidence and knowledge', *Analytic Philosophy*, 45(4): 296–305.

Judge, K., Mulligan, J. and Benzeval,M. (2001) 'Income inequality and population health', *Social Science & Medicine*, 46: 567–79.

Kandpal, E., Baylis, K. and Arends-Kuenning, M. (2012) *Empowering Women Through Education and Influence: An Evaluation of the Indian Mahila Samakhya Program*, Discussion Paper No 6347. Bonn, Germany: IZA.

Kaner, E. and McGovern, R. (2013) 'Training practitioners in primary care to deliver lifestyle advice', *BMJ*, 346: f1763.

Kaplan, G. (2004) 'What's wrong with social epidemiology, and how can we make it better?' *Epidemiological Review*, 26: 124–35.

Katikireddi, S., Higgins, M., Bond, L., Bonell, C. and Macintyre S. (2011) 'How evidence based is English public health policy?', *BMJ*, 343. doi:10.1136/bmj.d7310

Kawachi, I., Daniels, N. and Robinson, E. (2005) 'Health disparities by race and class: why both matter', *Health Affairs*, 24: 343–352.

Kawachi, I., Kennedy, B., Lochner, K. and Prothrow-Stith, D. (1997) 'Social capital, income inequality, and mortality', *American Journal of Public Health*, 87: 1491–8.

Kawachi, I., Subramanian, S. and Almeida–Filho, N. (2002) 'A glossary for health inequalities', *Journal of Epidemiology & Community Health*, 56: 647–52.

Kay, T. and Spaaij, R. (2012) 'The mediating effects of family on sport in international development contexts', *International Review for the Sociology of Sport*, 47(1): 77–94.

Kearney, M., Bradbury, C., Ellahi, B., Hodgson, M. and Thurston, M. (2005) 'Mainstreaming prevention: prescribing fruit and vegetables as a brief intervention in primary care', *Public Health*, 19: 981–86.

Kearns, R. and Moon, G. (2002) 'From medical to health geography: novelty, place and theory after a decade of change', *Progress in Human Geography*, 26(5): 605–25.

Keen, E. (2012) 'Health and human rights in the UK', *Health Equalities: Trends and Innovations in Health and Social Care*, 1: 21–22. Available online at http://issue.com/thebha/docs/healthe-qualities1 (accessed 21 February 2012).

Kelly, M. (2012) 'Public health at National Institute for Health and Clinical Excellence from 2012', *Perspectives in Public Health*, 132(3): 111–13.

Kelly, M. and Moore, T. (2012) 'The judgement process in evidence-based medicine and health technology assessment', *Social Theory & Health*, 10(1): 1–9.

Kelly, M., Morgan, A., Ellis, S., Younger, T., Huntley, J. and Swann, C. (2010) 'Evidence-based public health: a review of the experience of the National Institute of Health and Clinical Excellence (NICE) of developing public health guidance in England', *Social Science & Medicine*, 71: 1056–62.

Kendall, G. and Li, J. (2005) 'Early socialization and social gradients in adult health: a commentary on Singh Manoux and Marmot's "Role of socialization in explaining social inequalities in health"', *Social Science & Medicine*, 61: 2272–76.

Kepp, M. (2008) 'Cracks appear in Brazil's primary health-care programme', *The Lancet*, 372: 877.

Kerrison, S. and Macfarlance, A. (eds) (2000) *Official Health Statistics. An Unofficial Guide*, London: Arnold.

Kibirige, J. (1997) 'Population growth, poverty and health', *Social Science & Medicine*, 45(2): 247–59.

Kickbusch, I. (1986) 'Introduction to the journal', *Health Promotion International*, 1(1): 3–4.

Kickbusch, I. (2003) 'The contribution of the WHO to a new public health and health promotion', *American Journal of Public Health*, 93(3): 383–8.

Kickbusch, I. (2007) 'The move towards a new public health', *Promotion & Education*, 14(6): 9.

Kickbusch, I. (2013) 'Health in all policies', *BMJ*, 347: f4283. doi:19.1136/bmjf4283

Kickbusch, I. and Maag, D. (2008) 'Health literacy', in K. Heggenhougen and S. Quah, (eds) *International Encyclopedia of Public Health, Vol. 3* (pp. 204–211), San Diego: Academic Press.

Kickbusch, I. and Seck, B. (2007) 'Global public health', in J. Douglas, S. Earle, S. Handsley, C. Lloyd, and S. Spurr (eds) *A Reader in Promoting Public Health. Challenge and Controversy* (pp. 159–168), Milton Keynes: Open University Press.

Kickbusch, I., Silberschmidt, G. and Buss, P. (2007) 'Global health diplomacy: the need for new perspectives, strategic approaches and skills in global health', *Bulletin of the World Health Organization*, 85(3): 230–2.

Kiernan, K. (1995) 'Social backgrounds and post–birth experiences of young parents. Summary', *Social Policy Research*, 80, York: Joseph Rowntree Foundation.

Killoran, A. (2010) 'A synopsis: effectiveness and efficiency in public health', in A. Killoran and M. Kelly (eds), *Evidence-Based Public Health. Effectiveness and Efficiency* (pp. 459–474), Oxford: Oxford University Press.

Kingdon, J. (1984) *Agendas, Alternatives and Public Policies*, Boston: Little Brown & Co.

Kirby, T. (2012) 'Farmers outcry at plans to reduce land for tobacco farming', *The Lancet*, 380: 1575–82.

Kleinman, A. and Mendelsohn, E. (1978) 'Systems of medical knowledge: a comparative approach', *The Journal of Medicine and Philosophy*, 3(4): 314–30.

Klepp, K-I. (2010). *Health Promotion: Achieving Good Health for All*, Oslo: Helsedirektoratet.

Klugman, J. (2011). *Human Development Report 2011. Sustainability and Equity: a Better Future for All*, Basingstoke: Palgrave Macmillan.

Knox, K., Conwell, Y. and Caine, E. (2004) 'If suicide is a public health problem, what are we doing to prevent it?', *American Journal of Public Health*, 94: 37–45.

Kohler, P., Manhart, L. and Lafferty, W. (2008) 'Abstinence only and comprehensive sex education and the initiation of sexual activity and teen pregnancy', *Journal of Adolescent Health*, 42: 344–51.

Kondo, N., Kawachi, I., Subramanian, S., Takeda, Y. and Yamagata, Z. (2008) 'Do social comparisons explain the association between income inequality and health? Relative deprivation and perceived health among male and female Japanese individuals', *Social Science & Medicine*, 67: 982–7.

Koplan, J., Bond, C., Merson, M., Merson, M., Reddy, K., Rodriguez, M., Sewankambo, N. and Wasserheit, J. (2009) 'Towards a common definition of global health', *The Lancet*, 373: 1993–5.

Korjonen, H. and Ford, J. (2013) *Grey Literature in Public Health: Valuable Evidence?* London: UK Health Forum. Available online at http://nhfshare.heartforum.org.uk/RMAssets/NHFreports/Grey_literature.pdf (accessed 11 May 2013).

Kotler, P. and Zaltman, G. (1971) 'Social marketing: an approach to planned social change', *Journal of Marketing*, 35: 3–12.

Kretzmann, J. and McKnight, J. (1993) *Building Communities from the Inside Out: a Path Towards Finding and Mobilising a Community's Assets*, Chicago: ACTA Pubs.

Kretzmann, J., McKnight, J., Dobrowolski S., and Puntenney, D. (2005) *Discovering*

Community Power: A guide to Mobilizing Local Assets and your Organization's Capacity, Illinois: ABCD Institute.

Krieger, N. (1999) 'Sticky webs, hungry spiders, buzzing flies, and fractal metaphors: on the misleading juxtaposition of "risk factor" versus "social" epidemiology', *Journal of Epidemiology & Community Health*, 53: 678–80.

Krieger, N. (2001) 'A glossary for social epidemiology', *Journal of Epidemiology & Community Health*, 55: 693–700.

Krieger, N. (2003) 'Place, space and health: GIS and epidemiology', *Epidemiology*, 14(4): 384–5.

Krieger, N. (2008) 'Proximal, distal, and the politics of causation: what's level got to do with it?', *American Journal of Public Health*, 98(2): 221–30.

Kromm, J., Frattaroli, S., Vernick, J. and Teret, S. (2009) 'Public health advocacy in the courts: opportunities for public health professionals', *Public Health Reports*, 124(6): 889–94.

Krugman, P. (2013) 'Zombie economics', Global edition of *The New York Times*, 16–17 February, 9.

Labonté, R. and Laverack, G. (2001) 'Capacity building in health promotion, part 1: for whom? And for what purpose?', *Critical Public Health*, 11(2): 111–37.

Lalonde, M. (1974) *A New Perspective on the Health of Canadians: a Working Document*, Ottawa: Minster of Supply and Service Canada.

Lancucki, L., Sasieni, P., Patnick, J., Day, T. and Vessey, M. (2012) 'The impact of Jade Goody's diagnosis and death on the NHS Cervical Screening Programme', *Journal of Medical Screening*, 19: 89–93.

Lang, T. and Raynor, G. (2012) 'Ecological public health: the 21st century's big idea? An essay by Tim Lang and Geof Raynor', *BMJ*, 345: e5466. doi:10.1136bmj.e5466

Lareau, A. (2002) 'Invisible inequality: social class and childrearing in black and white families', *American Sociological Review*, 67: 747–76.

Larkin, M. (1999) 'Globalization and health', *Critical Public Health*, 9(4): 335–45.

Laverack, G. (2001) 'An identification and interpretation of the organizational aspects of community empowerment', *Community Development Journal*, 36(2): 134–45.

Lawler, D., Frankel, S., Shaw, M., Ebrahim, S. and Davey Smith, G. (2003) 'Smoking and ill health: does lay epidemiology explain the failure of smoking cessation programs among deprived populations?', *American Journal of Public Health*, 93(2): 266–70.

Lawn, J., Rohde, J., Rifkin, S., Were, M., Paul, V. and Chapra, M. (2008) 'Alma-Ata 30 years on: revolutionary, relevant, and time to revitalise', *The Lancet*, 372: 917–27.

Lazarus, J. (2008) 'Participation in poverty reduction strategy papers: reviewing the past, assessing the present and predicting the future', *Third World Quarterly*, 29(6): 1205–21.

Le Fanu, J. (2012) 'Mathematics is bad for you: population risk reduction medicalizes us all', *BMJ*, 344: e2612. doi:10.1136/bmje2612

Leandro, G. (2005) *Meta-Analysis in Medical Research*, Oxford: Blackwell Publishing.

Lee, K. (2010) 'How do we move forward on the social determinants of health: the global governance challenges', *Critical Public Health*, 20(1): 5–14.

Leon, D. (2011) 'Trends in European life expectancy: a salutary view', *International Journal of Epidemiology*, 40(2): 271–7.

Leone, T. (2010) 'How can demography inform health policy?', *Health Economics, Policy and Law*, 5: 1–11.

Levitas, R. (2000) 'Community, utopia and New Labour', *Urban Economy*, 15(3): 188–97.

Levitas, R. and Guy, W. (eds) (1996) *Interpreting Official Statistics*, London: Routledge.

Li, Y. (2007) 'Social capital, social exclusion and wellbeing', in A. Scriven and S. Garman (eds) *Public Health: Social Context and Action* (pp. 60–75), Maidenhead: Open University Press/McGraw Hill.

Li, Y. (2010) 'Measuring social capital: formal and informal activism, its socio–demographic determinants and socio–political impacts', in M. Bulmer, J. Gibbs and L. Hyman (eds) *Social Measurement Through Social Surveys: An Applied Approach* (pp. 173–194), Farnham: Ashgate Publishing.

Link, B. and Phelan, J. (1995) 'Social conditions as fundamental causes of disease', *Journal of Health & Social Behaviour*, 35: 80–94.

Lithell, U., Rosling, H. and Hofvander, Y. (1992) 'Children's deaths and population growth', *The Lancet*, 339: 377–8.

Lloyd, C., Mete, C. and Grant, M. (2009) 'The implications of changing educational and family circumstances for children's grade progression in rural Pakistan: 1997–2004', *Economics of Education Review*, 28: 152–260.

Loewenstein, G., Asch, D., Friedman, J., Melichar, L. and Volpp, K. (2012) 'Can behavioural economics make us healthier?' *BMJ*, 344: e3482. doi:10.1136/bmj.e.3482

Loft, C. (2010) 'The enforcement role of local government as a tool for health', in F. Campbell (ed.) *The Social Determinants of Health and the Role of Local Government*, (pp. 68–69), London: IDeA.

Logan, R., Patnick, J., Nickerson, C., Coleman, L., Rutter, M. and von Wagner, C. (2011) 'Outcomes of the Bowel Cancer Screening Program (BCSP) in England after the first 1 million tests', *Gut*, 61(10). doi:10.1136/gutjnl-2011-300843

London Health Observatory (2012) *Marmot Indicators 2012: Summary Results for London.* Available online at http://lho.org.uk/LHOTopics/National_Lead_Areas/Marmot/Marmot indicators.aspx (accessed 21 April 2013).

Long, A. (1997) 'The Leeds Declaration: three years on – a symbol or a catalyst for change?', *Critical Public Health*, 7: 73–81.

Lorenc, T., Clayton, S., Neary, D., Whitehead, M., Petticrew, M., Thomson, H., Cummins, S., Sowden, A. and Renton, A. (2012) 'Crime, fear of crime, environment, and mental health and wellbeing: mapping review of theories and causal pathways', *Health & Place*, 18: 757–65.

Lorenc, T., Petticrew, M., Welch, V. and Tugwell, P. (2013) 'What types of interventions generate inequalities? Evidence from systematic reviews', *Journal of Epidemiology and Community Health*, 67(2): 190–3.

Loue, S. (2006) 'Community health advocacy', *Journal of Epidemiology & Community Health*, 60: 458–63.

Louw, Q., Manilall, J. and Grimmer, K. (2007) 'Epidemiology of knee injuries among adolescents: a systematic review', *British Journal of Sports Medicine*, 42(2): 2–10.

Lovett, K., Mackey, T. and Liang, B. (2012) 'Evaluating the evidence: direct-to-consumer screening tests advertised online', *Journal of Medical Screening*, 19: 141–53.

Low, A. and Low, A. (2006) 'Importance of relative measures in policy and health inequalities', *BMJ*, 332(7547): 967–9.

Lucia, A. and Ruiz, J. (2011) 'Exercise is beneficial for patients with Alzheimer's disease: a call for action', *British Journal of Sports Medicine*, 45(6): 468–9.

Ludbrook, A. (2009) 'Minimum pricing of alcohol', *Health Economics*, 18: 1357–60.

Lui, Q., Wang, B., Kang, Y. and Cheng, K. (2011) 'China's primary health–care reform', *The Lancet*, 377: 2064–5.

Lupton, R. (1995) *The Imperative of Health*, London: Sage.

Lynch, J., Due, P., Muntaner, C. and Davey Smith, G. (2000) 'Social capital: is it a good invest-ment strategy for public health?', *Journal of Epidemiology & Community Health*, 54: 404–8.

Lyons, M. (2007) *Place-Shaping: a Shared Ambition for the Future of local Government. Lyons Inquiry into Local Government*, London: The Stationery Office.

Ma, J., Lu, M. and Quan, H. (2008) 'From a national, centrally planned health system to a system based on the market: lessons from China', *Health Affairs*, 27(4): 937–48.

Macdonald, A. (2009) *Independent Review of the Proposal to Make Personal, Social, Health and Economic (PSHE) Education Statutory*, Nottingham: Department for Children, Schools and Families.

Machin, S. and Vignobles, A. (2004) 'Educational inequality: the widening socio–economic gap', *Fiscal Studies*, 25(2): 107–28.

Macinko, J. and Starfield, B. (2001) 'The utility of social capital in research on health determinants', *The Millbank Quarterly*, 79(3): 387–427.

Macinko, J., Starfield, B. and Shi, L. (2003) 'The contribution of primary care systems to health outcomes within Organisation for Economic Co-operation and Development (OECD) countries, 1970–1998', *Health Services Research*, 38(3): 831–64.

Macintyre, S., Ellaway, A. and Cummins, S. (2002) 'Place effects on health: how can we conceptualise, operationalise and measure them?', *Social Science & Medicine*, 55: 125–39.

Mackay, D., Nelson, S., Haw, S. and Pell, J. (2012) 'Impact of Scotland's smoke-free legislation on pregnancy complications: retrospective cohort study', *PLoS Medicine*, 9(3): e1001175. doi:10.1371/journal.pmed.1001175

Mackenbach, J. (1996) 'The contribution of medical care to mortality decline: McKeown revisited', *Journal of Clinical Epidemiology*, 49: 1207–13.

Mackenbach, J. (2006) *Health Inequalities: Europe in Profile. An Independent, Expert Report Commissioned by the UK Presidency of the EU*, London: Department of Health.

Mackenbach, J. (2009) 'Politics is nothing but medicine at a larger scale: reflections on public health's biggest idea', *Journal of Epidemiology & Community Health*, 63: 181–4.

Mackenbach, J. (2011a) 'Can we reduce health inequalities? An analysis of the English strategy (1997–2010)', *Journal of Epidemiology & Community Health*, 65: 568–75.

Mackenbach, J. (2011b) 'Public health and welfare', *European Journal of Public Health*, 22(1): 1.

Mackenbach, J. (2012) 'The persistence of health inequalities in modern welfare states: the explanation of a paradox', *Social Science & Medicine*, 75:761–9.

Mackenbach, J, Karanikolos, M. and McKee, M. (2013) 'Health policy in Europe: factors critical to success', *BMJ*, 2013; 346:f533. doi:10.aa36/bmj.f533

Mackenbach, J., Stirbu, I., Roskam, A., Schaap, M., Menvielle, G., Leinsalu, M. and Kunst, A. (2008) 'Socioeconomic inequalities in health in 22 European countries', *New England Journal of Medicine*, 358: 2468–81.

Mackey, T. and Liang, B. (2013) 'United Nations global health panel for global health governance', *Social Science & Medicine*, 76: 12–15.

Magnusson, R. (2009) 'Rethinking global health challenges: towards a "global compact" for reducing the burden of chronic disease', *Public Health*, 123: 265–74.

Mahtani, K., Protheroe, J., Slight, S., Demarzo, M., Blakeman, T., Barton, C., Brijnath, B. and Roberts, N. (2013) 'Can the London 2012 Olympics "inspire a generation" to do more physical or sporting activities? An overview of systematic reviews', *BMJ Open*, 3(1). doi:10.1136/bmjopen–2012–002058

De Maio, F. (2012) 'Advancing the income inequality-health hypothesis', *Critical Public Health*, 22(2): 39–46.

Major, L. (2011) 'The widening gap', *Society Now*, 11: 10.

Malik, K. (2013) *The Rise of the South: Human Progress in a Diverse World. Human Development Report 2013*, New York: United Nations Development Programme.

Mann, J. (1997) 'Medicine and public health, ethics and human rights', *The Hastings Centre Report*, 27(3): 6–13.

Manuel, D., Rosella, L., Tuna, M., and Bennett, C. (2010) *How many Canadians will be Diagnosed with Diabetes between 2007 and 2017? Assessing Population Risk*, Toronto: Institute for Clinical Evaluative Sciences.

Marks, L., Cave, S. and Hunter, D. (2010) 'Public health governance: views of key stakeholders', *Public Health*, 124: 55–9.

Marlow, L., Sangha, A., Patnick, J. and Waller, J. (2012) 'The Jade Goody effect: whose cervical screening decisions were influenced by her story?', *Journal of Medical Screening*, 19: 184–8.

Marmot, M. (2001) 'From Black to Acheson: two decades of concern with inequalities in health. A celebration of the 90th birthday of Professor Jerry Morris', *International Journal of Epidemiology*, 30: 1165–71.

Marmot, M. (2005) 'Social determinants of health inequalities', *The Lancet*, 365: 1099–104.

Marmot, M. (2010) *Fair Society, Healthy Lives: The Marmot Review*, London: University College London.

Marshall, A. (2011) *Radstats Population Studies Group – Population Ageing*. Available online at www.radstats.org.uk/popgroup/Radstats-Population-ageing-summary-of-issues.pdf (accessed 16 July 2013).

Marston, C. and King, E. (2006) 'Factors that shape young people's sexual behaviour: a systematic review', *The Lancet*, 368: 1581–6.

Martin, G., Grant, A. and D'Agostino, M. (2012) 'Global health funding and economic development', *Globalization and Health*, 8(8). doi:10.1186/1744-8603-8-8

Martin, T. (1995) 'Women's education and fertility: results from 26 demographic and health surveys', *Studies in Family Planning*, 26(4): 187–202.

Mason, R. (2013) 'David Cameron given a lecture on "debt" and "deficit" by top statistics official', *The Telegraph*, 1 February. Available online at http://telegraph.co.uk/news/politics/9842553/ (accessed 14 July 2013).

Massey, D. (1991) 'A global sense of place', *Marxism Today*, June: 24–29.

Matthews, R. (2000) 'Storks deliver babies (p=008)', *Teaching Statistics*, 22(2): 36–8.

Mayhew, L. and Smith, D. (2012) *Gender Convergence in Human Survival and the Postponement of Death*, Report No 200, London, UK: Cass Business School.

McCartney, M. (2012) 'What companies don't tell you about screening', *BMJ*, 344. doi:10.1136/bmj.e2311

McCoy, D., Kembhavi, G. and Luintel, A. (2009) 'The Bill and Melinda Gates Foundation's grant making programme for global health', *The Lancet*, 373: 1645–53.

McCreanor, T., Greenaway, A., Barnes, H., Borell, S. and Gregory, A. (2005) 'Youth identity formation and contemporary alcohol marketing', *Critical Public Health*, 15(3), 251–62.

McCulloch, A. and Joshi, H. (2001) 'Neighbourhood and family influences on the cognitive ability of children in the British National Child Development Study', *Social Science & Medicine*, 53: 579–91.

McDonagh, M., Whiting, P., Wilson, P., Sutton, A., Chestnutt, I., Cooper, J. Misso, K., Bradley, M. Treasure, E. (2000) 'Systematic review of water fluoridation', *BMJ*, 321: 855–9. doi:10.1136/bmj.321.7265.855

McGrady, M., Ellwood, R., Maguire, A., Goodwin, M., Boothman, N. and Pretty, I. (2012) 'The association between social deprivation and the prevalence and severity of dental caries and fluorosis in populations with and without water fluoridation', *BMC Public Health*, 12: 1122.

McKay, S. (2004) 'Poverty or preference: what do "consensual deprivation indicators" really measure?', *Fiscal Studies*, 25(2): 201–23.

McKee,M. and Raine, R. (2005) 'Choosing health? First choose your philosophy', *The Lancet*, 365: 369–71.

McKeown, T. (1976) *The Role of Medicine. Dream, Mirage or Nemesis?*, London: Nuffield Provincial Hospitals Trust.

McKinlay, E., Plumridge, L., McBain, L. McLeod, D., Pullon, S. and Brown, S. (2005) '"What sort of health promotion are you talking about?": a discourse analysis of the talk of general practitioners', *Social Science & Medicine*, 60: 1099–106.

McKinlay, J. (1981) 'A case for refocusing upstream: the political economy of illness', in J.

Gartley (ed.) *Patients, Physicians and Illness: A Sourcebook for Behavioural Science and Health* (pp. 9–25), New York: Free Press.

McMunn, A., Kelly, Y., Cable, N. and Bartley, M. (2012) 'Maternal employment and child socio-emotional behaviour in the UK: longitudinal evidence from the UK Millennium Cohort Study', *Journal of Epidemiology & Community Health*, 66: e19. doi:10.1136/jech.2010.109553

McPherson, K. (1998) 'Wider "causal thinking in the health sciences"'. *Journal of Epidemiology & Community Health*, 52: 612–13.

Meadows, P. (2011) *National Evaluation of Sure Start Local Programmes: an Economic Perspective*, London: Department for Education.

Meessen, B., Gilson, L. and Tibouti, A. (2011) 'User fee removal in low-income countries: sharing knowledge to support managed implementation', *Health Policy & Planning*, 26: ii1–ii4.

Mello, M. (2009) 'New York City's war on fat', *New England Journal of Medicine*, 360(19): 2015–20.

Mielewczyk, F. and Willig, C. (2007) 'Old clothes and an older look: the case for a radical makeover of health behaviour research', *Theory & Psychology*, 17: 811–37.

Milbourne, L. (2009) 'Remodelling the third sector: advancing collaboration or competition in community–based initiatives', *Journal of Social Policy*, 38(2): 277–97.

Milio, N. (1981) *Promoting Health Through Public Policy*, Philadelphia: F. A. Davies.

Milio, N. (1988) 'Making healthy public policy; developing the science by learning the art: an ecological framework for policy studies', *Health Promotion International*, 2(3): 263–74.

Miller, D. (2003) 'What's left of the welfare state?', *Social Philosophy & Policy*, 20: 92–112.

Miller, W. and Rollnick, S. (2012) 'Meeting in the middle: motivational interviewing and self–determination theory', *International Journal of Behavioural Nutrition and Physical Activity*, 9: 25–6.

Mills, C. W. (1959) *The Sociological Imagination*, New York: Simon & Schuster.

Mitchell, W., Crawshaw, P., Bunton, R. and Green, E. (2001) 'Situating young people's experiences of risk and identity', *Health, Risk & Society*, 3(2): 217–33.

Mogford, E., Gould, L. and Devoght, A. (2010) 'Teaching critical health literacy in the US as a means to action on the social determinants of health', *Health Promotion International*, 26(1): 4–13.

Mooney, G. (2012) *The Health of Nations: Towards a New Political Economy*, London: Zed Books.

Moore, S., Haines, V., Hawe, P. and Shiell, A. (2006) 'Lost in translation: a genealogy of the "social capital" concept in public health', *Journal of Epidemiology & Community Health*, 60: 729–34.

Morgan, A. and Ziglio, E. (2007) 'Revitalising the evidence base for public health: an assets model', *Promotion & Education*, 14(S2): 17–22.

Morgan, L. (2001) 'Community participation in health: perpetual allure, persistent challenge', *Health Policy & Planning*, 16(3): 221–30.

Morgan, O. and Baker, A. (2006) 'Measuring deprivation in England and Wales using 2001 Carstairs scores', *Health Statistics Quarterly*, 31: 28–33.

Morris, P., Aber, J., Wolf, S. and Berg, J. (2012) *Using Incentives to Change How Teenagers Spend their Time. The effects of New York City's Conditional Cash Transfer Program*, New York: MDRC.

Mowbray, M. (2005) 'Community capacity building or state opportunism?', *Community Development Journal*, 40(3): 255–64.

MRC Vitamin Study Research Group (1991) 'Prevention of neural tube defects: results of the Medical Research Council Vitamin Study (1991)', *The Lancet*, 338: 131–7.

Muldoon, L., Hogg, W. and Levitt, M. (2006) 'Primary care (PC) and primary health care (PHC). What is the difference?', *Canadian Journal of Public Health*, 97(5): 409–11.

Murphy, P. (1998). 'Reflections on the policy process', *M.Sc. in the Sociology of Sport and Sports Management*, Module 4, Unit 7, Part 15 (pp. 85–104), Leicester: Centre for Research into Sport and Society.

Naidoo, J. (1986) 'Limits to individualism' in S. Rodmell and A. Watt (eds) *The Politics of Health Education: Raising the Issues* (pp. 17–37), London: Routledge & Kegan Paul.

Narayan, K., Ali, M., and Koplan, J. (2010) 'Global non-communicable diseases: where worlds meet', *New England Journal of Medicine*, 363(13): 1196–8.

National Evaluation of Sure Start Team (2010) *The Impact of Sure Start Local Programmes on Five Year Olds and their Families*, London: Department for Education.

National Institute for Health and Care Excellence (2013) *Physical Activity: Brief Advice for Adults in Primary Care*. NICE Public Health Guidance 44, London: NICE.

Navarro, V. (2009) 'What we mean by the social determinants of health', *International Journal of Health Services*, 39(3): 423–41.

Navarro, V. (2011) 'The importance of politics in policy', *Australian and New Zealand Journal of Public Health*, 35(4): 313.

Needle, J., Petchey, R., Benson, J., Scriven, A., Lawrenson, J. and Hilari, K. (2011) 'The allied health professions and health promotion: a systematic literature review and narrative synthesis', *Service Delivery and Organization programme*, London: NIHR, 75. Available online at http://openaccess.city.ac.uk/931/ (accessed 10 May 2013).

Ness, R. and Rothenberg, R. (2007) 'Critique of epidemiology: changing the terms of the debate', *Annals of Epidemiology*, 17(12): 1011–12.

Nettleton, S. (1995) *The Sociology of Health and Illness*, Cambridge: Polity Press.

Neylan, J. (2008) 'Social policy and the authority of evidence', *Australian Journal of Public Administration*, 67(1): 12–19.

Nilsen, S., Bjørngaard, J., Ernstsen, L., Krokstad, S. and Steiner, W. (2012) 'Education-based health inequalities in 18,000 Norwegian couples: the Nord-Trøndelag Health Study (HUNT)', *BMC Public Health* 12: 998. doi:10.1186/1471-2458-12-998

Nnoaham, K., Frater, A., Roderick, P., Moon, G. and Halloran, S. (2010) 'Do geodemographic typologies explain variations in uptake in colorectal cancer screening? An assessment using routine screening data in the south of England', *Journal of Public Health*, 32(4): 572–81.

Noble, H. (2011) 'Comments on the Spirit Level controversy', *Radical Statistics*, 104: 49–60.

Norwegian Ministry of Foreign Affairs (2011) *Towards Greener Development: a Coherent Environment and Development Policy*. (Meld. St. 14, 2010–2011). Report to the Storting (White Paper). Available online at www.regjeringen.no/en/dep/ud/documents/propositions-and-reports/reports-to-the-storting/2010-2011/meld-st-14-2010-2011-2.html?id=655152 (accessed 1 February 2013).

Norwegian Ministry of Foreign Affairs (2012) *Global Health in Foreign and Development Policy*. (Meld. St. 11, 2011–2012) Report to the Storting (White Paper). Available online at www.regjeringen.no/pages/36968001/PDFS/STM201120120011000EN_PDFS.pdf (accessed 16 November 2012).

Nuffield Council on Bioethics (2007) *Public Health: Ethical Issues*, London: Nuffield Council on Bioethics.

Nugus, P., Greenfield, D., Travaglia, J., Westbrook, J. and Braithwaite, J. (2010) 'How and where clinicians exercise power: interprofessional relations in health care', *Social Science & Medicine*, 71: 898–909.

Nunn, A., Massard da Fonseca, E., Bastos, F. and Gruskin, S. (2009) 'AIDS treatment in Brazil: impacts and challenges', *Health Affairs*, 28(4), 1103–13.

Nussbaum, M. (2011), *Creating Capabilities: the Human Development Approach*, Cambridge, MA: Harvard University Press.

Nutbeam, D. (1998) *Health Promotion Glossary*, Geneva: World Health Organization.

Nutbeam, D. (2000) 'Health literacy as a public health goal: a challenge for contemporary health education and communication strategies into the 21st century', *Health Promotion International*, 15(3): 259–67.

Nutbeam, D. (2008) 'The evolving concept of health literacy', *Social Science & Medicine*, 67: 2072–8.

Nutbeam, D. (2009) 'Defining and measuring health literacy: what can we learn from literacy studies?', *International Journal of Public Health*, 54: 303–5.

Nutley, S., Davies, H. and Walter, I. (2002) *Evidence Based Policy and Practice: Cross Sector Lessons from the UK*, Working Paper 9, Swindon: ESRC UK Centre for Evidence based Policy and Practice, Research Unit for Research Utilization.

O'Leary, T., Burkett, I. and Braithwaite, K. (2011) *Appreciating Assets*, Dunfermline, Scotland: Carnegie, UK Trust. Available online at www.iacdglobal.org/publications/IACD–Reports (accessed 23 October 2012).

Oakley, A., Strange, V., Bonell, C., Allen, E., Stephensen, J., RIPPLE Study Team (2006) 'Process evaluation in randomised controlled trials of complex interventions', *BMJ*, 332: 413–16.

Office for National Statistics (2010a) *Final Recommended Questions for the 2011 Census in England and Wales: Health*. Available online at www.ons.gov.uk/census2011/health (accessed 12 July 2013).

Office for National Statistics (2010b) *Standard Occupational Classification 2010. Volume 3. The National Statistics Socio–economic Classification: (Rebased on the SOC2010) User Manual*. Basingstoke: Palgrave Macmillan.

Office for National Statistics (2011) *Life Expectancy at Birth and at Age 65 by Local Areas in the United Kingdom, 2004–2006 to 2008–2010*, London: Office for National Statistics.

Office for National Statistics (2012) *2011 Census: Frequently Asked Questions*. Available online at www.ons.gov.uk/ONS/guide-method/census/2011/census-date/2011-census-user-guide/faqs/index.html (accessed 2 April 2013).

Okie, S. (2006) 'Fighting HIV: lessons from Brazil', *New England Journal of Medicine*, 354(19): 1977–81.

Ollila, E. (2005) 'Global health priorities: priorities of the wealthy?', *Globalization and Health*, 1(6). doi:10.1186/1744–8603–1–6

Organisation for Economic Co-operation and Development (2011a) *Divided we Stand. Why Inequality Keeps Rising. An Overview of Growing Income Inequalities in OECD Countries*. OECD Publishing. doi:10.1787/9789264119536-EN

Organisation for Economic Co-operation and Development (2011b) *Health at a Glance 2011: OECD Indicators*. OECD Publishing. doi:10.1787/health_glance-2011-4-en

Organisation for Economic Co-operation and Development (2012) *Social Spending after the Crisis*. Available online at www.oecd.org/els/social/expenditure (accessed 2 April 2013).

Orme, J., Viggiani, N., Naidoo, J. and Knight, T. (2007) 'Missed opportunities? Locating health promotion within multidisciplinary public health', *Public Health*, 121, 414–19.

Orrow, G., Kinmouth, A., Sanderson, S. and Sutton, S. (2012) 'Effectiveness of physical activity promotion based in primary care: systematic review and meta-analysis of randomised controlled trials', *BMJ*, 344. doi:10.1136/bmj.e1389

Orton, L., Lloyd Williams, F., Taylor-Robinson, D., O'Flaherty, M. and Capewell, S. (2011) 'The use of research evidence in public health decision making processes: systematic review', *Public Library of Science*, 6(7): e21704.

Pang, T. and Weatherall, D. (2012) 'Genomics and world health: a decade on', *The Lancet*, 379: 1853–4.

Pantazis, C., Townsend, P. and Gordon, D. (1999) *Poverty and Social Exclusion Survey of Britain*. Working Paper No 1. *The Necessities of Life in Britain*, Bristol: Townsend Centre for International Poverty Research. Available online at www.bris.ac.uk/poverty/pse/99PSE-WP1.pdf (accessed 8 November 2012).

Parascandola, M. (2003) 'Objectivity and the neutral expert', *Journal of Epidemiology & Community Health*, 57: 3–4.

Parascandola, M. and Weed, D. (2001) 'Causation in epidemiology', *Journal of Epidemiology & Community Health*, 55: 905–12.

Parry, J., Mathers, J., Laburn–Peart, C., Orford, J. and Dalton, S. (2007) 'Improving health in deprived communities. What can residents teach us?', *Critical Public Health*, 17(2): 123–26.

Patnick, J. (2013) 'Benefits of cancer screening take years to appreciate', *BMJ*, 346: f299. doi:10.1136/bmj.f299

Paton, K., Sengupta, S. and Hassan, L. (2005) 'Settings, systems and organization development: the healthy living and working model', *Health Promotion International*, 20(1): 81–9.

Pawson, R. and Sridharan, S. (2010) 'Theory-driven evaluation of public health programmes' in A. Killoran and M. Kelly (eds) *Evidence-Based Public Health: Effectiveness and Efficiency* (pp. 43–62), Oxford: Oxford University Press.

Pawson, R. and Tilley, N. (1997) *Realist Evaluation*, London: Sage.

Peckham, S. and Hann, A. (2008) 'General practice and public health: assessing the impact of the new GMS contract', *Critical Public Health*, 18(3): 347–56.

Peerson, A. and Saunders, M. (2009) 'Health literacy revisited: what do we mean and why does it matter?' *Health Promotion International*, 24(3): 285–96.

Pega, F., Blakely, T., Carter, K. and Sjöberg, O. (2012) 'The explanation of a paradox? A commentary on Mackenbach with perspectives from research on financial credits and risk factor trends', *Social Science & Medicine*, 75: 770–3.

Pell, J., Haw, S., Cobbe, S., Newby, D., Pell, A., Fischbacher, C. McConnachie, A., Pringle, S., Murdoch, D., Dunn, F., Oldroyd, K., MacIntyre, P., O'Rourke, B. and Borland, W. (2008) 'Smoke-free legislation and hospitalizations for acute coronary syndrome', *Journal of the American Medical Association*, 359: 482–91.

Percy-Smith, J. (ed.) (1996) *Needs Assessment in Public Policy*, Buckingham: Open University Press.

Perkins, N., Smith, K., Hunter, D., Bambra, C. and Joyce, K. (2010) '"What counts is what works"? New Labour and partnerships in public health', *Policy & Politics*, 8(1): 101–17.

Perry, C., Thurston, M. and Osborn, T. (2008) 'Time for me: the arts as therapy in postnatal depression', *Complementary Therapies in Clinical Practice*, 14(1): 38–45.

Persson, G. (2006) 'Demography and public health', *Scandinavian Journal of Public Health*, 34(Suppl 67): 19–25.

Peter, F. (2001): Health equity and social justice', *Journal of Applied Philosophy*, 18(2): 159–70.

Peters, E., Baker, D., Dieckmann, N., Leon, J. and Collins, J. (2010) 'Explaining the effect of education on health: a field study in Ghana', *Psychological Science*, 21(10): 1369–76.

Peters, G-J., Kok, G. and Schaalma, H. (2008) 'Careers in ecstacy use: do ecstasy users cease of their own accord? Implications for intervention development', *BMC Public Health*, 8: 376–86.

Petrie, A., and Sabin, C. (2000) *Medical Statistics at a Glance*, Oxford: Blackwell Science.

Pettersson, B. (2007) 'Transforming Ottawa Charter health promotion concepts into Swedish public health policy', *Promotion & Health*, 14, 244–9.

Petticrew, M., Tugwell, P., Welch, V., Ueffing, E., Kristjansson, E., Armstrong, R., Doyle, J. and Waters, E. (2009) 'Better evidence about wicked issues in tackling health inequities', *Journal of Public Health*, 31(3): 453–6.

Phillimore, P., Beattie, A., Townsend, P. (1994) 'Widening inequality of health in northern England, 1981–91', *BMJ*, 308: 1125–35.

Plavinski, S., Plavinskaya, S. and Klimov, A. (2003) 'Social factors and increase in mortality in Russia in the 1990s: prospective cohort study', *BMJ*, 326: 1240–2.

Ploug, T., Holm, S. and Brodersen, J. (2012) 'To nudge or not to nudge: cancer screening programmes and the limits of libertarian paternalism', *Journal of Epidemiology & Community Health*, 66: 1193–6.

Pollitt, C. (2003) 'Joined-up Government: a survey', *Political Studies Review*, 1: 34–49.

Pollock, A. and Price, D. (2003) 'The public health implications of world trade negotiations on the general agreement on trade in services and public services', *The Lancet*, 362: 1072–5.

Popay, J. and Williams, G. (1998) 'Qualitative research and evidence-based healthcare', *Journal of the Royal Society of Medicine*, 91(31): 32–7.

Popay, J., Whitehead, J. and Hunter, D. (2010) 'Injustice is killing people on a large scale: but what is to be done about it?', *Journal of Public Health*, 32(2): 148–9.

Popham, F., Dibben, C. and Bambra, C. (2013) 'Are health inequalities really not the smallest in the Nordic welfare states? A comparison of mortality inequality in 37 countries', *Journal of Epidemiology & Community Health*, 67: 412–18.

Porta, M. (ed.) (2008) *A Dictionary of Epidemiology*, 5th edn, New York: Oxford University Press.

Portes, A. (1998) 'Social capital: its origins and applications in modern sociology', *Annual Review of Sociology*, 24: 1–24.

Potvin, L., Juneau, C., Jones, C. and McQueen, D. (2011) 'How is evidence used for planning, implementation and evaluation of health promotion? A global collection of case studies', *Global Health Promotion*, 18(1): 7–8.

Povlsen, L., Borup, I. and Fosse, E. (2011) 'The concept of "equity" in health-promotion articles by Nordic authors: a matter of some confusion and misconception', *Scandinavian Journal of Public Health*, 39: 50–6.

Powell, K., Thurston, M. and Perry, C. (2008) *The National Bowel Cancer Screening Programme in Cheshire and Merseyside: Perspectives of People with a Sensory Impairment*, Chester: University of Chester.

Powell, M. and Moon, G. (2001) 'Health Action Zones: the "third way" of a new area-based policy?', *Health and Social Care in the Community*, 9(1): 43–50.

Prättälä, R. and Puska, P. (2012) 'Social determinants of health behaviours and social change', *European Journal of Public Health*, 22(2): 166.

Preston, S. (2007) 'The changing relation between mortality and level of economic development', *International Journal of Epidemiology*, 36: 484–90.

Pring, R. (2011) Education for all. Evidence from the past, principles for the future. Twelve challenges. Seminar held at the University of Chester, Faculty of Education and Children's Services, 19 October.

Prochaska, J. and Diclemente, C. (1983) 'Stages and processes of self–change in smoking: towards an integrative model of change', *Journal of Consulting and Clinical Psychology*, 51: 390–5.

Public Health Resource Unit/Skills for Health (2008/2009) *Public Health Skills and Career Framework: Multi-Disciplinary, Multi-Agency, Multi-Professional*. Available online at http://phorcast.org.uk/document_store/1318357881_bNP_public_health_skills_and_career_framework.pdf (accessed 9 July 2012).

Public Health Wales (2013) *Vaccine Uptake in Children in Wales, October to December 2012*. Available online at www.wales.nhs.uk/sites3/page.cfm?orgid=457&pid=54144 (accessed 6 April 2013).

Purcal, C., Muir, K., Patulny, R., Thomson, C. and Flaxman, S. (2011) 'Does partnership funding improve coordination and collaboration among early childhood services? Experiences from the Communities for Children programme', *Child and Family Social Work*, 16: 474–84.

Puska, P. (2008) 'The North Karelia Project: 30 years successfully preventing chronic disease', *Diabetes Voice*, 53: 26–9.

Putnam, R. (1993) *Making Democracy Work: Civic Traditions in Modern Italy*, Princeton, NJ: Princeton University Press.

Putnam, R. (1995) 'Bowling alone: America's declining social capital', *Journal of Democracy*, 6: 65–78.

Pykett, J., Jones, R., Whitehead, M., Huxley, M. Strauss, K., Gill, N., McGeevor, K., Thompson, L. and Newman, J. (2011) 'Interventions in the political geography of libertarian paternalism', *Political Geography*, 30(6): 301–10.

Radical Statistics (2013) 'Statistical policy in Argentina', *Radical Statistics*, 108: 53–7.

Raeburn, J. and Rootman, I. (1989) 'Towards an expanded health field concept: conceptual and research issues in a new era of health promotion', *Health Promotion International*, 3(4): 383–92.

Rahman, A. (1999) 'Micro-credit initiatives for equitable and sustainable development: who pays?', *World Development*, 27(1): 6–82.

Ramos, A., Matida, L., Hearst, N. and Heukelbach, J. (2011) 'AIDS in Brazilian children: history, surveillance, antiretroviral therapy, and epidemiological transition 1984–2008', *AIDS Patient Care and STDs*, 25(4): 245–55.

Ranis, G., Stewart, F. and Ramirez, A. (2000) 'Economic growth and human development', *World Development*, 28(2): 197–219.

Rao, V. (2012) 'Law on infant foods inhibits the marketing of complementary foods for infants, furthering undernutrition in India', *BMJ*, 345: e8131.

Raphael, D. (2013a) 'The political economy of health promotion: Part 1, national commitments to provision of the prerequisites of health', *Health Promotion International*, 28(1): 95–111.

Raphael, D. (2013b) 'The political economy of health promotion: Part 2, national provision of the prerequisites of health', *Health Promotion International*, 28(1): 112–32.

Rasanathan, K., Montesinos, E., Matheson, D., Etienne, C. and Evans, T. (2011) 'Primary health care and the social determinants of health: essential and complementary approaches for reducing inequities in health', *Journal of Epidemiology & Community Health*, 65: 656–60.

Rawaf, S., De Maeseneer, J. and Starfield, B. (2008) 'From Alma-Ata to Almaty: a new start for primary health care', *The Lancet*, 372: 1365–6.

Rawlins, M. and Culyer, A. (2004) 'National Institute for Clinical Excellence and its value judgements', *BMJ*, 329: 224–6.

Rawls, J. (1971) *A Theory of Justice*, Cambridge, MA: Harvard University Press.

Raynor, D. (2012) 'Health literacy: is it time to shift our focus from patient to provider?', *BMJ*, 344: e2188. doi:10.1136/bmj.e2188

Reay, D. (2004) 'Education and cultural capital: the implications of changing trends in education policies', *Cultural Trends*, 13(2): 73–86.

Reay, D. (2006) 'The zombie stalking English schools: social class and educational inequality', *British Journal of Educational Studies*, 54(3): 288–307.

Reay, D., Crozier, G. and Clayton, J. (2010) '"Fitting in" or "standing out": working-class students in UK higher education', *British Educational Research Journal*, 36(1): 107–24.

Regidor, E., de la Fuente, L., Gutiérrez–Fisac, J., Mateo, S., Pascual, C., Sánchez-Payá, J. and Ronda, E. (2007) 'The role of the public health official in communicating public health information', *American Journal of Public Health*, 91(1): S93–S97.

Reubi, D. (2011) 'The promise of human rights for global health: a programmed deception? A commentary on Schrecker, Chapman, Labonté and De Vogli (2010) "Advancing health equity in the global market place: How human rights can help"', *Social Science & Medicine*, 73: 625–8.

Ribbens McCarthy, J. and Edwards, R. (2011) *Key Concepts in Family Studies*, London: Sage.

Richens, J., Imrie, J. and Copas, A. (2000) 'Condoms and seat belts: the parallels and the lessons', *The Lancet*, 355: 400–3.

Ring, N., Ritchie, K., Mandava, L. and Jepson, R. (2011) *A Guide to Synthesising Qualitative Research for Researchers Undertaking Health Technology Assessments and Systematic*

Reviews. Available online at www.nhshealthquality.org/nhsqis/8837.html (accessed 27 May 2013).

Rissel, C. (1994) 'Empowerment: the holy grail of health promotion?', *Health Promotion International*, 9(1): 39–47.

Rittel, H. and Webber, M. (1973) 'Dilemmas in a general theory of planning', *Policy Sciences*, 4: 155–69.

Roberts, H., Petticrew, M., Liabo, K. and Macintyre, S. (2012) '"The Anglo-Saxon disease": a pilot study of the barriers to and facilitators of the use of randomised controlled trials of social programmes in an international context', *Journal of Epidemiology & Community Health*, 66: 1025–1029.

Roberts, K. (2009) *Key Concepts in Sociology*, Basingstoke: Palgrave MacMillan.

Roberts, K. (2012) *Sociology. An Introduction*, Cheltenham: Edward Elgar.

Roberts, K. and Brodie, D. (1992) *Inner City Sport. Who Plays and What are the Benefits?*, The Netherlands: Giardano Bruno Culemborg.

Roberts, K., Pollock, G., Tholen, J. and Tarkhnishvili, L. (2009) 'Young leisure careers during post-communist transition in the South Caucasus', *Leisure Studies*, 28(3): 261–77.

Robertson, A. (1998) 'Critical reflections on the politics of need: implications for public health', *Social Science & Medicine*, 47(10): 1419–30.

Robertson, R. (2008) *Using Information to Promote Healthy Behaviours*, London: The King's Fund.

Robertson, S. (2006) '"Not living in too much of an excess": Lay men understanding health and well-being', *Health*, 10(2): 175–89.

Rodmell, S. and Watt, A. (eds) (1986) *The Politics of Health Education: Raising the Issues*, London: Routledge & Kegan Paul.

Rogers, P., Petrosino, A., Huebner, T. and Hasci, T. (2000) 'Program theory evaluation: practice, promise and problems', *New Directions for Evaluation*, 87: 5–13.

Rogers, R. (1983) 'Cognitive and physiological processes in fear-based attitude change: a revised theory of protection motivation', in J. Caccioppo and R. Petty (eds) *Social Psychophysiology: a Sourcebook* (pp. 153–176) New York: Guildford.

Rollnick, S. and Miller, W. (1995) 'What is motivational interviewing?' *Behavioural and Cognitive Psychotherapy*, 23: 325–34.

Rollnick, S., Butler, C., Kinnersley, P., Gregory, J. and Mash, B. (2010) 'Motivational interviewing', *BMJ*, 340: 1242–5.

Rootman, I. and Gordon-El-Bihety, D. (2008) *A Vision for a Health Literate Canada: Report of the Expert Panel on Health Literacy*, Ottawa: Canadian Public Health Association.

Rootman, I., Goodstadt, M., Hyndman, B., McQueen, D. V., Potvin, L., Springett, J. and Ziglio, E. (2001) *Evaluation in Health Promotion. Principles and Perspectives*, Geneva: World Health Organization.

Rose, G. (1981) 'Strategy of prevention: lessons from cardiovascular disease', *BMJ*, 282: 1847–51.

Rose, G. (1985) 'Sick individuals and sick populations', *International Journal of Epidemiology*, 14: 32–8.

Rose, G. (2008) *Rose's Strategy of Preventive Medicine*, Oxford: Oxford University Press.

Roseboom, T., de Rooij, S. and Painter, R. (2006) 'The Dutch famine and its long-term consequences for adult health', *Early Human Development*, 82: 485–91.

Rosenstock, L. (1974) 'The health belief model and preventive health behavior', *Health Education Monographs*, 2: 354–86.

Ross, C. and Wu, C. (1995) 'The links between education and health', *American Sociological Review*, 60: 719–45.

Ross, E. (1991) 'The origins of public health: concepts and contradictions', in. P. Draper (ed.) *Health Through Public Policy: The Greening of Public Health* (pp. 26–40), London: Green Print.

Rowlands, G. (2012) 'Health literacy and public health: a framework for developing skills and empowering citizens', *Perspectives in Public Health*, 132: 23–4.

Royal College of Physicians (2010) *How Doctors can Close the Gap: Tackling the Social Determinants of Health through Culture Change, Advocacy and Education*. RCP Policy Statement 2010, London: Royal College of Physicians.

Rudd, R. (2010) 'Improving America's health literacy', *New England Journal of Medicine*, 363: 2283–5.

Rummery, K. (2009) 'Healthy partnerships, healthy citizens? An international review of partnerships in health and social care and patient/use outcomes', *Social Science & Medicine*, 69: 1797–804.

Rychetnik, L., Hawe, P., Waters, E., Barratt, A. and Frommer, M. (2004) 'A glossary of evidence based public health', *Journal of Epidemiology & Community Health*, 58: 538–45.

Rycroft Malone, J. (2006) 'The politics of the evidence based practice movement', *Journal of Research in Nursing*, 11(2): 95–108.

Sabatier, P. (1998) 'The advocacy coalition framework: revisions and relevance to Europe', *Journal of European Public Policy*, 5(1): 98–130.

Sackett, D., Rosenburg, W., Gray, J., Haynes, R. and Richardson, W. (1996) 'Evidence-based medicine: what it is and what it isn't', *BMJ*, 312: 71–2.

Salomon, J., Wang, H., Freeman, M., Vos, T., Flaxman, A., Lopez, A. and Murray, C. (2012) 'Healthy life expectancy for 187 countries, 1990–2010: a systematic analysis for the Global Burden Disease Study 2010', *The Lancet*, 380: 2144–62.

Samb, B., Desai, N., Nishtar, S., Mendis, S., Bekedam, H., Wright, A. Hsu, J., Martiniuk, A., Celletti, F., Patel, K., Adshead, F., McKee, M., Evans, T., Alwan, A. and Etienne, C. (2010) 'Prevention and management of chronic disease: a litmus test for health systems strengthening in low-income and middle-income countries', *The Lancet*, 376: 1785–97.

Sanders, D., Baum, F., Benos, A. and Legge, D. (2011) 'Revitalising primary healthcare requires an equitable global economic system: now more than ever', *Journal of Epidemiology & Community Health*, 65: 661–5.

Sant, M., Allemani, C., Santaquilani, M., Knijn, A., Marchesi, F., Capocaccia, R. (2009) 'EUROCARE-4. Survival of cancer patients diagnosed in 1995–1999. Results and commentary', *European Journal of Cancer*, 45: 931–91.

Saracci, R. (2010) 'Introducing the history of epidemiology', in J. Olsen, R. Sarraci and D. Trichopoulos (eds) *Teaching Epidemiology* (pp. 3–23), New York: Oxford University Press.

Sassi, F., Le Grand, J. and Archard, L. (2001) 'Equity versus efficiency: a dilemma for the NHS', *BMJ*, 323: 762–3.

Saunders, P. and Naidoo, Y. (2009) 'Poverty, deprivation and consistent poverty', *The Economic Record*, 85(27): 417–32.

du Sautoy, P. (1966) 'Community development in Britain?', *Community Development Journal*, 1(1): 54–6.

Schell, C., Reilly, M., Rosling, H., Peterson, S. and Ekstrom, A. (2007) 'Socioeconomic determinants of infant mortality: a worldwide study of 152 low-, middle-, and high-income countries', *Scandinavian Journal of Public Health*, 35: 288–97.

Schoen, C., Osborn, R., Huynh, P., Doty, M., Davis, K., Zapert, K. and Peugh, J. (2004) Primary care and health system performance: adults' experiences in five countries. *Health Affairs*, W4:487–503. doi:10.1377/hlthaff.W4.487

Schoon, I. and Bynner, J. (2003) 'Risk and resilience in the life course: implications for interventions and social policies', *Journal of Youth Studies*, 6(1): 21–31.

Schrecker, T., Chapman, A., Labonté and De Vogli, R. (2010) 'Advancing health equity in the global marketplace: how human rights can help', *Social Science & Medicine*, 71: 1520–26.

Schrecker, T., Labonté, R. and De Vogli, R. (2008) 'Globalisation and health: the need for a global vision', *The Lancet*, 372: 1670–6.

Scott-Samuel, A. (1998) 'Health impact assessment: theory and practice', *Journal of Epidemiology & Community Health*, 52: 704–5.

Scott-Samuel, A. and Springett, J. (2007) 'Hegemony or health promotion? Prospects for reviving England's lost discipline', *Journal of the Royal Society for the Promotion of Health*, 127(5): 211–14.

Seaman, P. and Ikegwuonu, T. (2010) *Drinking to Belong: Understanding Young Adults' Alcohol Use within Social Networks*, York: Joseph Rowntree Foundation.

Secretary of State for Health (2010) *Healthy Lives, Healthy People: Our Strategy for Public Health in England*. Cm7985, London: The Stationery Office.

Secretary of State for the Home Department (2012) *The Government's Alcohol Strategy*. Cm 8336, London: The Stationery Office.

Sefton, T., Byford, S., McDaid, D., Hills, J. and Knapp, M. (2002) *Making the Most of it: Economic Evaluation in the Social Welfare Field*, York: Joseph Rowntree Foundation.

Sen, A. (1983) 'Poor, relatively speaking', *Oxford Economic Papers*, 35(2): 153–69.

Sen, A. (2004) 'Elements of a theory of human rights', *Philosophy and Public Affairs*, 32(4): 315–56.

Seymour, D. (2009) *Reporting Poverty in the UK: A Practical Guide for Journalists*, York: Joseph Rowntree Foundation.

Shaheen, F. (2011) *Ten Reasons to Care about Economic Inequality*, London: New Economics Foundation.

Shaw, I. (2002) 'How lay are lay beliefs?', *Health*, 6(3): 287–99.

Shaw, M., Galobardes, B., Lawler, D., Lynch, J., Wheeler, B. and Davey Smith, G. (2007) *The Handbook of Inequality and Socioeconomic Position: Concepts and Measures*, Bristol: The Policy Press.

Sheron, N., Hawkey, C. and Gilmore, I. (2011) 'Projections of alcohol deaths: a wake–up call', *The Lancet*, 377: 1297–9.

Shi, L., Starfield, B., Politzer, R. and Regan, J. (2002) 'Primary care, self-rated health, and reductions in social disparities in health', *Health Services Research*, 37(3): 529–50.

Shilton, T., Sparks, M., McQueen, D., Lamarre, M. and Jackson, S. (2011) 'Proposal for new definition of health', *BMJ*, 343: d5359.

Shucksmith, J., Carlebach, S., Riva, M., Curtis, S., Hunter, D., Blackman, T. and Hudson, R. (2010) *Health Inequalities in Ex-Coalfield/Industrial Communities*, London: IDeA.

Sigerist, H. (1961) *A History of Medicine: Early Greek, Hindu and Persian Medicine*, Oxford: Oxford University Press.

Sims, M., Maxwell, E., Bauld, L. and Gilmore, A. (2010) 'Short-term impact of smoke-free legislation in England: retrospective analysis of hospital admissions for myocardial infarction', *BMJ*, 340: c2161.

Sinclair, S. (2011) 'Partnership or presence? Exploring the complexity of community planning', *Local Government Studies*, 3(1): 77–92.

Singh, S., Darroch, J. and Frost, J. (2009) *Teenage Sexual Reproductive Behavior in Developed Countries: Can More Progress be Made?* Occasional Report No 3, New York: Guttmacher Institute. Available online at http://dspace.cigilibrary.org/jspui/handle/123456789/19715 (accessed 12 March 2013).

Singh-Manoux, A. and Marmot, M. (2005) 'Role of socialization in explaining social inequalities in health', *Social Science & Medicine*, 60: 2129–33.

Skrabanek, P. (1990) 'Why is preventive medicine exempted from ethical constraints?', *Journal of Medical Ethics*, 16: 187–90.

Slater, T. (2013) 'Your life chances affect where you live: a critique of the "cottage industry" of neighbourhood effects research', *International Journal of Urban and Regional Research*, 37(2): 367–387.

Sloggett, A. and Joshi, H. (1994) 'Higher mortality in deprived areas: community or personal disadvantage?', *BMJ*, 309: 1470–4.

Sloggett, A. and Joshi, H. (1998) 'Deprivation indicators as predictors of life events 1981–1992 based on the UK ONS longitudinal study', *Journal of Epidemiology & Community Health*, 52: 228–33.

Smith, B., Tang, K. and Nutbeam, D. (2006) 'WHO health promotion glossary: new terms', *Health Promotion International*, 21(4): 340–5.

Smith, K. (2012) 'Institutional filters: the translation and re-circulation of ideas about health inequalities within policy', *Policy and Politics*, 41(1): 81–100.

Smith, K. and Katikreddi, S. (2013) 'A glossary of theories for understanding policy making', *Journal of Epidemiology & Community Health*, 67: 198–202.

Smith, K., Bambra, C., Joyce, K., Perkins, N., Hunter, D., Bleinkinsopp, E. (2009a) 'Partners in health? A systematic review of the impact of organisational partnerships on public health outcomes in England between 1997 and 2008', *Journal of Public Health*. 21(2): 210–21.

Smith, K., Jerrett, M., Anderson, H., Burnett, R., Stone, V., Derwent, R., Atkinson, R., Cohen, A., Shonkoff, S., Krewski, D., Pope, C., Thun, M. and Thurston, G. (2009b) 'Public health benefits of strategies to reduce greenhouse-gas emissions: health implications of short-lived greenhouse pollutants', *The Lancet*, 374: 2091–103.

Smith, M. (1997/2002) 'Paolo Freire and informal education', *The Encyclopaedia of Informal Education*. Available online at www.infed.org/thinkers/et–freir.htm (accessed 10 March 2013).

Social Exclusion Unit. (2001) *A New Commitment to Neighbourhood Renewal: National Strategy Action Plan*, London: Cabinet Office.

Sondhi, A. and Turner, C. (2011) *The Influence of Family and Friends on Young People's Drinking*, York: Joseph Rowntree Foundation.

Sørensen, K. and Brand, H. (2013) 'Health literacy lost in translation? Introducing the European Health Literacy Glossary', *Health Promotion International*. doi:10.1093/heapro/da013

Sørensen, K., Van den Broucke, S., Fullam, J., Doyle, G., Pelikan, J., Slonska, Z. and Brand, H. (2012) 'Health literacy and public health: a systematic review and integration of definitions and models', *BMC Public Health*, 12:80. Available online at www.biomedcentral.com/147–2458/12/80 (accessed 3 June 2013).

Sparkes, M. (2011) 'Building healthy public policy: don't believe the misdirection', *Health Promotion International*, 26(3): 259–62.

Spijkers, W., Jansen, D. and Reijneveld, S. (2011) 'The impact of area deprivation on parenting stress', *European Journal of Public Health*, 22(6): 760–5.

Springett, J. (2001) 'Appropriate approaches to the evaluation of health promotion', *Critical Public Health*, 11(2): 139–51.

Stacey, D., Bennett, C., Barry, M., Col, N. F., Eden, K., Entwistle, V., Fiset, V., Holmes-Rovner, M., Khangura, S., Llewellyn-Thomas, H. and Rovner, D. (2012) 'Decision-aids for people facing health treatment or screening decisions (review)', *Cochrane Database of Systematic Reviews* 2011, 10, art.: CD001431. doi:10.1002/14651858.CD001431.pub3

Ståhl, T., Wismar, M., Ollila, E., Lahtinen,e. and Leppo, K. (2006) *Health in all Policies: Prospects and Potentials*. Finland: Ministry of Social Affairs and Health/European Observatory on Health Systems and Policies.

Starfield, B. (2011) 'Politics, primary healthcare and health: was Virchow right?', *Journal of Epidemiology & Community Health*, 65(8): 653–5.

Starfield, B., Shi, L. and Macinko, J. (2005) 'Contribution of primary care to health systems and health', *The Millbank Quarterly*, 83(3): 457–502.

Steger, M. and Wilson, E. (2012) 'Anti-globalization or alter-globalization? Mapping the political ideology of the global justice movement', *International Studies Quarterly*, 56: 439–54.

Stephens, C. (2008) 'Social capital in its place: using social theory to understand social capital and inequalities in health', *Social Science & Medicine*, 66: 1174–84.

Stern, N. (2006) *The Economics of Climate Change: The Stern Review*, Cambridge: Cambridge University Press.

Stevens, A. (2011) 'Telling policy stories: an ethnographic study of the use of evidence in policy-making in the UK', *Journal of Social Policy*, 40(2): 237–55.

Stewart, H. and Elliott, L. (2013) 'Nicholas Stern: 'I got it wrong on climate change: it's far, far worse', *The Observer*, 26 January. Available online at www.guardian.co.ukenvironment/2013/jan/27/nicholas-stern-climate-change-d (accessed 1 February 2013).

Stockwell, T., Auld, M., Zhao, J. and Martin, G. (2011) 'Does minimum pricing reduce alcohol consumption? The experience of a Canadian province', *Addiction*, 107: 912–20.

Stott, N. and Davis, R. (1979) 'The exceptional potential in each primary care consultation', *Journal of the Royal College of General Practitioners*, 29: 201–5.

Strong, K., Wald, N., Miller, A., Alwan, A., on behalf of the WHO Consultation Group (2005) 'Current concepts in screening for non-communicable disease: World Health Organization Consultation Group Report on methodology of non-communicable disease screening', *Journal of Medical Screening*, 12(1): 12–19.

Stuckler, D., Basu, S., Suhrcke, M., Coutts, A. and McKee, M. (2011) 'Effects of the 2008 recession on health: a first look at European data', *The Lancet*, 378: 124–5.

Susser, M. (1998) 'Does risk factor epidemiology put epidemiology at risk? Peering into the future', *Journal of Epidemiology & Community Health*, 52: 608–11.

Susser, M. (2001) 'Glossary: causality in public health science', *Journal of Epidemiology & Community Health*, 55: 376–8.

de Swann, A. (2001) *Human Societies: An Introduction*, Cambridge: Polity Press.

Sykes, S., Wills, J., Rowlands, G. and Popple, K. (2013) 'Understanding critical health literacy: A concept analysis', *BMC Public Health*, 13: 150. Available online at www.biomed-central.com/1471-2458/13/150 (accessed 3 June 2013).

Szreter, S. (1997) 'Economic growth, disruption, deprivation, disease, and death: on the importance of the politics of public health for development', *Population and Development Review*, 23(4): 693–728.

Szreter, S. (2002) 'Rethinking McKeown: the relationship between public health and social change', *American Journal of Public Health*, 92(5): 722–5.

Szreter, S. and Woolcock, M. (2004) 'Health by association? Social capital, social theory, and the political economy of public health', *International Journal of Epidemiology*, 33: 650–67.

Tam, C. and Lopman, B. (2003) 'Determinism versus stochasticism: in support of long coffee breaks', *Journal of Epidemiology & Community Health*, 57: 477–8.

Taub, A., Allegrante, J., Barry, M. and Sakagami, K. (2009) 'Perspectives on terminology and conceptual and professional issues in health education and health promotion credentialing', *Health Education & Behaviour*, 36(3): 439–50.

Taylor, M. (2000) 'Communities in the lead: power, organisational capacity and social capital', *Urban Studies*, 37(5–6): 1019–35.

Taylor, M. (2011) 'Low wage or no wage', *Society Now*, 11: 11. Available online at www.esrc.ac.uk/_images/society_now_issue11_tcm8-18756.pdf (accessed 3 June 2013).

Taylor, P. (1993) *The Texts of Paolo Freire*, Buckingham: Open University Press.

Taylor-Gooby, P. (2012) 'Root and branch restructuring to achieve major cuts: the social policy programme of the 2010 UK coalition government', *Social Policy & Administration*, 46(1): 61–82.

Tesh, S. (1988) *Hidden Arguments: Political Ideology and Disease Prevention Policy*, New Brunswick: Rutgers University.

Thaler, R. and Sunstein, C. (2008) *Nudge: Improving Decisions about Health, Wealth and Happiness*, London: Yale University Press.

Thomas, J. (2009) 'Using social marketing to address obesity: the ongoing "Liverpool Challenge" social marketing programme', *Journal of Communication in Healthcare*, 2(3): 216–27.

Thomas, J., Sage, M., Dillenberg, J. and Guillory, V. (2002) 'A code of ethics for public health', *American Journal of Public Health*, 92(7): 1057–9.

Thurston, M. (2006) *The National Healthy Schools Programme: A Vehicle for School Improvement? Case Studies from Cheshire*, Chester: University of Chester.

Thurston, M. and Green, K. (2004) 'Adherence to exercise in later life: how can exercise on prescription be made more effective?', *Health Promotion International*, 19(3): 379–87.

Thurston, M., Alford, S. and Hughes, D. (2010). *An Evaluation of the Cheshire & Merseyside Public Health Network 'Drink a Little Less, see a Better You' Social Marketing Campaign*, Chester: University of Chester.

Thygesen, L., Andersen, G. and Andersen, H. (2005) 'A philosophical analysis of the Hill criteria', *Journal of Epidemiology & Community Health*, 59: 512–16.

Titmuss, R. (1974) *Social Policy: an Introduction*, B. Abel-Smith and K. Titmuss (eds), London: Allen & Unwin.

Tomlinson, M. and Kelly, G. (2013) 'Is everybody happy? The politics and measurement of national wellbeing', *Policy & Politics*, 41(2): 139–57.

Tomlison, M., Walker, R. and Wiliams, G. (2008) 'Measuring poverty in Britain as a multi-dimensional concept, 1991 to 2003', *Journal of Social Policy*, 37(4): 597–620.

Tones, K. (1986) 'Health education and the ideology of health promotion: a review of alternative approaches', *Health Education Research*, 1(1): 3–12.

Tones, K. (1996) 'The anatomy and ideology of health promotion: empowerment in context', in A. Scriven and J. Orme (eds) *Health Promotion. Professional Perspectives* (pp. 9–21), Milton Keynes: The Open University.

Tones, K. (2002a) 'Health literacy: new wine in old bottles?', *Health Education Research*, 17(3): 287–90.

Tones, K. (2002b) 'Reveille for radicals! The paramount purpose of health education?', *Health Education Research*, 17(1): 1–5.

Tones, K., and Tilford, S. (2001) *Health Promotion: Effectiveness, Efficiency, Equity*, London: Nelson Thornes.

Townsend, P. (1985) 'A sociological approach to the measurement of poverty: a rejoinder to Professor Amartya Sen', *Oxford Economic Papers*, 37: 659–68.

Townsend, P. (1987) 'Deprivation', *Journal of Social Policy*, 16(2): 125–46.

Tranter, P. and Pawson, E. (2001) 'Children's access to local environments: a case study of Christchurch, New Zealand', *Local Environment*, 6(1): 27–48.

Travis, A. (2013) 'Public health statistics could cease to be published amid wave of budget cuts', *The Guardian*, 10 July. Available online at www.guardian.co.uk/society/2013/jul/10/public-health-statistics-publish-cuts-cameron?CMP=twt_gu (accessed 11 July 2013).

Tuffin, R., Quinn, A., Ali, F. and Cramp, P. (2009) 'A review of the accuracy of death certification on the intensive care unit and the proposed reforms to the Coroner's system', *Journal of the Intensive Care Society*, 10(2): 134–7.

Tunstall, H., Shaw, M. and Dorling, D. (2004) 'Places and health', *Journal of Epidemiology & Community Health*, 58: 6–10.

Tutton, R. (2012) 'Personalizing medicines: futures present and past', *Social Science & Medicine*, 75: 1721–8.

UK National Screening Committee (2012) *Screening in the UK 2011–2012*, London: UK National Screening Committee.

UN Millennium Project (2005) *Investing in Development: A Practical Plan to Achieve the Millennium Development Goals*, London: Earthscan.

United Nations (1992) *United Nations Framework Convention on Climate Change*. Available online at http://unfcc.int/essential_background/convention/items/6036.php (accessed 31 July 2013).

United Nations (2010) *The Millennium Development Goals Report 2010*, New York: United

Nations. Available online at www.un.org/millenniumgoals/pdf/MDG%20Report%202010%20En%20r15%20-low%20res%2020100615%20-.pdf (accessed 8 June 2013).

United Nations (2012) *Population Facts No 2012/1*, New York: United Nations.

United Nations Development Programme (1990) *Human Development Report 1990*, New York: Oxford University Press.

United Nations Development Programme (2009) *Human Development Report 2009. Overcoming Barriers: Human Mobility and Development*, New York: United Nations. Available online from http://hdr.undp.org (accessed 11 May 2013).

Valentine, G., Jayne, M., Gould, M. and Keenan, J. (2010). *Family Life and Alcohol Consumption: A Study of the Transmission of Drinking Practices*, York: Joseph Rowntree Foundation.

Vallgårda, S. (2007) 'Health inequalities: political problematizations in Denmark and Sweden', *Critical Public Health*, 17: 45–56.

Vallgårda, S. (2010) 'Tackling social inequalities in health in the Nordic countries: targeting a residuum or the whole population', *Journal of Epidemiology & Community Health*, 64: 495–96.

Vallgårda, S. (2011) 'Why the concept of "lifestyle disease" should be avoided', *Scandinavian Journal of Public Health*, 39: 773–75.

Vallgårda, S. (2012) 'Nudge: a new and better way to improve health?', *Health Policy*, 104: 200–3.

Van der Maesen, L. and Nijhuis, H. (2000) 'Continuing the debate on the philosophy of modern public health: social quality as a point of reference', *Journal of Epidemiology & Community Health*, 54: 134–42.

Velleman, R. (2009) *Children, Young People and Alcohol: How They Learn and How to Prevent Excessive Use*, York: Joseph Rowntree Foundation.

Verheul, E. and Rowson, M. (2001) 'Poverty reduction strategy papers', *BMJ*, 323: 120–21.

Verweij M. and Dawson A. (2007) 'The meaning of "public" in public health', in A. Dawson and M Verweij (eds) *Ethics, Prevention and Public Health* (pp.13–29), Oxford: Oxford University Press.

de Viggiani, N. (2007) 'Unhealthy prisons: exploring structural determinants of prison health', *Sociology of Health & Illness*, 29(1): 115–35.

Vineis, P. (1997) 'Proof of observational medicine', *Journal of Epidemiology & Community Health*, 51: 9–13.

Waddington, I. (2000) *Sport, Health and Drugs. A Critical Sociological Perspective*, London: E. & F. N. Spon.

Wagner, E. (1982) 'The North Karelia Project: what it tells us about the prevention of cardiovascular disease', *American Journal of Public Health*, 72(1): 51–3.

Wald, D. and Wald, N. (2010) 'The polypill in the primary prevention of cardiovascular disease', *Fundamental & Clinical Pharmacology*, 24: 29–35.

Wald, N. (2008) 'Guidance on terminology', *Journal of Medical Screening*, 15: 50.

Wallace, J. and Schmuecker, K. (2012) *Shifting the Dial: From Wellbeing Measures to Policy Practice*, Dunfermline: Carnegie UK Trust/IPPR North.

De Walque, D., Dow, W. H., Nathan, R., Abdul, R., Abilahi, F., Gong, E., Isdahl, Z., Jamison, J., Jullu, B., Krishnan, S., Majura, A., Miguel, E., Moncada, J., Mtenga, S., Mwanyangala, M., Packel, L., Schachter, J., Shirima, K. and Medlin, C. (2012) 'Incentivising safe sex: a randomised trial of conditional cash transfers for HIV and sexually transmitted infection prevention in rural Tanzania', *BMJ Open*, 2e 000747. doi:10.1136/bmjopen-2011-00747

Walsh, D., Rudd, R., Moeykens, B. and Maloney, T. (1993) 'Social marketing for public health', *Health Affairs*, 12(2): 104–19.

Walt, G. (1994) *Health Policy: An Introduction to Process and Power*, London: Zed Books.

Walt, G. (1998) 'Globalisation of international health', *The Lancet*, 351: 434–37.

Wanless, D. (2004) *Securing Good Health for the Whole Population: Final Report*, London: The Stationery Office.

Wassertheil-Smoller, S. (2004) *Biostatistics and Epidemiology. A primer for Health and Biomedical Professionals*, New York: Springer.

Watts, G. (2009) 'The health benefits of tackling climate change. An executive summary for *The Lancet* series'. Available online at http://download.thelancet.com/flatcontentassets/series/health-and-climate-change.pdf (accessed 31 January 2013).

Weed, D. and Mckeown, R. (2003) 'Science, ethics, and professional public health practice', *Journal of Epidemiology & Community Health*, 57: 4–5.

Weed, D. and Mink, P. (2002) 'Roles and responsibilities of epidemiologists', *Annals of Epidemiology*, 12: 67–72.

Weiss, C. (1995) 'Nothing as practical as good theory: exploring theory-based evaluation for comprehensive community initiatives for children and families', in J. Connell, A. Kubisch, L. Schorr and C. Weiss (eds) *New Approaches to Evaluating Community Initiatives: Concepts, Methods and Contexts* (pp. 65–92), Washington DC, The Aspen Institute.

Weller, S. and Campbell, C. (2009) 'Uptake in cancer screening programmes: a priority in cancer control', *British Journal of Cancer*, 101: S55–S59.

Welshman, J. (2008) 'The cycle of deprivation: myths and misconceptions', *Children & Society*, 22: 75–85.

Werner, D. (1984) 'The village health worker: lackey or liberator?', in N. Black, D. Boswell, A. Gray, S. Murphy, and J. Popay (eds) *Health and Disease: A Reader* (pp. 176–182), Milton Keynes: Open University Press.

Werner, D. (1995) 'Who killed primary healthcare?' *New Internationalist*, 272. Available online at http://newint.org/features/1995/10/05/who (accessed 7 March 2013).

West, R. (2005) 'Time for a change: putting the Transtheoretical (Stages of Change) Model to rest', *Addiction*, 100: 1036–39.

Whitehead, M. (1992) 'The concepts and principles of equity and heath', *International Journal of Health Services*, 22(3): 429–45.

Whitehead, M. and Dahlgren, G. (2006) *Concepts and Principles for Tackling Social Inequities in Health: Levelling up Part 1*, Copenhagen: World Health Organization.

Whitehead, M., Dahlgren, G. and Evans, T. (2001) 'Equity and health sector reforms: can low-income countries escape the medical poverty trap?', *The Lancet*, 358: 833–36.

Wilkinson, P., Smith, K., Davies, M., Adair, H., Armstrong, B., Barrett, M., Bruce, N., Haines, A., Hamilton, I., Oreszczyn, T., Ridley, I., Tonne, C. and Chalabi, Z. (2009) 'Public health benefits of strategies to reduce greenhouse-gas emissions: household energy', *The Lancet*, 374: 1917–29.

Wilkinson, R. (1996) *Unhealthy Societies: The Afflictions of Inequality*, London: Routledge.

Wilkinson, R. and Pickett, K. (2006) 'Income inequality and population health: a review and explanation of the evidence', *Social Science & Medicine*, 62: 1768–84.

Wilkinson, R. and Pickett, K. (2010) *The Spirit Level. Why Equality is Better for Everyone*, London: Penguin Books.

Williams, G. (2003) 'The determinants of health: structure, context and agency', *Sociology of Health & Illness*, 25: 131–54.

Williams, S. and Calnan, M. (1996) 'The "limits" of medicalization? Modern medicine and the lay populace in "late" modernity,' *Social Science & Medicine*, 42(12): 1609–20.

Williamson, D. and Carr, J. (2009) 'Health as a resource for everyday life: advancing the conceptualization', *Critical Public Health*, 19(1): 107–22.

Wills, J. (2009) 'Health literacy: new packaging for health education or radical movement?', *International Journal of Public Health*, 54: 3–4.

Wills, J., Evans, D. and Scott-Samuel, A. (2008) 'Politics and prospects for health promotion in England: mainstreamed or marginalised?', *Critical Public Health*, 18(4): 521–31.

Wilson, E., Dalberth, B., Koo, H. and Gard, J. (2010) 'Parents' perspectives on talking to preteenage children about sex', *Perspectives on Sexual and Reproductive Health*, 42(1): 56–63.

Wilson, G. and Schlam, T. (2004) 'The transtheoretical model and motivational interviewing in the treatment of eating and weight disorders', *Clinical Psychology Review*, 24: 361–78.

Wilson, J. (2009) 'Can disease prevention save health reform?', *Annals of Internal Medicine*, 151(2): 145–47.

Wilson, J., and Jungner, G. (1968) *Principles and Practice of Screening for Disease*, Public Health Papers No 34, Geneva: World Health Organization. Available online at http://whqlibdoc. who.int/php/WHO_PHP_34.pdf (accessed 28 May 2013).

Winkleby, M., Jatulis, D., Frank, E. and Fortmann, S. (1992) 'Socioeconomic status and health: how education, income and occupation contribute to risk factors for cardiovascular disease', *American Journal of Public Health*, 82(6): 816–20.

Winters, L. (2009) *Evaluation of the Phase 2 Snack Right Social Marketing Project: Final Report*, Liverpool: Liverpool Public Health Observatory.

Wolleswinkel-van Den Bosch, J., Van Poppel, F., Tabeau, E. and Mackenbach, J. (1998) 'Mortality decline in the Netherlands in the period 1850–1992: a turning point analysis', *Social Science & Medicine*, 47(4): 429–43.

Woodall, J., Dixey, R. and South, J. (2012) 'Prisoners' perspectives on the transition from the prison to the community: implications for settings-based health promotion', *Critical Public Health*, 23(2): 188–200.

Woodcock, J., Edwards, P., Tonne, C., Armstrong, B., Ashiru, O., Banister, D., Beevers, S., Chalabi, Z., Chowdhury, Z., Cohen, A., Franco, O., Haines, A., Hickman, R., Lindsay, G., Mittal, I., Mohan, D., Tiwari, G., Woodward, A. and Roberts, I. (2009) 'Public health benefits of strategies to reduce greenhouse-gas emissions: urban land transport', *The Lancet*, 374: 1930–43.

Woodhouse, J. and Ward, P. (2013) *Alcohol Minimum Pricing*. House of Commons Library. Available online at www.parliament.uk/briefing-papers/SN05021 (accessed 1 July 2013).

Wooley, H., Pattacini, L. and Somerset–Ward, A. (2009) *Children and the Natural Environment: Experiences, Influences and Interventions – Summary*. Natural England Commissioned Reports, Number 026, Sheffield: Natural England.

World Commission on Environment and Development (1987) *Our Common Future*, Oxford: Oxford University Press.

World Health Organization and the United Nations International Children's Fund (1978) *Declaration of Alma-Ata*. International Conference on Primary Health Care, Alma-Ata, USSR, 6–12 September.

World Health Organization (1986) *The Ottawa Charter for Health Promotion*, Ottawa: World Health Organization.

World Health Organization (1999) *Health21: the Health for all Policy Framework for the WHO European Region*, Copenhagen: WHO Regional Office for Europe.

World Health Organization (2005a) *The Bangkok Charter for Health Promotion in a Globalized World*. Available online at www.who.int/healthpromotion/conferences/6gchp/bangkok_ charter/en/ (accessed 16 November 2012).

World Health Organization (2005b) *WHO Multi-country Study of Women's Health and Domestic Violence against Women*. Geneva: World Health Organization.

World Health Organization (2006) *Constitution of the World Health Organization. Basic Documents, forty–fifth edition, Supplement*. Available online at www.who.int/governance/ eb/who_constitution_en.pdf (accessed 26 March 2012).

World Health Organization (2007) *The World Health Report 2007: A Safer Future. Global Public Health Security in the 21st Century*, Geneva: World Health Organization.

World Health Organization (2009) *Milestones in Health Promotion. Statements From Global Conferences*, Geneva: World Health Organization.

World Health Organization (2012) *International Statistical Classification of Diseases and Related Health Problems. 10th Revision.* Available online at http://apps.who.int/classification/icd10/browse/2010/en (accessed 5 September 2012).

World Health Organization (2013) *Civil Registration: Why Counting Births and Deaths is Important.* Available online at www.who.int/mediacentre/factsheets/fs324/en (accessed 6 September 2013).

Wright, J. and Polack, C. (2006) 'Understanding variation in measles-mumps-rubella immunization coverage: a population-based study', *European Journal of Public Health*, 16(2): 137–42.

Wright, J., Williams, R. and Wilkinson J. (1998) 'Development and importance of health needs assessment', *BMJ*, 316: 1310–13.

Wrong, D. (1961) 'The oversocialized conception of man in modern sociology', *American Sociological Review*, 26(2): 183–93.

Yach, D. and Bettcher, D. (1998) 'The globalization of public health, II: the convergence of self–interest and altruism', *American Journal of Public Health*, 88: 738–41.

Yarlagadda, S., Webster, P. and Haworth, E. (2012) 'The role of public health in climate change and sustainability: is the UK public health community's response adequate?', *Perspectives in Public Health*, 132(5): 207–8.

Zhu, N., Ling, Z., Lane, J. and Hu, S. (1989) 'Factors associated with the decline of the Cooperative Medical System and barefoot doctors in rural China', *Bulletin of the World Health Organization*, 67(4): 431–41.

Zola, I. (1972) 'Medicine as an instrument of social control', *The Sociological Review*, 20: 487–504.

INDEX

214

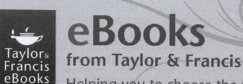
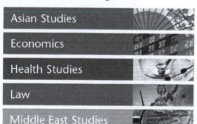